GW00538001

Second Edition

ENERGY PSYCHOLOGY

Explorations at the Interface of Energy, Cognition, Behavior, and Health

Second Edition

ENERGY PSYCHOLOGY

Explorations at the
Interface of Energy, Cognition,
Behavior, and Health

Fred P. Gallo

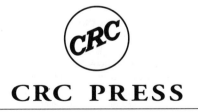

CRC PRESS

Boca Raton   London   New York   Washington, D.C.

Cover: Based on a design by Brigitte Goldenbaum, Hamburg, Germany.

Library of Congress Cataloging-in-Publication Data

Catalog record is available from the Library of Congress

Visit the CRC Press Web site at www.crcpress.com

© 2005 by CRC Press

No claim to original U.S. Government works
International Standard Book Number 0-8493-2246-4
Library of Congress Card Number
Printed in the United States of America 1 2 3 4 5 6 7 8 9 0
Printed on acid-free paper

Dedication

To Carolyn, our children, and grandchildren
To my parents, Mary Louise and Fred

Preface to the Second Edition

The first edition of *Energy Psychology* was released in July 1998. However, my learning and the writing began in late 1992 while I was studying kinesiology and later traveling the United States teaching professionals about the many wonders of energy psychology. I was on a mission to make this treatment approach widely available, not just for the people I treat at my clinical practice in Hermitage, Pennsylvania. And increasingly, this vision has become a reality not only in America but also throughout many areas of Canada, Europe, Australia, Central and South America, South Africa, Asia, and more. This proliferation has been due in part to the publication of the first edition of *Energy Psychology* as well as related articles and books, supportive research on the effectiveness of energy psychology, and the dedication of therapists and trainers who have been willing to take up the torch and run with it.

I have attempted to prepare this second edition to reflect significant aspects of the field, while remaining true to the original edition. However, energy psychology is growing so rapidly that no volume of this size can do it justice. There are many approaches that I am only marginally familiar with, since I have been spending much of my time teaching and developing the approaches that I refer to as energy diagnostic and treatment methods (EDxTM) and energy consciousness therapy (ECT). Yet my edited volume, *Energy Psychology in Psychotherapy* (2002), provides chapters on key approaches to energy psychology, theory, and applications. That book complements this one.

While the chapter titles in *Energy Psychology* remain the same, I have expanded the sections on scientific underpinnings, clinical research, manual muscle testing, related energy psychology approaches, and professional resources. Additional algorithms and descriptions of other energy psychology approaches also have been added.

Chapter 1 briefly discusses some psychological paradigms or models: psychodynamic, environmental–behavioral, cognitive, systemic–cybernetic, neurologic, and biochemical, and paves the way to the energy paradigm with a discussion of electrical neurotransmission, regeneration, L-fields, and quantum mechanics.

Chapter 2 explores four therapeutic methods that have demonstrated efficiently in treating post-traumatic stress disorder and phobias. Those methods are visual/kinesthetic dissociation (V/KD), eye movement desensitization and reprocessing (EMDR), traumatic incident reduction (TIR), and thought field therapy (TFT). Plausible active ingredients of these methods are discussed in some detail with particular focus on the active ingredient of bioenergy.

Chapter 3 investigates the body's energy system, primarily focusing on acupuncture and some of the research that is supportive of the existence of bioenergy systems. This chapter also explores morphogenetic fields, homeopathy, and flower remedies, as well as empirical investigations of prayer.

Chapter 4 covers the origins of energy psychology in applied kinesiology and traces a number of offshoots, including Touch for Health (TFH), clinical kinesiology (CK), and educational kinesiology (Edu-K). The influence of applied kinesiology in the work of John Diamond, M.D., and Roger J. Callahan, Ph.D., is also briefly reviewed.

Chapter 5 specifically highlights many aspects of the psychotherapeutic approach of John Diamond. His approach is the first to utilize applied kinesiology and the acupuncture meridian system to diagnose and treat psychological problems, combining this approach with psychodynamic understandings.

Chapter 6 discusses the system developed by Roger J. Callahan, which is referred to as thought field therapy. This chapter introduces the notion of therapeutic sequences or algorithms, energy diagnostic procedures, psychological reversal, energy toxins, and briefly touches on thought field therapy research. Additionally, a thought field therapy trauma treatment procedure is covered along with reviews of a few trauma cases.

Chapter 7 is entitled "The Energy Therapist's Manual." It covers client preparation and debriefing issues such as rapport, pacing, belief in the treatment, attunement, scaling, explaining the method, manual muscle testing, thought field therapy treatment points, psychological reversal, criteria-related reversals, neurologic disorganization corrections, energy toxins, etc. Additionally, sequences of treatment points, referred to as therapeutic algorithms, are offered for a wide array of clinical problems including specific phobias, trauma, addiction, anxiety, panic, obsessive-compulsive disorder, clinical depression, anger, guilt, and so on. This section includes many thought field therapy and related therapeutic algorithms. This chapter also provides an introduction to other energy psychotherapy methods including emotional stress release (ESR), frontal/occipital (F/O) holding, emotional freedom techniques (EFT), Tapas acupressure technique (TAT), energy diagnostic and treatment methods (EDxTM), negative affect erasing method (NAEM), neuro-energetic sensory technique (NEST), and healing energy light process (HELP).

Finally, Chapter 8 covers the current research on energy psychology and also explores clinical issues and proposes some avenues for future research. The question about the relevance of treatment point sequencing is raised, and approaches to evaluating thought field therapy and other energy psychotherapies are suggested with regard to phobias, trauma, addiction, generalized anxiety, dissociative identity disorder, anger-rage, and a number of other areas. Integration of energy psychotherapies into one's practice is also discussed.

I have included an appendix — "Manual Muscle Testing Uses and Abuses" — which explores this important topic in more depth than in the earlier chapters of the book. I have also added an energy psychology glossary, as well as information on other resources.

I originally wrote *Energy Psychology* with the intention of providing a professional introduction to the field that would be of interest and benefit to psychologists, psychiatrists, psychotherapists, other health care providers, and students. I also wanted to interest researchers in examining these treatment approaches that I have found to be so highly effective. These remain my sincere intentions with this second edition.

Years ago, when I was a college freshman, I read a book by Erich Fromm in which he expressed the hope of inspiring young people to enter the helping profession. His words encouraged and inspired me to enter the field of psychology and psychotherapy, and for this, I am grateful. Similarly, I am hopeful that this book will inspire and encourage young people to study, apply, and further advance the concepts and methods covered here for the welfare of all people. I'm optimistic that together we can help to make this world a healthier place.

Fred P. Gallo, Ph.D.

Acknowledgments to the Second Edition

This second edition of *Energy Psychology* reflects important aspects of my clinical work with clients and the training I offer to professionals throughout the world. I remain deeply appreciative to those acknowledged in the first edition and I would also like to express gratitude to others who have supported the therapeutic and scientific advancement of this work. Although I wish I had the space to list thousands, here's a very short list: Association for Comprehensive Energy Psychology (ACEP), Joaquin Andrade, Bill Becket, Gerrie Brooks, Ruth M. Buczynski, Lesley Hannell Corvino, Gary Craig, Donna Eden, David Feinstein, Phil Friedman, John Frisco, Mark Furman, Jeannie Galvin, Michael Galvin, David Gruder, John Hartung, Dagmar Ingwersen, Fide Ingwersen, Vann Joines, Willem Lammers, Wolfgang Lenk, Marie Macomber, Gary Peterson, Lee Pulos, Sandy Radomski, Anthony Robbins, Deanna Sager, David Santoro, Alfred Schatz, Gunther Schmidt, Eroca Shaler, Richard Simon, Toby Solomon, Loretta Sparks, Philip Streit, Dorney Thompson, Sharon Toole, Beate Walter, and Steve Wells.

For assistance with photographs, I would like to thank Amy Formica, Philip Gallo, Leah Mazzocca, Rachelle Misco, and Alissa Umbs.

Finally, I appreciate the wonderful professionals at CRC Press and Taylor & Francis Informa who made this edition possible, especially Barbara Norwitz, Patricia Roberson, Preethi Cholmondeley, Rachel Tamburri-Saunders, and Christine Andreasen.

Preface to the First Edition

The aspiration that has fueled the writing of this book is possibly the same that has drawn you to its pages. For my part, this began about 7 years ago when I discovered that many psychological problems can be treated consistently in quantum leaps, without the need to pass through laborious stages of discovery, emoting, and cognitive restructuring that are frequently considered to be the hallmarks of true psychotherapy. While this is not intended to be a disparaging comment about longer forms of therapy — as there are many conditions and life issues that do not, and perhaps should not, respond with such rapidity — when therapy can proceed rapidly, why not?!

While I have always been thrilled with assisting others in achieving profound, healthy change, frequently the metaphor of midwife had been all too painfully accurate. The image is one of I, the midwife, assisting the patient in painfully releasing trauma, transcending fear, depression, and other negative emotions, and giving birth to a healthier state of being. All too frequently, however, somebody needing to emerge would become stuck in the birth canal, and I would either attempt to pull the person out or otherwise encourage the patient to breathe deeply and push. No doubt all of us have been party to such painful midwifing.

This book is about an emerging, absolutely enthralling new perspective in psychology and psychotherapy. *Energy psychology* is defined as the branch of psychology that studies the effects of energy systems on emotions and behavior. These systems include, but are not limited to, the acupuncture meridians and morphic resonance. *Energy psychotherapy* consists of approaches to psychotherapy that specifically address bioenergy systems in the diagnosis and treatment of psychological problems. Just as Newtonian classical physics eventually gave way to modifications required by relativity and quantum mechanics, psychology as a whole and psychotherapy in particular will now come to reckon with a *new* set of variables, a *new paradigm*. Interestingly, the *new* perspective has existed in various forms for several millennia.

This shift, which David Kuhn (1962) could have easily predicted, is necessitated in that our current paradigms have not offered adequate solutions or accurate predictions in a number of important areas, such as post-traumatic stress disorder. The new view is that of *energy*, which is already taking hold in areas of medicine in light of magnetic resonance, electromagnetic treatments of various sorts, and even psychoneuroimmunology. Certainly, this was predated by other technologies that tap into bioenergy systems, including various types of biofeedback, such as electrocardiographs and electroencephalograms.

Now this understanding enters the fields of psychology and psychotherapy as we begin to notice that psychological problems can be understood as manifestations of energy disruptions or energy configurations that can be precisely diagnosed and treated with great dispatch. Suddenly midwifing becomes much easier for both therapist and patient alike.

This is not to say that what we have been doing up to now is not worthwhile. We should not want to throw out the baby with the bath water, to continue with our birthing metaphor. But some of our most cherished "commonsense" notions need not necessarily apply. How often have we heard ourselves and others parroting: *"No pain, no gain." "You didn't develop this problem overnight, so don't expect to get over it right away." "You've had this problem for a long time..." "Change takes time." "Change is difficult." "The patient wasn't ready yet." "I don't have a magic wand."*

Well it seems now that change readily can occur without pain. And it does not matter how long the problem has existed; it can be alleviated quickly. Change is often quite easy. And it is seldom an issue of the patient not being ready yet. And quite possibly the therapist does have access to a "magic" wand.

The purpose of this book is to assist you in creating a profound difference in your life and in the lives of the people who come to you in suffering. This is a book about therapy and change and about how to bring that change about suddenly. This is a book about a paradigmatic shift that can be utilized readily by clinician and researcher alike to treat and to investigate the treatment of psychological problems with protocols that are easily applied.

Chapter 1 reviews some of the paradigms or models that we have become accustomed to — environmental–behavioral, cognitive, systemic–cybernetic, neurologic, and biochemical — and paves the way to the energy paradigm with a discussion of electrical neurotransmission, regeneration, L-fields, and quantum mechanics.

Chapter 2 explores four therapeutic methods that have shown promise in efficiently treating post-traumatic stress disorder symptoms. Those methods are visual/kinesthetic dissociation (V/KD), eye movement desensitization and reprocessing (EMDR), traumatic incident reduction (TIR), and thought field therapy (TFT). Plausible active ingredients of these methods are discussed in some detail with particular focus on the active ingredient of bioenergy.

Chapter 3 investigates the body's energy system, primarily focusing on acupuncture and some of the research that is supportive of the existence of bioenergy systems. This chapter also explores morphogenetic fields, homeopathy, and flower remedies, as well as empirical investigations of prayer.

Chapter 4 discusses the origins of energy psychology in applied kinesiology and traces a number of offshoots, including Touch for Health (TFH), clinical kinesiology (CK), and educational kinesiology (Edu-K). The influence of applied kinesiology in the work of John Diamond, M.D., and Roger J. Callahan, Ph.D. is also briefly reviewed.

Chapter 5 specifically highlights many aspects of the psychotherapeutic approach of John Diamond, M.D. His is the first to utilize applied kinesiology and the acupuncture meridian system to diagnose and treat psychological problems, combining this approach with psychodynamic understandings.

Chapter 6 discusses the system developed by Roger J. Callahan, Ph.D., referred to as thought field therapy. This chapter introduces the notion of therapeutic sequences or algorithms, energy diagnostic procedures, psychological reversal, energy toxins, and briefly touches on thought field therapy research. Additionally, a thought field therapy trauma treatment procedure is covered along with reviews of a few trauma cases.

Chapter 7 is entitled "The Energy Therapist's Manual." It covers client preparation and debriefing issues such as rapport, pacing, belief in the treatment, attunement, scaling, explaining the method, manual muscle testing, thought field therapy treatment points, psychological reversal, criteria-related reversals, neurologic disorganization corrections, energy toxins, etc. Additionally, sequences of treatment points, referred to as therapeutic algorithms, are offered for a wide array of clinical problems including specific phobias, trauma, addiction, anxiety, panic, obsessive-compulsive disorder, clinical depression, anger, guilt, and so on. This section includes many therapeutic algorithms and related treatments outside the scope of "official thought field therapy." This chapter also provides an introduction to other energy psychotherapy methods including emotional stress release (ESR), frontal/occipital (F/O) holding, emotional freedom techniques (EFT), Tapas acupressure technique (TAT), and negative affect erasing method (NAEM).

Finally, Chapter 8 discusses the current research on thought field therapy and also explores additional clinical issues and proposes some avenues for future research. The question about the relevance of treatment point sequencing is raised, and approaches to evaluating thought field therapy and other energy psychotherapies are suggested with regard to phobias, trauma, addiction, generalized anxiety, dissociative identity disorder, anger-rage, and a number of other areas. Integration of energy psychotherapies into one's practice is also discussed.

Given this brief overview, the reader is encouraged to adopt a mental set that sets aside other well-practiced mental sets, to suspend judgment and to allow the empirical evidence of the senses to be one's guide. It is always possible to filter out that which is different from what we already "know," simply reinforcing what we believe to be so. The trick and the gift are to set aside the filter, the internal chatter that gets in the way of absorbing something new.

Acknowledgments to the First Edition

This book represents an important aspect of the clinical work that I have been doing over the past several years. I would like to acknowledge and express my gratitude to a number of people without whose contributions this book could never have come into being.

First of all, I thank Roger J. Callahan for introducing me to the exciting new field of energy psychotherapy. His contribution is one of the most significant ever. He has brought a measure of efficacy and empiricism to the area, as well as the willingness and courage to put his reputation on the line.

I am also grateful to John Diamond for his openness, adventure into uncharted waters, and willingness to delve so deeply into this paradigm. His seminal work has given birth to this field as applied to psychotherapy and human evolution. He has also helped me to begin to appreciate the workings of the ego–energy connection and the balance between specificity and global awareness through which creativity is possible.

Without the piercing perception and diligent work of George J. Goodheart, Jr., I do not know how we could have even gotten as far as we have. His contribution reaches way beyond the mind–body dualism, truly introducing the many health fields to holism. He has been one of our greatest teachers.

I have the utmost respect, appreciation, and gratitude for Charles Figley for encouraging me to conduct this project and for mentoring me through some tough spots along the way. As many recognize, he is one of the greatest ambassadors our field has to offer. His compassion knows no bounds.

I also acknowledge the dedication and work of a number of scientists who have contributed to our understanding of bioenergy and its interface with the known and unknown laws of physics. This list includes, but is not limited to, Robert O. Becker, Harold Saxon Burr, Samuel Hahnemann, Edward Bach, and David Bohm.

I express my gratitude to the colleagues who have attended my seminars. It has been through the opportunity of interaction with them that I have been able to think through much of what is covered in these pages.

Finally, I express my deepest appreciation and admiration to the anonymous personage of China who initially discovered that the body has a palpable energy system that can be harnessed for the benefits of our health and happiness.

About the Author

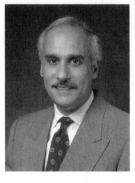

Fred P. Gallo, Ph.D., clinical psychologist, entered private practice in 1977. He began his professional career as a teacher and a counselor after undergraduate and graduate study in philosophy and psychology at Duquesne University in Pittsburgh, Pennsylvania. He attended graduate training in clinical psychology and child development and received his M.A. from the University of Dayton and his Ph.D. from the University of Pittsburgh. Prior to entering private practice, he worked in the fields of juvenile corrections, mental retardation, child welfare, and chemical dependency. He also taught at Pennsylvania State University. In addition to private practice, he is on staff at the University of Pittsburgh Medical Center (UPMC) at Horizon.

In addition to this second edition of *Energy Psychology*, Dr. Gallo has published five books that expand the field of energy psychology and psychotherapy. He has also written numerous articles that have appeared in professional publications and has contributed book chapters. Throughout his professional career he has studied and practiced a number of clinical methods applied to individuals, families, and groups, including client-centered therapy, Gestalt therapy, cognitive-behavioral therapies, neurolinguistic programming, Ericksonian hypnosis and psychotherapy, eye movement desensitization and reprocessing, behavioral kinesiology, and thought field therapy. He is also the founder of two therapeutic approaches — Energy Diagnostic and Treatment Methods (ED×TM) and Energy Consciousness Therapy (ECT) — and presents professional seminars, including his certification program, internationally.

Dr. Gallo is a member of the American Psychological Association, the Pennsylvania Psychological Association, and the Association for Comprehensive Energy Psychology.

He lives in New Wilmington, Pennsylvania, with his wife Carolyn.

Contents

1 Scientific Theaters (Or through the Looking Glass)

The significant problems in our lives cannot be solved at the same level of understanding that we were at when we created them.

— Albert Einstein

How many ways are there to enter a room? While there is the standard way of walking through the door, one might also enter in a variety of unusual ways, such as by climbing through a window or perhaps by breaking through or tunneling under a wall. By not limiting ourselves to the obvious, we can pursue our goal in other unorthodox ways: on tiptoes, crawling on hands and knees, balancing on both hands, scooting on our back, or doing somersaults; running, walking, skipping, or jumping; loudly, softly, or quietly; alone or with companions; dramatically, subdued, or discretely; and the list goes on.

How many ways are there to say hello and goodbye? Again, a wide variety of choices exist: say it; wave; yell it; leave a note; nod; smile; an accent on one aspect of the word or phrase — *hell*-o, hell-*o*, *good*-bye, good-*bye*; and so on.

Now what about psychotherapy? Just as there are many ways to get from here to there, from point "A" to point "B," treating psychological problems is no different. There must be several hundred navigational maps offering the therapist guidance in the art and science of behavior change. Admittedly, many of the *direct*ions are not as efficiently direct as one might desire, and often the guidelines appear to be restatements of essentially the same approach with different words. Thus, the wheel is reinvented again and again and again. One might even say that all too frequently it is impossible to even get from here to there in some·of those ways.

Psychological therapies are rooted in philosophical assumptions or viewpoints about the nature of humans and the nature of psychological problems, and their procedures emanate from such assumptions. We hope that therapies also stem from common sense, logic and empirical research, even though *relevant* research on many therapeutic approaches is quite limited. Medical practitioners, too, frequently employ substances and procedures in the absence of a firm theoretical basis and with limited understanding of the mechanisms of action. Examples include general anesthetics, quinine for malaria, colchicines for gout, citrus fruits to prevent and treat scurvy, and even aspirin (Harris et al., 1999). Upon reviewing the *Physician's Desk Reference,* we may easily add many more medications to the list. Also, it is common knowledge that while medications are subjected to multimillion dollar drug trials

1

before receiving Federal Drug Administration (FDA) approval, we never really know the far-reaching implications of a medication until it has been extensively prescribed. After an accumulation of negative experiences *in the field,* further cautions are published or the medication is recalled. In this sense, some might opine that the term *medical science* is an oxymoron?

Indeed, serendipity often plays a major role in the construction of these theories or theaters (*thea,* the root, meaning the *act of seeing*), as a discovery is stumbled upon (e.g., Pavlov's salivating dogs, Einstein's thought experiments, Fleming's petri dish, etc.) and then later paradigmized. It is obvious to the serious student of theory that the very act of constructing a theory or model is simultaneously inclusive and exclusive and a useful distortion.

We have no market on the truth with these theories or paradigms, although the effective ones in some respects point to the truth, which appears to be a forever unfolding process. As Korzybski aptly elucidated, "A map is not the territory it represents, but, if correct, it has a similar structure to the territory, which accounts for its usefulness" (Korzybski, 1958, p. 60). Whatever we say something is, it is not. Therefore, we ought to be cautious not to mistake the map for the territory. To do so would lead us to treat our patients and clients in the same manner that *Procrustes*, the son of *Poseidon* in Greek mythology, treated his captives. It is said that he stowed them precisely in his bed by stretching the legs of the short ones and trimming the legs of the tall ones. To behave similarly with our theories would be to ignore special circumstances, individual differences, and the evidence of the senses. We must make room in our theories to recognize anomalies and thus expand our vision and understanding of the truth.

Physicist William A. Tiller (1997) has expressed a similar viewpoint, highlighting the value of models in terms of guiding our evolving understanding through the questions that each model raises:

> In this quest for understanding and its utilization, we generate models or "visualizations" of the phenomena as aids to our efforts or, rather, as temporary vehicles via which we gain fuller understanding. In fact the models generally become targets against which we throw experiments in order to test the accuracy of our reasoning and our understanding. They are like the rungs of a ladder via which humankind climbs from one state of understanding to another. In any new area of inquiry, it is valuable to have a model with which to make prognostications that may be compared with the reality of experimental results. It is also important to remember that any model, no matter how seemingly successful, will eventually be proved incomplete in detail and that its primary purpose is to act as a vehicle that gives a sense of understanding that triggers the proper set of questions or experiments needed to probe deeper. Just as the classical Newtonian model had to give way to the classical Einsteinian model, the latter had to give way to the Relativistic Quantum Mechanical model — and so it goes as we ride the river of life onward into our future. (Tiller, 1997, pp. 41–42)

With these cautions in mind, we explore some of our principal *paradigms* (from the late Latin *paradigma*, meaning *to show alongside*). Please bear in mind that this book is not intended to represent an exhaustive exploration of all the aspects of these models or viewpoints, nor is it intended to cover the whole of contemporary approaches. Rather, here is a backdrop for that which follows.

PRE-SCIENTIFIC PARADIGMS

Superstition aside, preceding the advent of scientific paradigms, we have primarily theistic, mystical, and metaphysical inspirations about nature and humanity. By the term *pre*-scientific, in no way do I mean to imply that all of these views are inferior to our *scientific* ones. We might opt instead for a term such as *para*-scientific, suggesting that these positions occur alongside (or intermingle with) scientific ones (science denotes *having knowledge*). Such inclinations have not ceased nor can we ever expect to arrive at a time when humans will tire of them. As long as there is reason for us to wonder and as long as science is unable to provide answers to our most profound and pressing questions, we shall seek answers elsewhere — actually, anywhere we can find them. Even many scientific models are influenced, indeed driven, by imagination and mystical leanings. "Why is there something rather than nothing?" "What accounts for our existence?" "What is consciousness?" "What is self?" "Where is the way to the truth?" "What is Being?" "What drives us or draws us?" "What is the source of health and deviance?" "Where is the way to cure?" In answer to these and many other questions, people throughout the ages have posited gods and God, angels and devils and demons, free will vs. determinism or pawns of Mt. Olympus, sin, spirit, soul, heaven and hell, grace, exorcism, Messiah, and so on. Even in areas more akin to science we point to that which we cannot discern with our senses: big bang, quarks, electrons, protons, neutrons, atoms, molecules, energy, gravity, strong and weak forces, and so on.

Kant (1783) emphasized that we must place limits on *pure reason* and that this requirement, in turn, makes plenty of room for faith. Reason is applicable when we have the data of experience to guide it. In science, we attempt to organize the available data in order to make accurate predictions and to create theories that are testable and that make it possible to secure additional pertinent data. This approach is not applicable to matters of faith, although "logical" consistency in our faith is hopefully a virtue. Additionally, regardless of our scientific theories and procedures, we must remain open to intuition and inspiration, which leads the way to relevant application of our scientific models and toward new findings. At the basis of our theories is belief and faith. It is well known that we cannot prove or disprove a theory, although we can conduct experiments that may or may not support it. In addition to our nature as scientific beings, we are mystical and believing beings as well — beings of faith in search of our essence and what accounts for how nature works.

PSYCHODYNAMIC PARADIGM

One more or less scientific way to consider human behavior and psychopathology is from the perspective of the unconscious and development. Here we hypothesize hypothetical structures such as id, ego, superego, repression, fixation, symptom substitution, and so on. In his collaboration with Josef Breuer, Sigmund Freud explored hypnosis and later free association in the study of hysteria, concluding that this condition stemmed from repressed traumas that were symbolically represented as physical symptoms. The hysteric's blindness, deafness, voice paralysis (perhaps symbolic of not wanting to see, hear, or speak evil) is deemed undischarged emotional energy, the repressed aspects of an event that account for the trauma. Freud concluded that the fundamental emotional energy was sexual and aggressive in nature. While he explored various methodologies, including hypnosis and *laying of hands*, eventually he settled on *free association*, *interpretation*, and *catharsis* in an attempt to usher the unconscious into consciousness and thus free the patient from the tyranny of repressed material. Psychoanalysis may be seen as an archeological expedition that retrieves the artifacts of one's past, expands consciousness, and thus seeks to create space for healthy development. At core, however, Freud's approach led to and stemmed from rather negativistic beliefs about humanity — *flesh in love with itself.*

As we know, the psychodynamic model was variably explored by others who eventually parted from Freud. Alfred Adler looked to the relevance of the individual striving to quell the feeling of inferiority and to achieve power or superiority. He saw health as a function of common sense and social interest. Adler's view was more positive and much less deterministic than Freud's position. His therapeutic protocols were also quite distinct. Rather than having patients lie on a couch, he sat face to face with them. They talked.

Carl Jung delved into the mystical and expanded the theory of the unconscious to include the personal and collective variants, the latter including archetypes that show up in fantasy, dreams, symbols, and synchronicity. He also elucidated basic features of personality such as extroversion, introversion, and intuition. Jung concluded that harmony between the conscious and unconscious is the most significant task for the individual and society to achieve. Jung was also positive and saw the unconscious as a powerful consciousness that extended beyond the individual.

Wilhelm Reich maintained that sexual repression is the source of psychological and social problems and observed that psychological problems are energetically stored in the musculature and various sectors of the body. The therapy that emanated from this viewpoint did not require verbalization as much as procedures for releasing the energetic blocks by applying eye movements, breathing, etc. He also proposed the existence of an energy that is present throughout the universe — *Orgone* energy — that is also profoundly evident during orgasm. And the list goes on.

It seems obvious that in addition to having mystical and metaphysical leanings, we are conscious as well as unconscious beings. Intrapsychic material and processes also play an important role in our functioning.

BEHAVIORAL–ENVIRONMENTAL PARADIGM

Another way to view human behavior and psychopathology is from the standpoint of external behavior. Given this perspective, we do not entertain hypothetical internal constructs such as ego, mind, belief, motivation, and so forth. In concert with the radical behaviorist, we avoid peering inside the "black box," while not going so far as to conclude that there is nothing inside it. External behavior is the dependent variable, and a host of environmentally independent variables are introduced to produce behavior change. "The objective ... is to establish the relation between behavior and the context of its occurrences" (Overskeid, 1995, p. 517).

For example, acrophobia may be treated by exposing the phobic patient to gradually or rapidly increasing elevations, imaginary or *in vivo*, without the option of escape. Avoidance is negatively reinforcing or rewarding because the anxiety is diminished or alleviated as soon as the patient escapes from the fear-producing stimuli. It is assumed that avoidance serves to keep the stimulus–response (S-R) bond in tact and that the bond will be severed after a period of time that proves it to be of no value. Indeed, it has been demonstrated that *in vivo* exposure is significantly more effective than relaxation or cognitive restructuring in the treatment of acrophobia (Menzies and Clarke, 1995a, 1995b).

As another example, if a patient has post-traumatic stress disorder (PTSD), the behavioristic paradigm might guide us to determine the environmental contingencies that elicit the various symptoms including "flashbacks," nightmares, hypervigilance, heightened startle response, affective numbing, etc. The stimulus–response bonds can then be determined and subjected to our treatment efforts. Essentially, we conclude that the problem is one of conditioning history or learning. Extinction of the stimulus–response bonds is the desired outcome in effective therapy. Again, we may choose to expose the trauma victim to the various stimuli, predominantly in imagination, while preventing avoidance, thus promoting extinction of the symptoms.

In the tradition of Joseph Wolpe, M.D. (1958), the extinction procedure may be softened by introducing relaxation while the patient is exposed to the traumatic memory or phobic situation, thus reducing the level of anxiety during exposure. Relaxation inhibits the anxiety response that is associated with the various stimuli, including the memory of the trauma or, in the case of our patient with acrophobia, height. The assumption is that anxiety and relaxation cannot coexist at the same time in the same exact place (i.e., the patient being treated). "If a response inhibitory to anxiety can be made to occur in the presence of anxiety-evoking stimuli so that it is accompanied by a complete or partial suppression of the anxiety response, the bond between these stimuli and the anxiety response will be weakened" (Wolpe, 1961, p. 189). The conditions of such reciprocal inhibition may also be fulfilled with other anxiety-inhibiting states, such as sexual and aggressive responses, that compete with anxiety.

No doubt humans are behavioral beings and that environmental contingencies, extinction, and so on are relevant. Schedules of reinforcement and other variables outlined by the behaviorists are apparent facts at one level of description. Behavior therapies are variably effective, depending on the condition being treated. For example, home-based behavioral interventions have been found to be highly effective in the treatment of autism (Sheinkopf and Siegel, 1998). Also, in the case of post-traumatic stress disorder, of all the behavioral techniques, flooding has been shown to be effective in reducing anxiety symptoms (Cooper and Clum, 1989; Keane et al., 1989; Boudewyns and Hyer, 1990; Foa et al., 1991), although flooding is also associated with a number of undesirable side effects, which include panic episodes, depression, and alcoholic relapse (Pitman et al., 1991). Additionally, this therapeutic procedure can prove exceptionally uncomfortable for the patient, with several 60-

to 90-min. exposure sessions necessitated over 6 to 16 sessions in order to achieve noteworthy clinical effects. Still, the most significant clinical results have been within the 60% range after 15 desensitization sessions (Brom et al., 1989).

COGNITIVE PARADIGM

Yet another way to view human behavior and psychopathology is from the position of cognition. While the behaviorist explores the relationship between behavior and context, the cognitive psychologist "establishes the internal design, through whose functioning organisms are capable of behaving in context" (Overskeid, 1995, p. 517). In this respect, language is often seen as an important mediator of behavior, and it therefore becomes the primary focus of intervention.

Returning to our patient with acrophobia, while there is an obvious stimulus–response bond such that height produces anxiety symptoms, the cognitive paradigm would hold that internal processing is really what causes the anxiety. That is, rather than stimulus–response, we turn our attention to stimulus–integration–response (or S-I-R). From this perspective it is proposed that the person with acrophobia, while observing sign stimuli of the proximity of converging lines of perspective, namely, the visual cues that convey the sense of height, thereupon engages in such anxiety-provoking self-talk as "This is terribly dangerous, and I'm bound to slip and fall to my death." It might also be discovered that this internal dialogue is further embellished with an internal image or movie of falling helplessly to the death. The scenario is vivid, convincing, and profoundly frightening. However, the thoughts themselves may be seen as containing an irrational component.

The traditional, rationally oriented cognitive therapist will subsequently respond in either a forcefully directive manner, such as is often the case with Albert Ellis's *rational emotive behavior therapy* (REBT), or in a relatively nondirective, Socratic manner, which is characteristic of Aaron T. Beck's *cognitive therapy* (CT). Both approaches assist the patient in challenging the validity of these cognitive structures, images, and self-utterances. From Ellis's perspective, the patient would be instructed to dispute this irrational position by recognizing that this is merely *awfulizing* or catastrophic thinking, that "having a thought of falling helplessly to your death does not mean that it will inevitably happen," and so on. At the same time, the patient might receive relevant instruction in the fact that it is not the circumstance of being in high places (i.e., activating event or "A") that is causing the high level of anxiety (i.e., consequence or "C"), but rather the mediator that occurs between A and C (i.e., irrational belief or "iB"). That is, A iB C, whereby A represents the height and C represents the anxiety and avoidance, which is caused by iB, the internal irrational belief.

Some cognitive therapies do not focus so much on the issue of rationality as the internal narrative in which the patient engages and through which experience is created. The emphasis is still stimulus–integration–response; however, attention is directed at the constructionist narrative. The patient is assisted in altering the response by altering the narrative via reframing, relabeling, and so on (Epston and White, 1992; Meichenbaum, 1997).

Of course, a cognitively-oriented therapist might choose to attend to internal linguistic factors other than beliefs and narration. Attention to the internal imagery itself might be altered alone or in concert with the internal dialogue. Similarly, the internal tone of voice might be another variable to consider. For example, alteration of the tone from one of desperation to that of confidence and calm would produce a shift in one's emotional response.

A paradigm shift within the cognitive paradigm is found with a "neo-cognitive" approach referred to as *psychology of mind* (POM) and *health realization* (HR) (Pransky, 1992; Mills, 1995), and more recently as *philosophy of living* (POL). This approach focuses on the three principles of *mind, thought,* and *consciousness* in order to make sense of psychological phenomena and to guide the therapeutic process. While the source of psychological disturbance is perceived as a function of thought, these approaches do not venture into analyzing and disputing erroneous cognition, attending to narration, and so on. The very process of examining the pathological thought processes is not considered to be advisable, as it may actually serve to reinforce the pathology. In this respect it is felt that such a process gives the patient an erroneous idea, suggesting that thought is independently powerful, separate from the mind. Rather, the patient is led to a philosophic shift and understanding of the effect of thought itself, especially when one abdicates one's own power in relationship to thought. To perceive thought as having power in and of itself is concluded to be incorrect. So, too, feelings and memories are not independently powerful. With this approach to therapy, the patient is taught about the interaction of moods and thoughts, observing that a low mood elicits negative thoughts, emotions, and a basic sense of insecurity, whereas a high mood yields quite the opposite. In the spirit of St. Francis of Assisi, patients learn that while negative thoughts will inevitably fly through their heads like buzzards, "You don't have to let them make a nest in your head." Pransky (1992) depicts moods as being equivalent to internal weather. It is neither good nor bad. It is just weather — just moods. He recommends that we be grateful in our high mood and graceful in our lower ones. Psychology of mind/health realization holds that everyone has the ability to realize mental health and that simply coming from a state of health is a much more efficient and gratifying way to approach therapy for both the client and therapist. The therapist's mission is to assist the client in achieving greater understanding, to clear up the blind spots that fuel pathology.

Whereas the behaviorist primarily attends to causal factors in the environment, the cognitive therapist views the primary cause as within the behaving organism. Certainly the behaviorist recognizes that conditioning is an event that somehow manifests within the patient; however, the trigger or essential cause is determined to emanate from the environment. Again, the distinction of the cognitive paradigm is that the cause is internal processing and that linguistic processing and other forms of internal representation are involved.

SYSTEMIC–CYBERNETIC PARADIGM

Human functioning and psychological problems can also be conceptualized within the context of the family, the workplace, the community, internationally, etc. In this respect, disorders are seen as a function of interactions within relationships and systems. The symptoms are punctuated as responses to relationship problems, misguided solutions, ways of exercising control, structural interactions, and so forth. The treatment therefore addresses these variables to promote healthier human interactions and, consequently, mental health.

The initial impetus of the systemic approach was cybernetics (Wiener, 1948, 1954; Ashby, 1956), which was developed in part from premises that can be traced to the thinking of Georg Hegel (1770–1831). Hegel's philosophical system entailed a number of useful assumptions including the following (Philips, 1969):

1. The whole is greater than the sum of its parts.
2. The nature of the parts is determined by the whole.
3. The parts cannot be comprehended independent of the whole.
4. There is dynamic interdependence of the parts.

This philosophic position obviously lends itself more easily to a study of systems, rather than individuals as independent entities, although the internal processing and external behavior of the individual also can be studied cybernetically (Furman and Gallo, 2000).

Additionally, the systemic approach recognizes a cybernetic relationship such that cause-and-effect relationships are so dynamically interrelated that their roles reverse and demarcations are blurred. That is, what can be punctuated or perceived as causing a specific "effect" may just as well be reversed such that the "cause" becomes the "effect" and the "effect" becomes the "cause." This kind of relationship is readily evident with an air-conditioning system. After the temperature in the room rises above a set point, the thermostat "causes" the air conditioner to operate until the temperature has returned to the set point, which in turn "causes" the thermostat to turn off the air-conditioning unit. The room temperature can be seen as the "cause" of the thermostat activity, while the thermostat can be seen as the "cause" of the room temperature remaining within a certain range. The thermostat can also be seen as "causing" the air conditioner to turn on and off, while the air conditioner can be seen as "causing" the thermostat to turn on and off. Other systemic relationships can be designated.

From the standpoint of therapy, one may translate thermostat into daughter and air conditioner into mother and room temperature into family mood or other family members. From the standpoint of systems theory, any therapist wishing to operate effectively within this system should be cognizant of Ashby's *law of requisite variety* (Ashby, 1956). In essence, this law states that in order to control the system — that is to produce therapeutic change — the therapist must have available at least as many options or countermoves to the moves presented by the system. That element within the system that possesses the greatest requisite variety or versatility governs or controls the system.

Again, there is no question that we are social beings and that our relationships play a large role in our behavior and perception of self. We are apt to use the information gathered from our interactions with others to define ourselves as worthwhile, caring, needed, competent, etc. Likewise, we may define ourselves as victims, persecutors, guilty, angry, neglected, and so on. By altering the structure of the relationships, symptoms and even one's deeper sense of self can be altered according to this thesis. The whole is greater than the sum of its parts.

BIOCHEMICAL PARADIGM

Turning our attention to chemistry, it is clear that neurotransmitters, hormones, and blood levels of oxygen play a significant role in our functioning and in the manifestation of psychological dysfunction. The patient with acrophobia experiences a surge of adrenaline when he or she attempts to climb a ladder or lean over a balcony from a height of several stories. When our patient with post-traumatic stress disorder was exposed to the original traumatic event, the stress was accompanied by the release of various endogenous neurohormones, including cortisol, oxytocin, vasopressin, endogenous opioids, epinephrine, and norepinephrine (van der Kolk, 1994). Additionally, low levels of serotonin, a formidable neurotransmitter, have been shown to be instrumental in exaggerated startle response (Gerson and Baldessarini, 1980; Depue and Spoont, 1989), in impulsivity and aggression (Brown et al., 1979; Coccero et al., 1989), and with respect to the involuntary preoccupation with the trauma (van der Kolk and van der Hart, 1991). Low levels of serotonin are also known to be significant aspects of depression and obsessive-compulsive disorder (Jenike et al., 1990). With these factors in mind, the medical practitioner prescribes various psychotropic agents to regulate neurotransmitters and thus afford the client some level of relief from his or her symptoms. Although these medications generally only afford symptomatic relief while the patient is taking them, in some cases the patient is able to stop the medication after a period of use without a return of symptoms.

Again, it can be readily asserted that chemistry is also a relevant factor in the formula of psychological functioning and psychological problems. We are chemical beings as much as we are mystical, conscious, unconscious, systemic, cognitive, and behavioral beings.

NEUROLOGIC PARADIGM

Besides unconscious psychodynamics, consciousness, external behavior, effects from the environment, and chemical and cognitive factors, neurology clearly plays a significant role in behavior and the manifestation of psychological problems. Distinct brain structures have been shown to be relevant in various aspects of cognitive and emotional functioning. For example, the hypothalamus is instrumental in the regulation of basic drives such as hunger, thirst, sex, and aggression; the hippocampus is relevant in declarative or explicit (conscious) memory functioning; and the amygdala is involved in a variety of aspects of emotional responsiveness and nondeclarative or implicit (unconscious) memory.

With respect to the effects of trauma on brain functioning and integrity, LeDoux (1994; 1996; LeDoux et al., 1989) has proposed an indelibility hypothesis that states that post-traumatic stress disorder results in irreversible lesions or synaptic patterns in the amygdala, thus accounting for the resistance of post-traumatic stress disorder to varieties of therapeutic efforts. It has also been theorized that the personality or the "self" can be seen as a function of synaptic configurations: "patterns of inter-connectivity between neurons in [the] brain" (LeDoux, 2002, p. 2).

However, with regard to learning and memory in general, attempts to locate specific physiological changes in the brain — that is, the engrams of memory — have not proved fruitful (Lashley, 1950; Penfield and Perot, 1963). Therefore, Pribram (1962, 1969), on the basis of these findings and his own research, has postulated a holographic model of the brain, suggesting that memory and perception, as well as possibly many other aspects of psychological functioning, are holographically rather than engramatically localized. "In short, Pribram discovered that the brain [does] more than just simple digital data processing. In order to remember, imagine, problem-solve, or appreciate music, the brain creates large-scale interference patterns with information, distributing information content throughout the brain" (Pulos, 1990, p. 32). Even the universe as a whole, as well as our perception of it, has been posited to exist holographically (Bohm, 1980), although that aspect goes beyond our present focus. It should be noted that many neurophysiology studies have supported Pribram's holographic hypothesis (Talbot, 1991).

While many questions remain regarding how the brain and other aspects of the nervous system operate, obviously the hardware of our neurology plays a role in the manifestation of our behavior, psychological functioning, and disturbances. Human beings are also neurologic beings. This leads us to an even more essential component and an even more fundamental domain.

ENERGY PARADIGM

Energy resides at the most fundamental level of being. Einstein's dictum, $E = mc^2$ (where E is energy, m is mass, and c is the speed of light), asserts that mass (or matter) and energy are interconvertible aspects of the same reality, and therefore matter is essentially energy frozen in time. In a related sense, energy is matter waiting to happen or material potentiality. Since energy operates at the speed of light and thus within a realm outside of time (Young, 1976a), it poetically follows that energy is timelessness as yet to be frozen into matter. If we could send matter soaring through space at the speed of light, we would have infinite energy and, of course, infinite matter.* Essentially then, everything in our "material" reality can be reduced to energy, although it has been suggested that action (Young, 1976a,b, 1984) and consciousness (Goswami, 1993) are more fundamental yet. However, even though distinctions among these principles can be made, energy in some form must necessarily be involved with consciousness and action.

Energy exists in various states and forms, with some more readily detectable than others. Thus, standard instrumentation can easily measure electricity as long as the current is of sufficient amperes and volts. The same holds true of electrome-chanical, electro-optical, electro-acoustical, and electromagnetic forms of energy. It

---

* However, since matter and energy are equivalent, the energy of a moving object will add to its mass and make it difficult to increase its speed. According to Einstein, an object cannot reach the speed of light, since its mass would become infinite and it would therefore require an infinite amount of energy to achieve such a speed.

is feasible and highly probable, however, that there are degrees and types of energy so subtle that they cannot be detected or accurately measured by current instruments.

If everything in our material universe is essentially energy, it follows that this holds true for the hardware of our nervous system, the neurochemistry, and even thought and cognition. While therapy can be conducted at more obvious material levels, it is hypothesized that if therapy can be directed precisely at an energy level, it will prove more thorough and immediate in its effects.

ELECTRICAL NEUROTRANSMISSION

Concerning the essentiality of energy, there are relevant analogies in medicine. For example, consider the phenomena of reuptake of the neurotransmitter serotonin or 5-hydroxytryptamine (5-HT). When a patient is clinically depressed or prone to anxiety or obsessive-compulsive rituals, the availability of serotonin at nerve synapses is compromised. While serotonin can be made more available by decelerating the reuptake process with selective serotonin reuptake inhibitors (SSRIs) such as fluoxetine (Prozac), paroxetine (Paxil), and sertroline (Zoloft), with herbal remedies such as *Hypericum perforatum* (also called St. John's wort), or with amino acids such as 5-HTP, the question remains about what causes serotonin depletion in the first place. Clearly, neurologic, biochemical, and cognitive explanations can be offered in response to our query. However, could it be that an electrical, electromagnetic, or photoelectric process accounts for both normal as well as abnormal functioning at the synapse, let alone throughout our cells? Additionally, since serotonin is also fundamentally energy, might not an energy-based procedure regulate the production of serotonin and thus alleviate depression, obsessive-compulsive behaviors, anxiety, and such? In this respect, similar to the use of transcutaneous electrical nerve stimulation (TENS) to control pain, transcranial electrostimulators (not electroconvulsive therapy) have proved effective in treating insomnia and depression (Rubik, 1995) as well as addictive disorders (Schmitt et al., 1986; Becker, 1990). While these may be relatively gross procedures, they nonetheless point to the relevance of electrical aspects involved in neurotransmission.

CURRENT OF INJURY AND REGENERATION

Along similar lines, several researchers have found microamperes of electricity or even an electromagnetic field to be effective in stimulating the healing of nonunion fractures (Bassett et al., 1982; Becker and Selden, 1985; Becker, 1990; Bassett, 1995). This technology is consistent with the finding that when a broken bone heals there is a specific current of injury at the site of the lesion that is instrumental to any regeneration process. The natural or induced current causes the bone marrow to dedifferentiate, to essentially revert to fetal material, and then to transform into bone.

Becker's initial research with the current of injury involved comparisons of variable electrical potential at the site of limb amputation between frogs and salamanders. It is common knowledge that when a salamander loses a leg (or practically any body part, for that matter), it will completely regenerate. Not so for the frog, which pays the price of its "higher" evolutionary status. Why should this be the case? Becker observed a positive electrical potential at the amputation site on the frog that became neutral as healing occurred. The salamander, on the other hand (or leg if you will), initially evidences a positive electrical potential, which reverses to negative before gradually becoming neutral as the limb regenerates. To further evaluate the relevance of this phenomenon, Becker replicated the positive-to-nega-tive-to-neutral process with frogs and was able to regenerate new limbs (Becker and Selden, 1985).

These findings are predated by some other important discoveries. At the beginning of the last century, it was learned that the hydra is electrically polarized, with the head positive and the tail negative. In 1909, Owen E. Frazee found that he could enhance the regeneration of larval salamanders by an electrical current. In the early 1920s, University of Texas researcher Elmer J. Lund conducted research demonstrating that regeneration in hydra-like species could be affected by sending subtle direct current through the body. Regeneration could be augmented or even reversed in this manner.

> A current strong enough to override the creature's normal polarity could cause the head to form where a tail should reappear, and vice versa. Others confirmed his discovery, and Lund went on to study eggs and embryos. He claimed to have influenced the development of frog eggs not only with currents but also with magnetic fields (Becker and Selden, 1985, pp. 82–83).

In 1952, following up Lund's research, G. Marsh and H.W. Beams conducted some revealing research on electrical polarity in the freshwater turbellarian flatworms of the order tricladida (also known as the planarian or *platyhelminthes*) that led them to believe that biologic electrical fields govern morphogenesis. They discovered that this species, noted for its phenomenal regenerative capacities, manifests an electrical arrangement with the head negatively charged and the tail positively charged. They also discovered that the planarian's growth could be controlled in essentially the same way that Lund found with hydras. That is, normal polarity could be reversed by sending direct current through portions of a worm's body. Increasing the current would also cause the worm to rearrange itself such that a tail would form where the head "should" be, and vice versa (Becker and Selden, 1985).

L-Fields

At Yale University, Harold Saxon Burr (1972) also became so interested in Lund's findings that he and his associates began measuring electrical current, what he referred to as fields of life or *L-fields*, in and around practically every lifeform he could get his hands on. The list included molds, various mammals, worms, sala-manders, hydras, and humans. He even planted electrodes in trees for as long as a year, carefully monitoring electrical patterns. He found that the L-fields of trees varied with sunlight, sunspots, magnetic storms, darkness, and even cycles of the moon. Burr concluded that L-fields accounted for the stability of form of all life-forms in the same way that an electromagnetic field arranges iron filings in a specific order or form.

Something like this — though infinitely more complicated — happens in the human body. Its molecules and cells are constantly being torn apart and rebuilt with fresh material from the food we eat. But, thanks to the controlling L-field, the new molecules and cells are rebuilt and arrange themselves in the same pattern as the old ones.

> Until modern instruments revealed the existence of the controlling L-fields, biologists were at a loss to explain how our bodies "kept in shape" through ceaseless metabolism and changes of material. Now the mystery has been solved, the electrodynamic field of the body serves as a matrix, which preserves the "shape" or arrangement of any material poured into it, however often the material may be changed. (Burr, 1972, pp. 12–13)

To measure electrodynamic fields, Burr used a Hewlett-Packard direct current (DC) vacuum tube voltmeter. In one interesting series of studies, Louis Langman used this device to measure cervical electrical charges of women diagnosed with malignant, as compared to benign, gynecological conditions. Of 123 females between the ages of 21 and 61+ with malignant conditions, 118 subjects or 96% had a negative DC charge, whereas 5 subjects or 4% evidenced a positive DC charge. The reverse pattern was found with a sample of 78 females (ages 10 to 61+) with no gynecological condition: 74 subjects or 95% registered a positive cervical charge, and 4 subjects or 5% had a negative charge (Langman, 1972). Thus, regeneration as well as malignancy appears to operate electrically.

Quantum Mechanics

At the level of energy, the universe is mysterious and perplexing. It does not follow the classical notions of physics, which we are accustomed to in everyday life. Because we have incorporated the regularities and effects of this macro-external reality into our psychological functioning, the structure of reasoning, and perceptions, it becomes difficult to perceive the "rationality" of this other micro-reality of which our everyday reality is really a subset.

Highlighting this mystery are several quantum mechanical discoveries. Besides the paradoxical finding that photons and electrons appear to have a rudimentary level of consciousness (Bohm, 1986) and that they behave as both waves and particles, depending on the experiment conducted (that is, our interrelationship with "it," which really poses serious problems for the subject–object distinction), the results of experimental tests of a theorem developed by John Bell in 1964 — Bell's inequity theorem — pose yet another perplexing aspect of this more fundamental reality. This "theorem states that when two subatomic particles interact and then disperse in opposite directions, interference with one particle will instantly affect the other particle, regardless of the distance between them" (Pulos and Richman, 1990, p. 222). Bell's theorem, developed out of a test of the Einstein–Podolsky–Rosen (EPR) thought experiment, suggests that information can travel faster than the speed of light or, more to the liking of physicists who hold that light is the ultimate speed, that two "related" photons or other "related" subatomic "particles" are connected nonlocally. This is consistent with Bohm's notion of the holographic universe (Bohm, 1980, 1986; Bohm and Hiley, 1993), which was later taken up by Pribram (1986) in the field of neuroscience.

In 1972, Stuart Freedman and John Clauser of the University of California at Berkeley performed critical experiments that supported Bell's predictions of nonlocality (Clauser et al., 1978). Even more support was obtained by Alain Aspect and his team at the Institute of Optics at the University of Paris in 1982 (Aspect et al., 1982). And in 1998, even more definitive proof of nonlocality was provided by Nicolus Gisin and his team at the University of Geneva (Tittel et al., 1998). These experiments demonstrated remarkably that when the polarization of one of two "related" photons traveling in opposite directions was altered (e.g., positive to negative), the polarization of the other photon almost instantaneously shifted in kind. Since photons travel at the speed of light, and since the two photons were traveling away from each other in opposite directions, the speed of information transfer between the two photons would have to be nearly twice the speed of light. Yet this is impossible if the speed of light is constant and the ultimate speed. It follows from these experiments — especially those conducted by Gisin's team, which measured "communication" between photons separated by 11 km (approximately 7 miles) — that the photons could have been separated by a distance half that of the known universe and still the communication between them would have been nearly instantaneous. Obviously, the information transfer would be billions of times faster than twice the speed of light. "The results of [these] experiments provided unequivocal evidence that the correlations between detectors located in these space-like separated regions did not weaken as the distance increased. And this obliged physicists to conclude that nonlocality or nonseparability is a global or universal dynamic of the life of the cosmos" (Nadeau and Kafatos, 1999, p. 79). In view of the *Big Bang* (or the *Big Bloom*), because everything was integrally related at the time of the cosmological commencement, in a fundamental sense everything continues to be nonlocally connected. It appears that the new physics may apply to more than just the subatomic world; it applies to the macro-universe as well — including the mind. Therefore, the question immediately arises whether mind and matter are really all that distinct. Probably not!

ENERGY PSYCHOLOGY

Application of the energy paradigm to the field of clinical psychology* would follow the assumption that psychopathology can be treated by addressing subtle energy systems in the body. Additionally, such a technology might imply an even more profound paradigmatic shift, one that holds that, in essence, psychological problems are a function of energy structures or fields. That is, while psychological disturbance manifests psychodynamically, behaviorally, systemically, cognitively, neurologically, and chemically, at the most essential level there exists a structured or codified energy component that provides the instructions that catalyze the entire process. In Bohm's terms (1980), the energy code would therefore be consistent with the *implicate order*, which in turn manifests in the *explicate order*. That is, energy would

---

* Energy psychology is not limited to clinical areas. This approach is applicable to a number of areas, including peak performance, educational, vocational, sports, and industrial psychology and intervention.

entail the initial domino that sets the entire process of psychopathology into motion, into being. Energy is the fundamental fractal.

The introduction of the energy paradigm to clinical psychology, as well as to other branches of psychology and psychotherapy, is truly a major shift in perspective, directing our attention to an entirely unique set of variables. Yet, most of psychology and psychiatry has been oriented to classical Newtonian physics. The relationship of stimulus to response, whether the stimulus is environmental or cognitive, is still consistent with basic billiard ball cause–effect interactions. But within the realm of quantum physics, which is really the domain of subtle energy, photons, electrons, and so on, the universe does not operate as neatly as Newton proposed. Within this realm, change can occur instantaneously, without having to pass through the intermediary stages required in a Newtonian universe. Change can occur nonlocally and outside of time.

Assuming that thought exists in fields and that negative emotions are rooted in energy configurations, psychological phenomena are fundamentally quantum mechanical events or processes. They exist at low levels of inertia as compared to matter (Bohm and Hiley, 1993). Because energy is not highly inertially laden, if thought and psychological problems exist in energy-field form, then psychological problems can be resolved much more easily than one might assume, based on other paradigms. It would then be merely a matter of altering or collapsing the energy field.

We now turn our attention to some therapeutic methods that achieve profound results rapidly, and at least one of these approaches specifically highlights the relevance of energy in behavior and psychotherapeutic change. And it may well be that the changes facilitated by all of these methods operate fundamentally at the energy level.

2 Highly Efficient Therapies (Or Recipes for Rapid Relief)

Psychologists are open to new procedures and changes in expectations and values over time.

— Preamble to the Ethical Principles of the American Psychological Association

It is common knowledge among professionals and lay public alike that most psychotherapeutic approaches do not produce therapeutic results rapidly. Frequently, extended periods of time are required before the patient is pronounced "significantly improved" but hardly ever "cured."* Obviously, classical psychoanalysis, as well as many other versions of the old art, can involve years of many-sessions-a-week effort. Even relatively modern approaches such as flooding, *systematic desensitization, solution focused therapy, narrative therapy, rational emotive behavioral therapy* (REBT), and various other cognitive methodologies do not consistently produce significant results quickly (such as within the course of a few minutes or even as much as a single 45-min therapy session). Ordinarily, a number of sessions are required before one can even be certain that something noteworthy has happened. Is this a function of psychological change requiring extensive effort and time? Or could it be that therapies based on traditional notions are not entirely appropriate to the task of assisting patients in achieving change efficiently?

Recently, several therapies have emerged that reportedly produce rapid therapeutic results, often within a matter of minutes. Indeed, these methods significantly deviate from therapies based on traditional psychodynamic, behavioral, cognitive, developmental, systemic, neurologic, and chemical paradigms. Although most of the developers of the methods do not proffer an energy explanation of their methods' effectiveness, it is relevant to briefly explore each of these approaches before delving in greater depth into the energy paradigm. The reality of efficacious effects demands

---

* Beginning in 1993, I presented a series of seminars throughout the United States on thought field therapy, with one of my flyers announcing, "There Is a Cure." Even though the techniques presented were amazingly simple, effective, and efficient in treating trauma and many other conditions, I decided to soften the claims because of the ire of some professionals who believed that these were the claims of charlatans, did not believe in cure, or may have been threatened by such a possibility. Understandably, paradigm shifts are not easily accepted.

our attention, especially because methods that produce such results are likely in close proximity with the most immediate or fundamental cause of psychological problems.

ACTIVE INGREDIENTS PROJECT*

Four therapies for the treatment of post-traumatic stress disorder (PTSD) were presented at the "Active Ingredients in Efficient Treatments of PTSD" Conference at Florida State University in Tallahassee on May 12–13, 1995. This conference was presided over by the principal investigators of the systematic clinical demonstration project by the same title (Carbonell and Figley, 1995, 1996, 1999; Figley et al., 1999). The therapeutic methods investigated were eye movement desensitization and reprocessing (EMDR) (Shapiro, 1995), visual/kinesthetic dissociation (V/KD) (Bandler and Grinder, 1979), traumatic incident reduction (TIR) (Gerbode, 1989), and thought field therapy (TFT) (Callahan, 1985).

In 1993, Carbonell and Figley requested "nominations" of highly effective and efficient therapies for post-traumatic stress disorder from clinicians experienced in the treatment of the disorder. The request was not limited to American Psychological Association (APA)-approved, efficacy-documented methods. The researchers were willing to explore any method, no matter how bizarre in appearance, as long as it fulfilled the criteria for inclusion in the study. This request was sent out to approximately 10,000 members of the Internet consortium InterPsych, as well as to many other therapists and researchers at seminars, conferences, and so forth.

More than a dozen nominations were received; however, only the four previously mentioned methods fulfilled the criteria for inclusion in the study. In this respect, each approach required verification of effectiveness by approximately 200 to 300 licensed or certified clinicians who regularly treat traumatized clients. It had to produce significant relief of post-traumatic stress disorder symptoms within a few sessions. Repeatability under laboratory conditions was also essential for the method to be evaluated at Florida State University. The method also had to be readily teachable to paraprofessionals, as a coordinated response to crises such as natural disasters is of obvious importance. Additionally, the principal developers and/or practitioners had to be willing to treat clients at Florida State University for a week under research conditions. Finally, the proponents had to be willing to present and defend their approach to academic clinical researchers at Florida State University.

The demonstration project secured subjects by advertising in local newspapers and other media in the Tallahassee area. They requested the participation of people suffering from the aftermath of trauma, including phobic reactions. The 51 subjects included in the study were interviewed and given an array of psychological tests and physiologic measures. Symptom inventories revealed the sample to be comparable to the typical outpatient mental health population. Each subject was allotted

---

* Although it has been expanded, most of this chapter previously appeared as "Reflections on active ingredients in efficient treatments of PTSD" in *The International Electronic Journal of Innovations in the Study of the Traumatization Process and Methods of Reducing or Eliminating Related Human Suffering*, Volume 2, Parts 1 and 2. It is reproduced here with permission from the *Electronic Journal of Traumatology*. See Reference Section.

TABLE 2.1
Florida State University Active Ingredients
Project Data[a]

Method	Subjects	Time (min)	Pre-SUD	Post-SUD
V/KD	8	113	4.75	3.25
EMDR	6	172	5.00	2.00
TIR	2	254	6.50	3.40
TFT	12	63	6.30	3.00

[a] These data have been updated since the first edition of this book.
See Carbonell and Figley (1999) for more extensive details.

a maximum of four sessions. In all, 39 completed the course of treatment, although not all complied to the letter. Some did not diligently keep a daily journal as requested, and 17 did not return for the 6-month evaluation.

Nonetheless, early follow-up evaluations within the 4- to 6-month range revealed that all of the approaches yielded sustained reduction in subjective units of distress (SUD) (i.e., subjects' ratings of their level of distress upon reviewing the traumatic memories), although minimal rebound in distress level was evident in many cases. The average pretreatment subjective units of distress rating on a 0 to 10 scale were between 8 and 9. Although follow-up evaluation time frames and the number of subjects varied considerably across treatment conditions, notably imposing variables, respective mean group treatment times, and post-treatment follow-up subjective units of distress ratings are shown in Table 2.1.

Although strict comparisons among the methods would not be valid due to varying client selection criteria across methods as well as other variables, preliminary results nonetheless supported the contention of the nominating professionals that the methods are effective in reducing distress associated with trauma, including nightmares, intrusive recollections, phobic responses, and so on.

With this in mind, we turn now to a description of the four methods that were studied in this demonstration project. This is followed by an attempt to glean some of the feasible active ingredients that may account for the power of these seemingly diverse methodologies.

VISUAL/KINESTHETIC DISSOCIATION

Visual/kinesthetic dissociation assists the client in therapeutically dissociating from the negative feelings associated with the traumatic memory, phobic situation, or any situation that induces negative emotion by visually reviewing the event from an altered visual perspective (Cameron-Bandler, 1978).

One approach to visual/kinesthetic dissociation when treating trauma, for example, is to direct the client to visualize a snapshot of a moment immediately prior to the traumatic event when the individual was feeling safe or not experiencing anything in particular. Next, dissociation is introduced by having the client visualize himself or herself in that past scene rather than "being" in that scene. Dissociation can be further enhanced by having the client maintain a perceptual position that entails an additional level of dissociation, as promoted through instructions such as the following: "Watch yourself watching the younger you way over there in the past going through (that trauma)." Most clients are able to achieve this perceptual shift with linguistic assistance on the part of the therapist. While therapeutic dissociation is maintained, the client is directed to allow the "movie" of the event to unfold and to become aware of understandings or resources needed to promote resolution. For example, it may become evident to the client that "it is over and I survived." The client is then asked to "share" this knowledge and understanding with the "past self," the one who suffered the trauma. Obviously the sharing takes place in imagery and internal dialogue. Once the client perceives his or her "younger self" feeling safe and secure, the client may be directed to follow up with a kinesthetic gesture of "reaching out and taking hold" of the younger self and "bringing the younger self into one's self" so that the client may feel forever safe. This entire procedure often results in a significant reduction or elimination of the negative affect with any future recall of the event.

Another approach to visual/kinesthetic dissociation is to have the client imagine that he or she is seated comfortably in a movie theater, viewing an achromatic snapshot of a scene immediately preceding the trauma. Once this scene is in mind, the therapist directs the client to the next level of dissociation by saying words such as the following: "And now float out of your body seated there in the theater, and float back here in the projection booth with me while we watch you down there seated in the theater, watching the younger you way over there in the past on the movie screen. And continue to remain safely and comfortably up here in the projection booth with me, as we observe you seated in the theater, watching the movie of that traumatic event unfold in slow motion."

The therapist continues with dissociative language to assist the client in maintaining distance while the movie plays all the way to the end. The client is asked to allow the scene to unfold to a point where he or she feels relatively safe, allowing that final scene to freeze into a snapshot. Next, the therapist asks the client to reassociate into the seated position in the theater: "And now float back down into your body seated there in the theater, continuing to observe that snapshot of the safe scene after the trauma is over."

After this phase of the procedure is completed, the client is asked to associate into the scene on the screen: "And now step into that safe moment up on the screen. I am going to ask you to do something that only sounds difficult as I describe it, but you will actually find it fairly easy to do. When I say 'begin,' allow the scene to become colorful and to rapidly proceed backward all the way to the beginning. Everything should be going in reverse: gestures, walking, moving, words, and so on. Allow this all to happen very quickly, taking no more than two or three seconds to complete. And when you are at the beginning of the scene, that safe place before it all began, I would like you to stop picturing the scene and to look out at me. Do you understand?... Ready?... Begin."

After the backward movie is completed, the therapist directs the client to look at the therapist, to stop internal visualization. Checking the client's emotional response to the memory generally reveals a significant reduction or elimination of distress. Sometimes this method needs to be repeated a few times to eliminate all distress associated with the traumatic event.

Developed by Bandler and Grinder (1979), visual/kinesthetic dissociation is a neurolinguistic programming (NLP) technique. Neurolinguistic programming is a method of modeling and not a theoretical position. It entails patterning the internal and external behaviors of people who have been able to achieve consistent results in various activities, including psychotherapy. Visual/kinesthetic dissociation is likely modeled from the behavior of renowned therapists such as hypnotists-psychiatrists Milton H. Erickson, M.D., and Frederick S. Pearls, M.D., Ph.D., founders of Gestalt therapy. It is based on the recognition of synesthesia patterns, which are stimulus–response (S-R) bonds between sensory systems. For example, an external or internal visual stimulus can result in an immediate unpleasurable or negative kinesthetic response. When employed to treat trauma, the focus of visual/kinesthetic dissociation is on interrupting the synesthesia pattern by introducing dissociation while the client attends to the memory of the event. This creates a revised stimulus–response bond. That is, since the individual no longer recalls the trauma in an associated manner, negative emotionality is removed from the memory. This process should not be confused with the global dissociation that is characteristic of conditions such as post-traumatic stress disorder and various dissociative disorders. While these conditions involve severe disruptions of various integrative functions, visual/kinesthetic dissociation merely entails a shift in one's perception of a memory from associated (i.e., as if one is reliving the experience) to disassociated (i.e., not experiencing the memory in an associated manner).

EYE MOVEMENT DESENSITIZATION AND REPROCESSING

Eye movement desensitization and reprocessing directs the client to attend to traumatic memories while "tracking" eye movements in response to the therapist's prompting. The client also attends to any associated negative belief (e.g., "I'm powerless.") and attends to emotional and physical factors stimulated during the process. Subjective units of distress are monitored while the therapist follows the client in a fairly nondirective manner, prompting eye movements as relevant material emerges. After this procedure results in significant reduction in subjective units of distress, the client may rehearse an appropriate positive belief (e.g., "I'm powerful since I survived.") during eye movements in order to "install" the new, healthier belief. It should be noted that during eye movement desensitization and reprocessing, associated memories, evidence of a greater memory network, often emerge and are treated in a similar manner. Other phases of treatment include "body scan" to evaluate progress and determine targets for additional sets of eye movements, if necessary, and "closure," which includes assessment of safety, client debriefing, etc. Forms of stimulation other than eye movements, including tones, light, and physical tapping, have also been found to be effective.

Shapiro believes that the bilateral stimulation triggers "a physiological mechanism that activates the information-processing system" (Shapiro, 1995, p. 30). She lists various mechanisms that may be responsible for activating and facilitating processing: "dual focus of attention … to present stimuli and the past trauma; a differential effect of neuronal bursts caused by the various stimuli, which may serve as the equivalent of a low-voltage current and directly affect synaptic potential; [and] de-conditioning caused by a relaxation response" (Shapiro, 1995, p. 30). The traumatic material is assumed to be processed to an adaptive resolution via accelerated information processing. It is proposed that this tends to occur naturally with lesser issues but is frequently blocked when one is exposed to intense experiences such as trauma. It is hypothesized that eye movement desensitization and reprocessing serves to activate this natural healing mechanism.

While eye movement desensitization and reprocessing may be the most popular and most extensively researched approach to employ eye movements in the treatment of trauma and some other psychological disorders, the reader may be interested to know that there are at least three other therapeutic approaches that utilized eye movements: Rapid eye technology (Johnson, 1994), eye movement integration (Andreas and Andreas, 1995), and one eye techniques (Cook and Bradshaw, 1999). However, as of this publication, little or no empirical research has been conducted on these approaches.

TRAUMATIC INCIDENT REDUCTION

Traumatic incident reduction is one of many methods subsumed under what is referred to as metapsychology, the development of psychiatrist Frank Gerbode, partly from his extensive experience in scientology and dianetics. Traumatic incident reduction is a specific process whereby the client, referred to as "viewer," visualizes the traumatic incident while the therapist provides instructions. The viewer locates an incident that is believed to be resolvable within the course of the session, which may require several hours. The viewer is instructed to choose a most "interesting" traumatic event, since it is assumed that "interest" signals the capacity and inclination to learn. Once an incident is located, the viewer is instructed to note any awareness just prior to the event unfolding. Next, the event is viewed silently from beginning to end, after which the viewer reports what was observed. This process is repeated until the viewer arrives at a resolution. It is assumed that there are gaps in the viewer's awareness and that by repeatedly viewing the event this information comes to the fore, thus resulting in alleviation of negative emotions and cognition associated with the event. The resolution of earlier associated trauma, the awareness of which may emerge during this process, is also assumed to be relevant in this regard, as is awareness of the intention that the person had at the time the traumatic event(s) occurred.

While traumatic incident reduction has many commonalties to flooding, it is nonetheless a significant departure from this traditional approach to exposure. Although the behavior therapist may also attend to his or her relationship with the client, the traumatic incident reduction therapist takes great "pains" and time establishing a deep relationship with the viewer. Gerbode (1989) notes that Carl Rogers was a significant influence on him in this regard. Additionally, traumatic incident reduction assumes that the trauma will be resolved within the course of a single session, even if the session requires several hours to complete.

THOUGHT FIELD THERAPY

Thought field therapy directs the client to attend to a disturbing traumatic memory or other emotionally charged condition while physically tapping on specific acupuncture meridian points. The therapist often follows a diagnostic process involving a manual muscle testing procedure to discern a specific sequence of meridian points needed to achieve therapeutic results. Another thought field therapy diagnostic procedure, the voice technology (VT™),* determines a sequence by evaluating the patient's voice. A standard thought field therapy trauma algorithm, derived from diagnostic procedures, has the client attune to the traumatic memory, determine subjective units of distress between 1 and 10, and then briefly tap on each of the following potent meridian points (i.e., major treatments) in sequence: beginning of an eyebrow above the bridge of the nose (the second acupoint on the bladder meridian), directly under an eye orbit (the first acupoint on the stomach meridian), approximately 6 in. under an armpit (the 21st or last acupoint on the spleen meridian), and under the collarbone next to the sternum (the 27th or last acupoint on the kidney meridian). After these treatments are completed, the distress rating generally dropping by several points, the client is directed through the nine gamut treatments (9G), which involve simultaneously tapping between the little and ring fingers on the back of a hand (the third acupoint on the triple heater meridian) while doing the following: eyes closed and opened, eyes down left and down right, eyes in clockwise and counterclockwise directions, humming notes, counting, and humming again. At this point the subjective units of distress are generally lower yet, and the client is directed to repeat the major treatments. Frequently, at this phase, all or most distress associated with the memory has been alleviated. If the distress rating is not down to a 1, repeating the treatments will often achieve the desired results.

Sometimes associated memories emerge when treating a targeted traumatic memory. The thought field therapy treatments are then merely directed at the new material, which is generally treated just as quickly and effectively as the target memory.

Also, at times a client evidences a condition referred to as psychological reversal (PR), which blocks the treatments from working. It is hypothesized that psychological reversal entails reversed energy flow in the meridians, which results in a negativistic, self-sabotaging state. Psychological reversal treatment often quickly corrects this condition so that therapy can proceed successfully. While a variety of psychological reversals have been identified, the most common form is corrected by having the client simultaneously tap on the little finger side of a hand (the third acupoint on the small intestine meridian) while repeating an affirmation. such as "I accept myself even though I have this problem."†

---

* The VT is a diagnostic method trademarked by Roger J. Callahan, Ph.D.
† While many therapists who employ treatments for psychological reversal continue to use affirmations in conjunction with tapping on specific acupoints, over the past several years Callahan has discontinued this practice, as the use of affirmations does not appear to be invariably essential for correcting psychological reversal. In addition, it is likely that Callahan has done this to clarify the distinction between thought field therapy and cognitive approaches to therapy. An affirmation such as "I deeply accept myself even though I have this problem" obviously involves cognition.

Thought field therapy is based on the assumption that psychological problems are manifestations of isolable active information (Bohm and Hiley, 1993) energetically coded within thought fields. Callahan defines a thought field as: "the specific thoughts, perturbations and related information which are active in a problem or treatment situation. In order to diagnose and treat effectively, the appropriate thought field must be attuned" (Callahan, 1994a, p. 7). Examples of thought fields include traumatic memories, thinking about or being in proximity of phobic object, or even the thought of an elephant. A perturbation is defined as "the fundamental and easily modifiable trigger containing specific information, which sets off the physiological, neurological, hormonal chemical, and cognitive events that result in the experience of specific negative emotions" (Callahan, 1995, p. 2). By removing the perturbation(s) from the thought field, distress associated with the traumatic memory, the phobia, or the thought about an elephant (if one is phobic of elephants) is alleviated.

FEASIBLE ACTIVE INGREDIENTS

It is evident that a significant contribution of the active ingredients project is in its exploration of several methods that appear to efficiently treat trauma and phobias. The methods are unique and are predicated on revolutionary theoretical positions. Therefore, it is clear that there are a variety of ways to efficiently treat the same condition. While this is hardly earth shattering, nonetheless it affords reference points for deciphering the ingredients responsible for the methods' efficacy. That is, what commonalties account for the efficiency of these methods? Perhaps more importantly, when a method excels in some respect, what are the particular ingredients that account for this?

With these questions and interests in mind, plausible active ingredients that may account for the effectiveness of these four therapies are explored. While detailed research is indicated toward clarifying the extent of the treatment effects, as well as the necessary ingredients involved, it momentarily allows some speculation regarding the active ingredients. The following is not intended to be a comprehensive compilation but rather a highlighting of some feasible ingredients. These points are simply offered for their possible heuristic value toward advancing the understanding of active ingredients, stimulating research, and promoting the evolution and utilization of effective means of treating trauma-based conditions.

EXPOSURE AND ATTUNEMENT

Exposure has been a primary method for treating trauma. Clinical experience and research supports the position that *in vivo* and exposure in imagination to relevant stimuli over an extended period of time can result in the extinguishing of negative affective responses. So, too, some degree of "exposure" appears to be an ingredient in the methods reviewed. Each requires the subject to "think about" the trauma. This is necessary for later desensitization or extinguishing of associated symptoms. While the developers of the methods proffer varying theoretical positions, not always favoring terms such as "extinguish" or "desensitization," this is understandable and permissible in light of the rapidity of treatment effects and the significant departure of these methods from traditional procedures. In this respect, it is evident that exposure alone cannot adequately account for the efficacy of these therapies; otherwise, flooding would prove equally efficient. Additionally, the degree of exposure induced with some of the methods is so minimal that "attunement," a term preferred by Callahan (1994a,b), should perhaps be substituted. This term does not indicate intense vivification that is generally implied by "exposure." In instances of exposure as generally understood, it should be borne in mind that the subject willingly maintains an unwavering level of attention to the trauma. This is entirely distinct from traumatic material emerging spontaneously when the subject is the victim of such events. Conscious choice in this manner may frequently serve to create a sense of self-efficacy that further figures into the resolution formula.

DISSOCIATED OBSERVATION

An "outside observer" position is promoted directly with visual/kinesthetic dissociation (Cameron-Bandler, 1978), while the other methods may provide this ingredient indirectly. In this respect, the subject is no longer "in" the memory, but is "outside" looking at it. Such a shift stimulates the acquisition of other understandings while emotionality is reduced. The associated distinction becomes clear as a memory is recalled in a similar manner in which the event was initially experienced. In this instance, the image is "seen" through the individual's eyes, as though it is then occurring. If the affect is associated with such a memory, its intensity is readily perceivable when associated. Dissociation, on the other hand, entails recalling the event with the internal image including the observer, an event that could not have occurred at the time of the original event. This position yields a significant decrease in affective intensity relative to associated recall. With visual/kinesthetic dissociation, this perceptual shift appears to be a primary causal factor in promoting relief from the trauma. It should be emphasized, however, that dissociation is a temporarily induced aspect of the procedure, as the patient is later directed to re-associate and maintain the "learnings" acquired during the dissociation phase.

SUBMODALITIES AND TRANSMODAL REATTUNEMENT

In addition to viewing from a disassociated position, trauma neutralization can also be promoted via change in other facets of internal sensory representations, referred to as "submodalities" (Bandler, 1985). For example, the visual modality can be analyzed in terms of elements such as perspective, proximity, movement, and so forth. Visual/kinesthetic dissociation induces alteration of such elements by having subjects see them seeing themselves in the scene. Given this shift, as well as others prescribed during the process, additional imagery changes frequently follow. This may entail the memory shifting from a movie to a snapshot, from colorful to achromatic, from clear to vague, etc. Also, changes in the visual modality often result in transmodal reattunement. For example, closer-appearing images may entail a louder auditory component as compared to more distant appearing images. The other methods often appear to produce similar shifts. Shapiro (1995) cites the case of a Vietnam veteran treated with eye movement dissociation and reprocessing reporting that the auditory component of the memory became silent, the visual aspects became like "a paint chip under water," and the affect calmed. I too have obtained similar reports from patients treated with thought field therapy as well as eye movement dissociation and reprocessing. For example, some patients report that the memory appears "more distant" or "vague" after treatment is completed. This is not a hard and fast rule, however, as others report being able to distinctly or even more distinctly recall the trauma, albeit without the previously reported negative affects. Of course, recalling a memory clearly does not exclude the possibility of other submodality alterations. Additionally, there may be a distinction between cause and effect regarding these factors, depending upon the method involved. These phenomena warrant closer scrutiny.

DUAL FOCUS OF ATTENTION

Dual focus of attention is assumed to be a primary ingredient of eye movement dissociation and reprocessing (Shapiro, 1995) and possibly thought field therapy as well, in that both entail physical stimulation while the subject attends to the traumatic memory. However, the manner in which such simultaneous stimulation occurs is significant. For a subject to attend to elements within the environment while simultaneously attending to a traumatic memory, a distraction that certainly occurs even when therapeutic efforts are not being made may not sufficiently provide this ingredient. Specific eye movements, hand tapping and finger snapping (Shapiro, 1995, p. 67), listening to unique bilateral sounds (Yourell, 1995), and tapping at specific acupuncture meridian energy points (Callahan, 1985) are modes of stimulation likely to be most effective in this regard.

A relevant feature of dual-focused attention is that it helps the client to remain focused in the here and now. Especially with regard to a trauma, there is a tendency for one to lose a significant amount of contact with the present moment and instead revivify or otherwise reexperience the past event. Given simultaneous stimulation, the tendency to age-regress is interrupted. This affords the patient the experience of present time, which necessarily alters the experience of the past time.

PARADOX

Choosing to recall a trauma entails paradoxical elements that have been observed to be curative among a variety of therapeutic systems. Consider Viktor Frankl's paradoxical intention, Milton Erickson's double binds (Erickson et al., 1976), and the Zen master's koans. As the subject attends to the disturbing memory, perhaps there is a suspension of the usual ways of experiencing, thus permanently altering the experience of the traumatic event. Bear in mind, however, that this may only be a side feature, since it does not appear that, in general, paradoxical procedures have been as rapidly effective as the methods presented.

COMFORT

Each method departs from pure exposure to varying degrees, assisting the client in feeling more comfortable during the course of attuning the trauma. The least divorced from flooding appears to be traumatic incident reduction, while the most removed and thus most comfortable for both client and therapist is thought field therapy. Comfort is an important aspect of the most rapid means of alleviating trauma. The more comfort experienced during the procedure, the more rapidly neutralization is likely to occur. Although it is not entirely accurate to compare the methods studied in the active ingredients project, as the study was not structured to yield such comparisons, the data nonetheless favor such a hypothesis in that results were most rapidly achieved with thought field therapy and least rapidly with traumatic incident reduction. (Although traumatic incident reduction represents a definite advancement over flooding in that it achieves results more efficiently by focusing on resolving the trauma within the context of a single session and by connecting the identified trauma with earlier associated traumas, it nonetheless appears to be in closest propinquity to flooding relative to the other methods.) While methods such as systematic desensitization inhibit anxiety via progressive relaxation while reviewing segments of the trauma (i.e., reciprocal inhibition), these newer therapies utilize other, more rapid means of interrupting associated negative emotionality. In many instances this might be referred to as rapid reciprocal inhibition or rapid desensitization. Bilateral eye movements, tapping, and sounds (eye movement dissociation and reprocessing); tapping on meridian energy points (thought field therapy); or therapeutic dissociation (visual/kinesthetic dissociation) each promote comfort by interrupting the intensity of negative affects. Comfort allows one to attend more easily to the trauma. Additionally, comfort becomes associated with the trauma, quelling its effects. Neurologically, these processes serve to soothe the amygdala and sever the stimulus–response bond between various sensory representations of the trauma or other issue and the emotional components. Again, the reader's attention is directed to the fact that, while comfort appears to be a most relevant factor, it can hardly account singularly for the results evidenced with these therapies or efficient therapy in general.

Positive Expectations

Expectations are promoted that the memory will be resolved within the context of the session, rather than perpetuating the notion that extended time is needed. This challenges the subject's belief to the contrary, reinforced by the fact that distress has existed over an extended period of time. As Rosenthal and Frank (1956) suggested, "It may well be that the efficacy of any particular set of therapeutic operations lies in the analogy to a placebo in that they enhance the therapist's and patient's conviction that something useful is being done" (p. 300). This may be a relevant ingredient with methods such as traumatic incident reduction and visual/kinesthetic dissociation, but it is possibly less likely that the odd-appearing thought field therapy and eye movement dissociation and reprocessing would be conducive to promoting placebo effects. Subjects may be less inclined to believe that moving their eyes or tapping at specific points on the body could neutralize trauma. While some may find this a plausible notion, most people in Western culture would be less inclined to experience positive expectations from such procedures. Nonetheless, we should not overlook the congruent expectations of the therapist, which may resonate positive expectations for the client at a conceivably unconscious level.

INTENTIONALITY

What is intention? Let us review some definitions from the *American Heritage Dictionary of the English Language,* 3rd ed.: 1. A course of action that one intends to follow. 2. An aim that guides action; an objective. 3. Purpose with respect to marriage: honorable intentions. 4. A concept arising from directing the attention toward an object. 5. The process by which or the manner in which a wound heals. 6. Archaic. import; meaning. [Middle English *entencioun,* from Old French intention, from Latin *intentio,* intention, from *intentus,* intent, from past participle of *intendere,* to direct attention.]

For our purposes, we are interested in definitions that relate to a course of action, guiding action, directing attention, and meaning. The intention of the therapist and the client is an instrumental aspect of guiding the attention, action, and meaning of the therapeutic process and procedures. It is proposed that a procedure in and of itself is insufficient to produce a therapeutic result. To simply provide a technique without directing or aiming it at an appropriate target (e.g., thought of a trauma, a phobia, etc.) would prove of little or no benefit. The technique must be directed toward a goal or outcome in mind. This active ingredient is especially prominent with the "power therapies" in that both the therapist and client are intentionally focused on the target (e.g., memory of the trauma), monitoring its every movement toward the intended goal of resolution, alleviation of negative emotionality, and perhaps adaptive insight. Inasmuch as other therapeutic relationships operate in a similar fashion, they also share in this active ingredient.

Another aspect of intentionality worth exploring is a resonance of positive energy from the therapist to the patient, as well as from the patient "into" the "locus" of the psychological problem. This effect is possibly related to the psi phenomenon of psychokinesis and prayer for which there is some empirical support (Dossey, 1993). Also, most therapists have discovered clients who therapeutically respond to practically any technique — likely a combination of intention and positive expectations on the part of the client. Most therapists have also discovered that the afterglow from attending a powerful training experience resulted in their achieving outstanding results with clients in the weeks immediately following the training. Again, we surmise that intentions and positive expectations may be significant operating principles in this respect.

BIOENERGY

Thought field therapy was the only therapy represented at the 1995 Florida State University active ingredients conference that addresses the bioenergy system directly by having the client tap on specific acupuncture meridian points in sequence while accessing the trauma (Callahan, 1985, 1995). This procedure is entirely distinct from other methods of simultaneous stimulation and may reasonably account for the rapid treatment effects of thought field therapy as compared to many other methods. Callahan's position is that such stimulation transduces kinetic energy into the bioenergy system, thus removing perturbations or "active information" (Bohm and Hiley, 1993) from the specific thought field, which includes a memory of the trauma.

Perturbations are hypothesized codes that cause the energy system to activate negative affects.

If all fundamental change entails transformation at the energy level, then other effective methods may also treat the energy system in distinct ways. Perhaps eye movement desensitization and reprocessing primarily stimulates a neurologic process that accelerates information processing while balancing the energy system, thus alleviating negative effect and other sequelae associated with the trauma. Visual/kinesthetic dissociation may accomplish this same effect via reframing and alteration of internal sensory representations, which are facilitated through reduction of negative effect via temporary therapeutic dissociation. The bioenergetic balance promoted through visual/kinesthetic dissociation serves to neutralize the perturbed bioenergetic state associated with the traumatic memory, phobia, etc. Traumatic incident reduction possibly accomplishes this same end by assisting the patient in accessing interest, maintaining a respectful and supportive interaction, and promoting the acquisition of repressed information.

PATTERN INTERRUPTION AND DISRUPTION

Each of these approaches also introduces a significant change in the way that the traumatic memory or other emotionally charged material is stored or represented. Obviously, prior to adding tapping or eye movements, the memory was recalled without those additional elements. The pattern or structure of the memory now becomes interrupted, disrupted, and thus changed. It is no longer stored in the nervous and energy systems in the same way that it was previously (or not at all for that matter). The information or memory has been altered or overwritten. Therefore, this new representation or new memory cannot include the associated negative emotions and cognition. Adding therapeutic dissociation as well as retrieving repressed material can also change the memory and thus the experience. Neurologically, activation of the amygdala is not associated with this new memory. Also, it is proposed that the trauma loses its form or structure — which includes synaptic configurations, energy fields, chemical structure — and thus entropy prevails, namely, a loss of order. The structure determines the effect, and since that structure is obliterated, the emotional charge is gone as well.

CONCLUSIONS

From an energy psychology perspective, the hypothesis offered is as follows: When thorough psychotherapeutic change occurs of necessity, it does so at the most fundamental level. Therefore, all fundamental psychotherapy entails change at the level of energy, an essential building block of our reality. Of course, there are a variety of ways to skin the proverbial Schrödinger cat. Tapping on specific meridian points, which shall be explored in depth in Chapters 6 and 7, appears to be one of them. Bilateral ocular, tactile, or auditory stimulation are others. Therapeutic dissociation and submodality alterations are still others. Not inferior in the least are methods that alleviate energy disruption in a more global manner by way of profound philosophical shifts and observational awareness of the thought at the basis of the problem, meditation, and so on. Thus, we can chunk up or chunk down in order to achieve therapeutic results.

However, efficacy in addition to effectiveness must certainly be a pragmatic criterion worth pursuing. The position offered here is that specificity and precision seem to be factors involved in the most rapid and efficient results. And the more precisely we direct our therapeutic efforts at the level of energy, the more efficient and rapid our therapeutic results will be achieved. Choosing a baseball metaphor, one stands a better chance of hitting a home run when the ball is hit at the "sweet spot" on the bat. With this in mind, let us attend more closely to the energy paradigm.

3 The Energy Paradigm (Or the Electric Patterns of Life)

Under this name, which conveys the experience of effort with which we are familiar in ourselves, physics has introduced the precise formulation of a capacity for action or, more exactly, for interaction. Energy is the measure of that which passes from one atom to another in the course of their transformations. A unifying power, then, but also, because the atom appears to become enriched or exhausted in the course of this exchange, the expression of structure.

— **Teilhard de Chardin,** *The Phenomenon of Man* **(1955)**

The Universe is vast. Nothing is more curious than the self-satisfied dogmatism with which mankind at each period of its history cherishes the delusion of the finality of its existing modes of knowledge. Skeptics and believers are all alike. At this moment scientists and skeptics are the leading dogmatists. Advance in detail is admitted: fundamental novelty is barred. This dogmatic common sense is the death of philosophical adventure. The Universe is vast.

— **Alfred North Whitehead,** *Essays in Science and Philosophy* **(1948)**

ACUPUNCTURE

Five thousand years ago, give or take a century or two, an anonymous person or persons in China discovered that the body has an energy system that follows specific pathways referred to as channels or meridians. Predating the Chinese findings by a couple of thousand years, the same bioenergy system, albeit with unique distinctions and treatment procedures, was elucidated in India. There is also evidence that similar knowledge sprang up previously in other parts of the world, including Egypt, Europe, Arabia, Brazil, among the Bantu tribes of Africa, and the Eskimos. Goodheart (1987) points out that "[t]he papyrus ebers of 1150 B.C., one of the most important of the ancient Egyptian medical treatises, refers to a book on the subject of muscles which would correspond to the 12 meridians of acupuncture" (p. 10).

The Chinese system elaborates 12 primary bilateral meridians, each of which passes through a specific organ of the body, including the lungs, heart, stomach, large intestine, liver, and so forth. It also details the collector meridians, which intersect the front and back of the body and enter the brain, the so-called governing vessel, and the central or conception vessel. Additionally, there are a number of lesser-known

31

collaterals and extraordinary vessels that connect with the primary meridians. The entire system is interconnected in such a way that the flow of energy, referred to by the Chinese as *qi* or *chi* (pronounced chee, as in cheese, and often written as *ch'i*), travels from one meridian to the next, circulating throughout the body.*

DISCOVERING THE MERIDIANS

How the meridians were discovered remains a mystery. Besides the likelihood of considerable trial and error, it has been proposed that perhaps the specifics of the bioenergy system were delineated as a result of observing the effects of injuries to soldiers in battle (Chang, 1976). The locations of the assaults were recorded and correlated with various positive and negative effects. On the positive side, if a soldier was injured at a specific location at the shoulder, for example, the vicinity of a significant point related to the lung meridian, possibly a respiratory condition that he had been struggling with for years would miraculously vanish. Many events of this nature could have led to an understanding of a relationship between the shoulders, as well as other bodily locations, and the lungs. Similarly, other organs were correlated with various locations on the body.

Another rather dubious theory is that the specifics of the energy system were discovered as a result of the haphazard activities of tailors who accidentally inflicted injuries upon themselves and their patrons. Possibly in time the precise locations of such injuries were compared among members of the garment industry, and this information eventually migrated into the medical establishment.

Still another theory, more or less palatable depending on one's orientation, is that the people who discovered the bioenergy system possessed higher sensory abilities that made it possible for them to see or palpate the energetic flow within the meridians, thus enabling them to precisely delineate the meridian geography. Today, while many acupuncturists employ specific therapeutic recipes for needle placement, still other more highly skilled practitioners are reported to detect the stagnant or overactive flow of chi via palpation of the relative strength or weakness in 12 specific pulses on the patient's wrists.

NEI CHING

Regardless of how the discoveries came about, an extensive compilation eventually appeared in the 24-volume *Nei ching*. This is the oldest writing on acupuncture, attributed to Huang Ti, the "Yellow Emperor," who, although it is debated, reportedly ruled China for 100 years from about 2697 to 2597 B.C. Modern-day acupuncture has deviated little from this text, suggesting that the system was developed and refined over the course of many preceding centuries.

---

* This subtle life energy has been referred to by many names throughout various cultures and traditions. In India it is *prana* and in Japan it is *ki*. Others have used the terms *vis medicatrix naturae, life energy, yesod, baraka, waken, orenda,* and *megbe*. In a very real sense, assuming that it is real, this energy system may not be considered to be directly a part of the physical body at all but rather a flow of energy that interacts with a number of energy fields that intersect within and surround the physical body. It is of interest to note that the Chinese term *chi* is also translated as influence, power, and mind.

In addition to providing information about the pathways themselves, the *Nei ching* text details information on specific acupoints. For example, along each meridian there is a *tonification* point, which, when stimulated, increases the availability of energy within the meridian. *Sedation* points, on the other hand, reduce overactive energy. Additionally, there are *luo* (pronounced low) points, which balance energy between meridians; *shi* (pronounced she) points, that are stimulated when energy is exceptionally deficient; *alarm* points, used for diagnosis and treatment; *source* points, that affect the meridian as a whole; and so on (Walther, 1988).

ACUPOINT STIMULATION

It is common to think of acupuncture as performed with needles, since the meridian acupoints can be stimulated with needles. However, the term acupuncture is actually a misnomer. It is perhaps better to refer to this treatment as meridian therapy, as there are many forms of stimulation that can be applied to affect the availability of chi within and between meridians. In addition to the simple insertion of needles, other means of stimulation include twirling the inserted acupuncture needle (*d'ai chi*); exerting pressure with the fingers or various acu-aids (acupressure — clearly a misnomer since the term denotes *needle pressure*); rubbing on acupoints; running one's hands in the direction of the meridian flow (running the meridian); creating a vacuum at the points with suction cups; using electricity or a cold laser; consuming specific herbs, vitamins, minerals, and glandular extracts; performing specialized exercises, such as Hatha Yoga routines; manipulating specific muscles associated with respective meridians; burning moxa (moxibustion, which is discussed in the *Nei Ching*, in addition to the use of needles); as well as a wide variety of additional means. Goodheart (1975) and Callahan (1985) have explored the effectiveness of tapping or percussion at acupoints. Diamond (1985) has elucidated affirmations, which he has found to be relevant toward balancing energy within meridians as well as in the person's life as a whole. For example, an imbalance associated with the large intestine meridian, which can be relevant to emotions such as guilt, has been effectively alleviated by having the client state an affirmation such as the following: "I am basically clean and good." A heart meridian imbalance, which may entail chronic feelings of anger, may be corrected by an affirmation such as "I have forgiveness in my heart." Diamond has also investigated the relevance of rhythmic percussion on the sternum over the thymus gland, which he considers to be the controlling gland of the bioenergy system (Diamond, 1980b, 1985), as well as the value of listening to specific performances of various kinds of music to enhance what he calls "life energy" (Diamond, 1981b, 1983, 1986). *Life energy* is Diamond's term for chi.

PROVING CHI AND MERIDIANS

Even though acupuncture and many other forms of meridian therapy have been employed for thousands of years and acupuncture is becoming increasingly accepted as an effective therapeutic approach with licensure granted in many jurisdictions, questions still remain regarding the reality of meridians and chi, the specificity of acupoints, and, most relevant, the effectiveness of such therapies. Anecdotal reports, while interesting and informative in many respects, just will not do.

One of the problems involved in accepting meridians has been the absence of any known anatomical structure. While de Vernejoul and his colleagues (1984, 1985) have provided radiological photographs of radioactive technetium-injected meridians, reportedly others have searched similarly in vain (Becker and Selden, 1985). Stux and Pomeranz (1995) report that most researchers who have attempted to replicate the de Vernejoul study have concluded that he was actually photographing the lymphatic system and not meridian pathways. However, for a moment let's take a closer look at this study, as it does provide some significant findings.

The de Vernejoul study involved a total of 330 subjects. The researchers injected radioactive tracers (isotopes), technetium 99m, at acupuncture points and a computerized gamma camera was used for image analysis. On each subject, the radioactive tracer was injected at control or sham points located outside any acupoint and additional injections were made at acupoints, specifically the seventh point on the kidney meridian (K-7) bilaterally. Both healthy subjects and those with kidney (renal) pathology were used and each subject trial was repeated several times. Those tracer migrations from acupoints in both healthy and ill subjects followed the identical pathways described as meridians in traditional Chinese medicine, which were distinct from vascular and lymphatic pathways. With injections at bilateral kidney-7, there was a faster diffusion on the healthy side and slower diffusion on the diseased side. In inflammatory organ disease, there was increased migration speed of the tracer in the meridian of the related organ. The researchers noted that the findings might be applicable to diagnosis and therapeutic evaluation. The laboratory experiments with cell membranes suggested that acupoint stimulation could be used to provoke constant and reproducible change in cellular physiology. They also concluded that the migration speed and patterns of the radioactive tracer along pathways that coincide with the acupuncture meridians demonstrate that these routes have neither a vascular nor a lymphatic origin and are likely related to the connective tissue (fascia) diffusion following the neurovascular bundles along the extremities.

Another study conducted in China suggests that a possible anatomical substrate for meridians is perivascular space (Ma et al., 2003). The authors note that perivascular space has been demonstrated to be a body fluid pathway in addition to blood vessels and lymphatics. They studied characteristics of the tissues around the blood vessels along the stomach and gallbladder meridians, with the goal of identifying anatomical structures corresponding to the meridians described in traditional Chinese medicine. Through perivascular dye injection and frozen section histology, they found perivascular space fluid pathways around the blood vessels along the meridians. Subsequent physiologic studies revealed that the perivascular space shows significantly greater electrical conductivity and significantly higher partial oxygen pressure compared to medial and lateral tissues. The researchers concluded that the perivascular space along the meridians has properties offering a feasible explanation for the meridian phenomena.

While Pomeranz (1996) corroborates the effectiveness of acupuncture on the basis of his extensive research, instead of support for the existence of chi, he offers an acupuncture-endorphin theory for the effects of acupuncture in light of 16 lines of evidence. He points out that although the traditional Chinese medicine paradigm is energetic in orientation, claiming that chi energy flows through the meridians, he has been unable to find evidence for the existence of this subtle energy. It should be noted, however, that while Pomeranz shows evidence that acupuncture stimulates the release of endorphins when the needles are inserted in nerves within specific muscles, he is not claiming that all of acupuncture's effects are due to endorphins. In an interview he stated, "There are a lot of [acupuncture] points that don't have muscles or nerves — you're going into tendons or into the ear lobe. But if you're doing those things, you're getting effects that are not [related to] endorphins. Only endorphin release requires nerve stimulation and *d'ai chi* [i.e., twirling the acupuncture needle]; but there's more to acupuncture than endorphins" (Pomeranz, 1996, p. 87).

Along these lines Gerber points out that while experiments have demonstrated that endorphin-blocking agents such as naloxone diminish the analgesic effects of acupuncture, both "needle-induced analgesia as well as the pain-relieving effects of low frequency electrostimulation of acupuncture points…. High frequency electrical stimulation of acupuncture points for pain relief seems to be relatively unaffected by naloxone, but is [instead] inhibited by the administration of serotonin antagonists" (Gerber, 1988, p. 94). Therefore, the effects of acupuncture and other meridian therapies cannot be comprehensively explained by an endorphin-releasing model.

Radiologist Bjorn Nordenstrom (1983), in his detailed support for the concept "that tissues polarize and interconnect via biologically closed electric circuits," suggests that such phenomena may account for the results of acupuncture (p. 328). His research, which is indicative of the presence of subtle electric currents that follow pathways along interstitial spaces and blood vessels, offers some support for the existence of meridians and chi, which is at least electrical or electromagnetic in makeup. In view of the research conducted by German biophysicist Fritz-Albert Popp and his associates (Popp and Beloussov, 2003), which shows that cells emit and apparently communicate via photons (i.e., biophotons), it is conceivable that light is also an integral aspect of chi. It is common knowledge among physicists that light carries an enormous amount of information and therefore, so would chi if it involves light. Similarly, French biologist Jacques Benveniste reports that molecules and cells emit specific audio frequencies (Benveniste et al., 1998).

Becker has conducted extensive research supportive of the existence of a primitive bodily energy system responsible for regeneration and that also accounts for the effects of acupuncture (Becker and Selden, 1985). With regard to regeneration, he provides convincing evidence that the current of injury that is observed at injury sites is not merely a by-product of injury to cells but is rather consistent with a primitive energy-control system that guides regeneration. In this respect, he has found that the direct current at the site of injury on frogs, which are not highly regenerative, is positively charged; in contrast, the current of injury on salamanders, for which regenerative capacities are paramount, is negatively charged. Even though these discoveries may not make it possible to draw unequivocal conclusions across animal species, they are nonetheless strongly indicative of an "evolutionarily ancient" electrical controlling system involved in healing, as well as in the total organization of the physical body. Because Becker's experiment "put electromagnetic energy back into biology as a controlling factor, this simple experiment is often referred to as the *beginning of the new scientific revolution*" [emphasis mine] (Becker, 1990, p. 38).

Variations of electrical charges, which are consistent with the directionality of the current, were observed earlier by Langman in his research on gynecological conditions, discussed in Chapter 1 (Burr, 1972, pp. 137–154). To summarize, in an extensive sample of women with cervical malignancies, 96% revealed a negative DC electrical charge as compared to 4% with a positive charge.

Becker also conducted research that offers support for the specificity of acupoints and for the existence of meridians (Reichmanis et al., 1975; Becker and Selden, 1985; Becker, 1990). He reports that he was initially approached in the early 1960s by an army colonel who was investigating the basis of acupuncture and exploring the possibility of an electrical basis. Although he did not have an opportunity to pursue research on acupuncture at that time, his chance came about a decade later. He notes that in the early 1970s research into acupuncture was encouraged by the National Institutes of Health (NIH) after President Nixon's visit to China serendipitously brought acupuncture into research vogue because Western journalist James Reston was effectively treated in China for postoperative pain with acupuncture following an emergency appendectomy (Becker and Selden, 1985).

Becker reports that many of the initial investigators hypothesized that acupuncture operated by way of the placebo effect and that it would therefore work approximately one third of the time and that needle placement would prove irrelevant. Obviously, the Chinese, as well as the U.S. military, had already disproved this theory. And as history would repeat itself, the earliest researchers merely corroborated these findings. However, Becker offered a more interesting hypothesis into the problem. He proposed that the meridians were essentially electrical conductors that operate in a cybernetic manner, relaying information between the injury site and the central nervous system. He suggested that the brain responded to the incoming message by producing the conscious perception of pain and by regulating the flow of electricity to the injury site, thus promoting healing in essentially the same way that regeneration was found to be activated electrically. He further hypothesized that the acupuncture needles prevented the pain message from traveling to the brain by short-circuiting the electric current. In this respect, he proposed that if the acupoints are truly electrical amplifiers, then the metal acupuncture needles would cause the short by connecting the acupoint to adjacent tissue fluid.

Noting that electric current degrades as it travels along metal cables and that this factor is compensated for by intermittently positioning booster amplifiers along the power line, Becker theorized that amplification might also be the essential function of acupoints. Since the electric current of the meridians would be of such low intensity (i.e., nanoamperes and microvolts), amplifiers would be needed within inches of each other, as is the case with the acupoints.

I envisioned hundreds of little DC generators like dark stars sending their electricity along the meridians, an interior galaxy that the Chinese had found and explored by trial and error over two thousand years ago. If the points really were amplifiers, then a metal needle stuck in one of them, connecting it with nearby tissue fluids, would short it out and stop the pain message. And if the integrity of health really was maintained by a balanced circulation of invisible energy through this constellation, as

the Chinese believed, then various patterns of needle placement might indeed bring
the current into harmony. (Becker and Selden, 1985, pp. 234–235)

Becker observed that Western medicine rejected acupuncture because cotermi-
nous anatomical structures for the meridians could not be found. To investigate this
and related aspects, he proposed that the skin at the acupoints would evidence
electrical variations that would be consistent with his hypothesis that the acupoints
were conductors and amplifiers: "Resistance would be less and electrical conductivity correspondingly greater, and a DC power source should be detectable right at
the point.... If we could confirm these variations ... and measure current coming
from the points, we'd know acupuncture was real in the Western sense" (Becker and
Selden, 1985, p. 235).

After Becker received the National Institutes of Health grant to investigate his hypothesis, he and his associate, biophysicist Maria Reichmanis, developed an electrode
device to measure electrical skin resistance. The instrument could be rolled along the
meridian lines, providing a reliable continuous reading:

We found that about 25 percent of the acupuncture points on the human forearm [the
large intestine and circulation-sex lines on the upper and lower surfaces of the arms]
did exist, in that they had specific, reproducible, and significant electrical parameters
and could be found in all subjects tested [emphasis mine]. (Becker, 1990, p. 46)

Even though most of the acupoints on these meridians were not detectable with
the Becker–Reichmanis device, the fact that all subjects tested revealed consistency
cannot be ignored. Becker suggests that the discrepancy could have been due to any
number of factors, including the fact that since "acupuncture is such a delicate blend
of tradition, experiment, and theory, the other points may be spurious; or they may
simply be weaker, or a different kind, than the ones our instruments revealed"
(Becker and Selden, 1985, p. 235).

On the basis of their experiments, Becker and Reichmanis concluded that there
is a subtle electric current generated within the meridians, and that, similar to the
system they observed and mapped out in their experiments with amphibians, the
current travels into the central nervous system.

Each point was positive compared to its environs, and each one had a field surrounding
it, with its own characteristic shape. We even found a fifteen-minute rhythm in the
current strength at the points, superimposed on the circadian ("about a day") rhythm
we'd found a decade earlier in the overall DC system. It was obvious by then that at
least the major parts of the acupuncture charts had, as the jargon goes, "an objective
basis in reality." (Becker and Selden, 1985, pp. 235–236)

Even though many of the acupoints were "hot," that did not necessarily mean that
there were meridians beneath the surface that connected the points. However, on the
basis of comparing skin surface resistance in various areas, Becker and Reichmanis
came to the following conclusions:

Next, we looked at the meridians that seemed to connect these points. We found that these meridians had the electrical characteristics of transmission lines, while nonmeridian skin did not. We concluded that the acupuncture system was really there, and that it most likely operated electrically. (Becker, 1990, p. 46)

MORPHOGENETIC FIELDS

In addition to the bioenergy systems discussed thus far, it has been hypothesized that various fields exist that account for the inherited physical forms and instinctual behaviors of organisms. These are referred to as morphogenetic fields (Sheldrake, 1981, 1988), and they serve the purpose of replicating systems much in the same way that a blueprint serves the purpose of guiding construction. Of the four levels of causality originally outlined by Aristotle (Young, 1976b), morphogenetic fields and the resonance that operates with them are akin to formal causality.

> Morphic resonance takes place through morphogenetic fields and … gives rise to their characteristic structures. Not only does a specific morphogenetic field influence the form of a system …, but also the form of this system influences the morphogenetic field and through it becomes present to similar systems. (Sheldrake, 1981, p. 96)

With regard to inherited characteristics, the phenomena of morphic resonance and morphogenetic fields stand in stark contrast to DNA-based inheritance, although the two avenues would appear to operate in concert with each other. This is not to be confused with the notion of Lamarkian inheritance (i.e., inheritance of acquired characteristics), for which there is little empirical support.

As an example in support of morphogenetic fields, Sheldrake cites psychological research initiated by W. McDougall at Harvard University in 1920 as a thorough evaluation of Lamarkian inheritance (Sheldrake, 1981). The experiment was a test of inherited learning among laboratory Wistar strain white rats that were inbred for generations. The task essentially involved training the rats to escape from a water maze via one of two gangways: a brightly lit one vs. a dimly lit one. The natural proclivity would be for the rats to attempt to leave by way of the brightly lit gangway, but rather they were trained to escape via the dimly lit one. When a rat would attempt to exit via the bright path, it would receive an electric shock. Sheldrake quotes McDougall:

> Some of the rats required as many as 330 immersions, involving approximately half that number of shocks, before they learnt to avoid the bright gangway. The process of learning was in all cases one which suddenly reached a critical point. For a long time the animal would show clear evidence of aversion for the bright gangway, or taking it with a desperate rush; but, not having grasped the simple relation of constant correlation between light and shock, he would continue to take the bright route as often or nearly as often as the other. Then, at last, would come a point in his training at which he would, if he found himself facing the bright light, definitely and decisively turn about, seek the other passage, and quietly climb out by the dim gangway. After attaining this point, no animal made the error of again taking the bright gangway, or only in very rare instances. (McDougall, 1927, p. 282)

> In each generation, the rats from which the next generation [was] to be bred were selected at random before their rate of learning was measured, although mating took place only after they were tested. This procedure was adopted to avoid any possible conscious or unconscious selection in favor of quicker-learning rats. (Sheldrake, 1981, p. 187)

After 15 years and 32 generations, it was evident that with each successive generation the rats learned the task more rapidly. The number of errors steadily decreased with each generation, and even the qualitative responses of later generations were noticeably different, as they approached the maze more cautiously. The results thus far supported Lamarkian theory.

Upon completion of this phase of the study, McDougall repeated the 15-year experiment, this time selecting subjects on the basis of learning scores. This experiment was conducted with an entirely different sample of rats categorized into quick and slow learner groups. As predicted, "the progeny of the quick learners tended to learn relatively quickly, while the progeny of the slow learners learned relatively slowly" (Sheldrake, 1981, p. 187). However, even the "dull" rats improved in learning scores with successive generations. Again, Lamarkian theory was supported.

As McDougall neglected to systematically assess the learning rate in offspring whose parents had not been trained, Crew (1936) conducted a similar experiment with similar inbred rats, including "a parallel line of 'untrained' rats, some of which were tested in each generation for their rate of learning, while others, which were not tested, served as parents of the next" (Sheldrake, 1988, p. 188). This "replication" experiment revealed no systematic rate of learning in either the experimental or untrained control groups. Although these results initially stood in stark contrast to those of McDougall, it was observed that Crew's rats learned the task more readily, with many of them learning the task without being exposed to electric shock. Even though this was a different batch of rats, the average learning score of Crew's rats was approximately that of McDougall's rats at the completion of more than 30 generations of training. Additionally, pronounced fluctuations in learning scores across generations among Crew's rats could have buried the magnitude of learning among later generations. Finally, intensive inbreeding among Crew's rats may have deleteriously affected the results in that later generations showed lower reproductive rates and a greater number of abnormalities.

Finally, a replication experiment was conducted over 20 years and 50 successive generations of rats by Agar and colleagues (1942, 1954) in Australia. Again, trained and "untrained" rats were studied, but Agar avoided Crew's design flaws. "In agreement with McDougall, they found that there was a marked tendency for rats of the trained line to learn more quickly in subsequent generations. *But exactly the same tendency was also found in the untrained line*" (Sheldrake, 1988, pp. 189–190). Apparently, McDougall had observed similar disconcerting trends upon occasional testing of untrained lines. However, Agar's systematic results firmly refuted a Lamarkian interpretation of McDougall's findings, since the untrained lines performed comparably to the trained rats.

Sheldrake suggests that the changes observed in the trained and untrained lines of the same species offer some support for the hypothesis of formative causation, which is consistent with the notions of morphogenetic fields and morphic resonance.* In essence, morphic resonance is akin to a television wave that serves to inform the receiver, thus producing specific visual and auditory effects. The picture and sound are replicated by millions of television receivers, which is analogous to a broad-spectrum morphogenetic field. It is suggested that behavior, as well as physical form, entails a field-based heritability component, possibly distinct from DNA. We might refer to this as ener*genetic* heredity.

THE POWER OF PRAYER

In some respects, intercessory prayer (or distant healing, as some would prefer) is related to morphic resonance and psychokinesis. However, prayer speaks of the power and resonating energy of intention, words, and God. The majority of us pray.† We pray for ourselves, loved ones, people in need, peace on earth, our crops, and our pets. Some people even pray to win the lottery. Although the word *pray* is from the Latin root *precari*, meaning "to ask" or "to request," not all prayers can be categorized in this way. In addition to requests for help or *intercession*, prayer can be used for *worship*, *celebration*, and *meditation*. Before covering empirical studies of *distant intercessory prayer*, however, first let us review these categories of prayer.

Prayers of *worship* may involve expressions of adoration, devotion, love, praise, surrender, or offering to God. For example, an aspect of Christian worship in the form of prayer includes: "Our Father, who art in heaven, hallowed be thy name." Or "Glory be to the Father and to the Son and to the Holy Spirit; as it was in the beginning, is now, and ever shall be, world without end. Amen." The Bahá'í faith also offers prayer of worship such as the following: "Bear witness, O my God, that Thou hast created me to know Thee and to worship Thee. I testify, at this moment, to my powerlessness and to Thy might, to my poverty and to Thy wealth. There is none other God but Thee, the Help in Peril, the Self-Subsisting." Every religious practice includes prayers of worship to the Creator. This is the greatest form of prayer, since its purpose is to honor and give pleasure to God.

Prayers of *celebration* involve thanksgiving, blessing, initiation, etc. For example, while pouring water over an infant's forehead, the priest or minister offers a baptismal prayer: "I baptize thee in the name of the Father, and of the Son, and of the Holy Spirit." Thanking God for your blessings is a celebration prayer: "Bless us oh Lord and these Thy gifts, which we are about to receive from Thy bounty, through Christ our Lord. Amen." Another standard mealtime prayer: "God is great, God is good, and we thank Him for His food. Amen."

Prayer can also be used in *meditation* in the same way that *mantras* are employed. Mantra is derived from the Sanskrit words, *manas* (meaning *mind*) and *trai* (meaning *to protect* or *liberate from*). *Mantra* may be translated literally as "to protect (or liberate) from the mind." This is a technique used with the mind in order to free oneself from certain effects of the mind. A standard yoga mantra is simply *Om*. Mahatma Gandhi used the following mantra: *Om Sri Rama Jaya Rama, Jaya, Jaya*

---

* Sheldrake offers experimental designs to test the hypothesis of formative causation.

† A 1996 national survey found that 82% of Americans believe in the healing power of prayer and 95% avowed a belief in God or a higher power (Gallup and Lindsay, 1999).

Rama. Instead of traditional mantras, however, people may use expressions more in line with their religious beliefs, such as "My Lord and my God," "Jesus, my savior," "Yahweh," "Hashem," or "Praise Allah, bless me." These mantra prayers involve adoration while helping to clear the mind of intrusive thoughts that interfere with getting in touch with our spiritual core.

Finally, there are prayers that involve asking God to intercede — *intercessory* prayer: "Give us this day our daily bread." Or, "Dear God, I implore you to cure my sister of her health problems." A Buddhist intercessory prayer states, "May all beings everywhere, Seen and unseen, Dwelling far off or nearby, Being or waiting to become: May all be filled with lasting joy." A prayer for the king in the book of *Psalms* says, "May Yahweh answer you in time of trouble; may the name of the God of Jacob protect you!" Then there is the renowned 13th century intercession prayer of St. Francis of Assisi:

Lord, make me an instrument of Thy peace;
where there is hatred, let me sow love;
where there is injury, pardon;
where there is doubt, faith;
where there is despair, hope;
where there is darkness, light;
and where there is sadness, joy.
O Divine Master,
grant that I may not so much seek to be consoled as to console;
to be understood, as to understand;
to be loved, as to love;
for it is in giving that we receive,
it is in pardoning that we are pardoned,
and it is in dying that we are born to eternal life. Amen

A similar prayer of intercession was offered by Mother Teresa of Calcutta:

Make us worthy, Lord, to serve our fellow men
throughout the world who live and die in poverty and hunger.
Give them through our hands this day their daily bread,
and by our understanding love, give peace and joy.

Although intercessory prayer is generally thought of as imploring God for help, it can take other forms. Many Hindu prayers are directed to various gods. And many Roman Catholics pray to Mary and to various saints including St. Jude, St. Theresa the Flower, and St. Francis of Assisi to intervene on their behalf. However, in these instances, the healing intervention is believed to ultimately come from God.

Dossey (1993, 2001) has covered research on distant intercessory prayer, although many of the studies cited might be better categorized as psychokinesis, which has received extensive empirical support. For example, well-designed studies have demonstrated the effects of "distant prayers" (related to psychokinesis) in promoting or inhibiting the growth of bacteria and fungi (Barry, 1968; Tedder and

Monty, 1981; Nash, 1982). Also, Radin and Nelson (1989) conducted a meta-analysis of 832 studies on the distant effects of human consciousness (psychokinesis) on microelectronic systems and found significant, robust, repeatable results.

There are plenty of anecdotal reports on the beneficial effects of prayer. The Roman Catholic Church, for example, canonizes saints on the basis of prayers being answered in the form of miracle cures. While the miracle claims are investigated thoroughly, obviously these are not experimental studies.

In a related sense, Lawlis (2003) reports on a number of informal "experiments" that he conducted on the physiological effects of prayer:

> Between 10 and 15 patients admitted for the treatment of cancer care participated in each study group. In each experiment one member of the group was selected as the focus patient. The focus patient would then leave the group and go into a separate room, where he or she was hooked up to a biofeedback monitor. ... At random times and unbeknownst to the subject, the prayer group would focus on the patient, sending him or her love and support. At these times the biofeedback devises measured an elevated skin temperature, indicating a physical change in the subject. Subjects reported an increased sense of well being indicating a physiological change. (p. 241)

Lawlis also discussed various extraordinary effects and "spontaneous remissions" that the patients experienced as a result of these experiments. In some instances, tumors dissolved. One patient experienced the healing of nonunion neck bone fractures in 1 week despite the fact that the fractures had been present for years. Another patient who had a leg fracture healed in 3 weeks, although she had gone through 3 years of surgery and electrical attempts to no avail.

Although a number of clinical trials of intercessory prayer have reported positive medical effects (Byrd, 1988; Harris et al., 1999; Leibovici, 2001; Sicher et al., 1998), many of the studies contain methodological problems and not all studies of intercessory prayer support its effectiveness (Joyce and Wellson, 1965; Collipp, 1969; Aviles et al., 2001).

Byrd (1988) reported on his pioneering prospective randomized, double-blind study conducted at San Francisco General Medical Center between August 1982 and May 1983 on the effects of remote intercessory prayer to the Judeo-Christian God for the health of coronary care unit (CCU) patients. Over the 10 months of the study, 393 patients admitted to the CCU were randomly assigned to an intercessory prayer group (192 patients) or to a control group (201 patients). During hospitalization, the experimental group received intercessory prayer by "born again" Christian participants praying outside the hospital. Initial statistical analysis revealed no difference between the groups. After entry, all patients had follow-up for the remainder of their admission. The results revealed that the prayer group had a significantly lower severity score based on the hospital course after entry ($P = 0.01$). Multivariate analysis separated the groups on the basis of the outcome variables ($P = 0.0001$). The control group required ventilator assistance, antibiotics, and diuretics more frequently than the intercessory prayer group.

While this study yielded noteworthy statistically significant results, there are a number of methodological flaws that cannot be ignored. For example, Byrd acknowledged that possibly the control group also was prayed for by friends and family. Therefore, prayer was not thoroughly controlled for except for the fact that three to seven intercessors prayed daily for the experimental patients. Also, there was no effort to control for the psychological status of the patients. Further, while the prayer group evidenced statistically significantly results on some factors, no significant differences were found among 20 of the health categories evaluated, including days spent in CCU, total hospital stay, and mortality rate. Multivariate analysis revealed six variables that accounted for statistical significance. Of the six variables, four were of borderline significance and two were clearly significant. Also, the study did not provide information on the patients' physicians. As some physicians may tend to use antibiotics and to intubate patients more readily than others, this may have been a primary variable that accounted for the difference between the two groups. One final problem was that the study coordinator, who also collected the data, knew which patients were being prayed for and she interacted regularly with the patients in the study. Therefore, it is possible that the double-blind was inadvertently pierced by the coordinator.

Harris (1999) and his group of the Mid America Heart Institute conducted a randomized, controlled, double-blind, prospective, parallel-group trial on the effects of intercessory prayer, drawing from 1019 patients admitted to a coronary care unit at Saint Luke's Hospital, Kansas City, Missouri, a private, university-associated hospital. The study was purported to be a replication of Byrd's study. After eliminating patients who were in CCU for less than 24 hours, there were 524 patients in the usual care group and 466 in the experimental group — a larger n than in the Byrd study. The investigators concluded that the experimental (prayed for) patients evidenced better healthy outcomes than the controlled (not prayed for) patients. The prayer group had significantly lower CCU scores than the usual care group ($P = 0.04$). Although the CCU score (comprising 34 items as compared to 26 items in the Byrd study) was intuitively devised and not validated, it was nonetheless evenly applied to both experimental and control groups.

Harris's study was superior to Byrd's in that it appeared to be thoroughly blinded and it involved a significantly greater number of patients. However, again there are a number of methodological problems. As noted, the CCU scoring system was not validated and the drop-out rate in the prayer group was significantly higher than the control group ($P = 0.001$). Because the mortality rate of the two groups was equivalent, perhaps the prayer group as a whole was not as ill, since so many were discharged before prayer was initiated. Although this study was equivalent to Byrd's in that there were no differences regarding days spent in CCU, days in the hospital, and mortality rate, it was not a true replication, as none of the six items found significant in Byrd's study was significant in Harris's study.

Between 1997 and 1999, Aviles and her group (2001) conducted a well-designed, randomized, controlled trial on intercessory prayer and cardiovascular disease progression in a coronary care unit population at the Mayo Clinic. The objective was to evaluate the effects of complementary therapy on cardiovascular disease progression after hospital discharge. The study was conducted on a total of 799 CCU patients randomized at discharge to an intercessory prayer or control group. The prayer was administered by one or more persons on behalf of each patient in the prayer group at least once a week for 26 weeks. After 26 weeks the primary end point was concluded as a result of death, cardiac arrest, hospitalization for cardiovascular disease, coronary revascularization, or an emergency department visit for cardiovascular disease. Patients were divided into a high-risk and a low-risk group. Although a primary end point occurred in 25.6% of the prayer group as compared to 29.3% of the control group, these results were not significant ($P = 0.25$). Significant differences did not occur among high-risk and low-risk patients either. Among high-risk patients, 31.0% in the prayer group and 33.3% in the control group experienced a primary end point ($P = 0.60$). And among low-risk patients, a primary end point occurred in 17.0% in the prayer group vs. 24.1% in the control group ($P = 0.12$). Remote intercessory prayer, as delivered in this Mayo Clinic study, yielded no statistically significant effect on medical outcomes after hospitalization in a coronary care unit. Aviles concluded that the results "do not suggest a contraindication to prayer, and further study is warranted to define the role of [intercessory prayer] on qualitative and quantitative outcomes and to identify end points that best measure the efficacy of prayer in a variety of patient populations" (p. 1198).

A rather perplexing methodological twist on prayer was conducted by Leibovici (2001), who reported on a randomized, controlled trial on the effects of remote, *retroactive* intercessory prayer on 2000 adult inpatients with bloodstream infections. Between 1990 and 1996, 3393 adult patients with bloodstream infection were identified at a hospital. In July 2000, the patients were randomized to intervention and control groups and a remote, retroactive prayer was said for the well-being and full recovery of the intervention group. The main measures were mortality, duration of hospitalization, and duration of fever. Mortality rate of the intervention group was 28.1% (475/1691) and the control group was 30.2% (514/1702), significance at the 0.04 level. Length of hospital stay was significantly shorter for the intervention group ($P = 0.01$) as was duration of fever ($P = 0.04$). What this study ultimately means is anyone's guess. However, the significant results and the flawless design demonstrate that something did happen. Are we able to reach back in time, pray for things to turn out differently than they "actually" did and have them turn out differently? Doubtful, but of course, how would we ever know? Perhaps these results merely reflect coincidence, a chance occurrence, an example of a Type II statistical error (when a false hypothesis is accepted as true).

One of the most thorough studies to date on the positive effects of distant healing or prayer was conducted by Sicher et al. (1998). In 1995 and 1996, the researchers conducted a double-blind pilot study on the medical and psychological benefits of distant healing (i.e., prayer and other spiritual practices) for patients with advanced acquired immunodeficiency syndrome (AIDS). At the completion of the study, four of the ten control subjects died; no deaths occurred in the treatment group. While this was amazingly significant, the results were confounded by age, as those who died were older. Given the possible benefits of distant healing for patients with AIDS, a randomized, controlled, double-blind study followed. A pair-matched design was used to control for factors shown to be associated with poorer prognosis: age, T-cell count, and illness history. Additionally, for the replication study an important intervening medical factor changed the study design regarding end point (i.e., morality). The pilot study was conducted before the introduction of "triple drug therapy" (simultaneous use of a protease inhibitor and at least two antiretroviral drugs), which has been shown to have a significant effect on mortality. Thus, differences in mortality were not expected and different end points were used in the study design. Based on results from the pilot study, the researchers hypothesized that the distant healing treatment would be associated with improved disease progression (fewer and less severe AIDS-defining diseases and improved CD4+ level*); decreased medical utilization; and improved psychological well-being. In all, 40 patients were involved in the study over a 6-month period. Patients were pair-matched for age, CD4+ count, and number of AIDS-defining illnesses and randomized either to receive 10 weeks of prayer or to be in a control group. Prayer was provided by self-identified "healers" representing many different healing and spiritual traditions. Healers were located throughout the United States during the study, and patients and healers never met. Patients were assessed by psychometric testing — i.e., profile of mood states (POMS), Wahler physical symptom inventory (WPSI), and medical outcomes survey (MOS) for HIV — and blood draw at enrollment and followed for 6 months. At 6 months, blind medical chart review found that the prayed-for patients acquired significantly fewer new AIDS-defining illnesses (0.1 vs. 0.6 per patient, $P = 0.04$), exhibited lower illness severity (severity score 0.8 vs. 2.65, $P = 0.03$), required significantly fewer doctor visits (9.2 vs. 13.0, $P = 0.01$), fewer hospitalizations (0.15 vs. 0.6, $P = 0.04$), and fewer days of hospitalization (0.5 vs. 3.4, $P = 0.04$). Treated patients also showed significantly improved mood compared to controls (change in POMS −26 vs. +14, $P = 0.02$). There were no significant differences in CD4+ counts. These data supported the possibility of a distant healing effect and the researchers suggested that the results indicated the value of further research.

Although numerous studies have reported on the effects of distant healing, a critical review of 23 studies that met strict scientific criteria concluded that 57% of the studies demonstrated a positive treatment effect (Astin et al., 2000). So while positive effects related to distant intercessory prayer are evident, not all well-designed investigations of intercessory prayer have yielded significant results. This discrepancy warrants further investigation.

If the prayer in these studies involved requests of God to intervene, then possibly the studies that did not show positive effects of prayer were flawed if Holmes (1938) is correct in stating in *The Science of Mind* that God never fails to answer prayers. Of course, I imagine that it is God's prerogative to answer prayers by saying "no" and the intention and commitment of the person who offers the prayer also must be significant factors. Further, do we have the option of requiring that prayers to be answered within the time frame of an experimental study in order for them to count? And should we dare discount the potential power of prayer simply because experimental studies have not unequivocally demonstrated its effectiveness?

---

* T cells are a type of white blood cell (lymphocyte), which is an important part of the immune system. There are two main types of T cells. T-4 cells, also called CD4+, are "helper" cells that lead the attack against infections. T-8 cells, also called CD8+, are "suppressor" cells that end the immune response. CD8+ cells can also be "killer" cells that kill cancer cells and cells infected with a virus. T cells can be distinguished by specific proteins on the cell surface. A T-4 cell has CD4 molecules on its surface. This type of T cell is also called "CD4 positive," or CD4+.

There is a story about a man who was blessed with the opportunity to meet God. After regaining his composure, one of the first questions out of the man's mouth was, "God, what is a billion dollars worth to you?" To this God replied that a billion dollars was insignificant. As the man persisted, however, God obliged him by saying that a billion dollars might be comparable to a penny. Next the man asked what a billion years was like to God, to which God said that since he is eternal, a billion years is essentially nothing. However, to offer a comparison to satisfy the man, God likened a billion years to a second. The man then implored God to let him have a billion dollars, to which God replied with a nod and a smile, "Sure! Just give me a second."

Some studies point to the effectiveness of intercessory prayer; some do not. Given the studies available, however, it is impossible to determine if the positive results are related to divine or saintly intervention; to belief; to the effects of consciousness, intentionality, and subtle energy; to chance; or to flawed methodology. Certainly empirical studies might be designed to clarify these queries further and we can expect to see such studies bless the pages of our medical and psychological journals within the near future. Nonetheless, even if science cannot offer definitive proof, many people steadfastly believe in the healing power of prayer. After all, many practices found to be helpful, therapeutic approaches included, have not been and probably never will be empirically validated to the satisfaction of science. Although we ought to strive for scientific validation as much as possible, if we limit ourselves to this the advancement of our fields will be gravely limited.

HOMEOPATHY

Also of relevance to bioenergy and biofields* is homeopathy. Developed by German physician Samuel Hahnemann (1755–1843), homeopathy is based in part on principles employed by early Greek physicians, dating to Hippocrates in the fifth century B.C. Among these principles is the *law of similarities* or that of "like curing like," which is antithetical to the *law of contraries* upon which most medicine of the time was based. The law of contraries prescribes treatment of illnesses with substances that produce opposite symptoms in healthy people. For example, diarrhea can be treated with agents that constipate, such as aluminum hydroxide. The law of similarities, on the other hand, is based on treating illnesses with substances that produce similar symptoms in healthy people. For example, the root of the *Veratrum album* (white hellebore), which causes severe vomiting and dehydration in high doses, can be used in low doses to treat cholera. High doses of quinine, which cause malaria-like symptoms, can be used in low doses to treat malaria.

Like Hippocrates, Hahnemann also held that cures should be chosen that support the patient's healing potential. While the internal healing tendency is recognized by medicine in general, it is one of the hallmarks of homeopathic medicine.

Hahnemann often used substances that were so highly toxic that he had to dilute them in an alcohol/water mixture before giving them to patients. However, even

---

* The term "biofields" is offered as a reference for biologically related fields, subsuming morphogenetic fields, thought fields, subtle field effects of homeopathy, and so on.

when diluted, he frequently found that the symptoms worsened before remitting. Therefore, he experimented with increasing levels of dilution to the degree that not a single molecule of the mother tincture was left in the mixture. To his surprise he found that the greater the dilution, the greater the potency of the medicine!

This process of diluting the substance to increase its potency is referred to as "potentization." In order to potentize a substance, Hahnemann employed a procedure referred to as "succussing," which involves vigorously shaking and banging the container of the remedy on a hard surface during the stages of dilution. He maintained that this procedure caused the remedy's energy to be released into the water/alcohol mixture.

Hahnemann reasoned that there is a subtle energy force in the body — the vital force — that responds "to the tiny provocations of the remedies and enable[s] the body to heal itself" (Lockie and Geddes, 1995, p. 18). In this respect, homeopathy is compatible with meridian therapies in that both are professed to treat an inherent bioenergy system.

Toward a more detailed theory of homeopathy's effectiveness, Gerber (1988) offers an interesting comparison between the behavior of energy within atoms and the human energy system:

> Homeopathic theory suggests that humans are somewhat like the electrons of an atom. Electrons within an atom occupy energy shells or spatial domains which are known as orbitals. Each orbital possesses certain frequency and energetic characteristics depending on the type and molecular weight of the atom. In order to excite or move an electron into the next highest orbital, one needs to deliver to it energy of a specific frequency. Only a quantum of the exact energetic requirements will cause the electron to jump to a higher orbital. This is known as the principle of resonance, in which tuned oscillators will only accept energy in a narrow frequency band. Through the process of resonance, energy of the proper frequency will excite the electron to move to a higher level or energy state in its orbit around the nucleus.
>
> Human beings may be similar to electrons in that their energetic subcomponents occupy different vibrations modes, which we might call health orbits and disease orbits. For the human being whose energetic systems are in an orbit of dis-ease, only subtle energy of the proper frequency will be accepted to shift the body into a new orbit or steady state of health. Homeopathic remedies are able to deliver that needed quantum of subtle energy to the human system through a type of resonance induction. (Gerber, 1988, pp. 84–85)

Homeopathy is so profoundly distinct from contemporary medicine that many allopathic physicians, true to their paradigm, are inclined to reject it as a viable approach to medicine. However, some homeopathic remedies have been subjected to methodologically sound experimental studies, demonstrating their effectiveness in the treatment of cholera, mustard gas burns, asthma (Lockie and Geddes, 1995), and hay fever (Reilly, 1986). Also, while a recent uncontrolled, open treatment study suggests that "homeopathy may be useful in the treatment of some patients with anxiety or depression, either as adjunctive or as a sole treatment," a placebo control study is needed to evaluate these results thoroughly (Davidson et al., 1997). More extensive research is needed to verify the benefits of homeopathy and to possibly convince the medical establishment of homeopathy's effectiveness. Reporting on the study that documented the effectiveness of homeopathy in treating hay fever (Reilly, 1986), Becker offered the following summary and observation of the effects that the established paradigm can have on the members of the profession:

> A truly scientific evaluation of the clinical effectiveness of homeopathy was not done until 1986, when Dr. David Reilly and his co-workers at the Glasgow Homeopathic Hospital reported in the prestigious British journal *Lancet* on an impeccable, double-blind study of the efficacy of a homeopathic preparation for hay fever with an ineffective placebo. They reported that "the homeopathically treated patients showed a significant reduction in patient- and doctor-assessed symptom scores." In addition, they found that "the significance of this response was increased when results were corrected for actual pollen counts, and the response was associated with a halving of the need for antihistamines." Obviously, the homeopathic preparation had a definite physiological effect that cannot be completely explained by the placebo effect. This occurred despite the fact that the medicine was diluted to the point at which, theoretically, none of the original medication remained.

> The publication of this paper elicited a storm of letters to the editor, which were interesting for what they revealed about the mind-set of the modern "scientific" physician. Despite the study's having been an exceptionally well-planned and well-executed scientific evaluation, one writer called it "the first randomized, double-blind trial of one placebo against another," and went on to state that "the homeopathic potency used contained not one molecule of the original extract." The objections raised by the critical letters came down to one point: homeopathy simply cannot work. If the results of a scientifically valid study are at variance with established theory, the study must be incorrect. The idea that one should consider revising the theory was not mentioned, except by a few correspondents. (Becker, 1990, pp. 119–120)

Although caution is certainly indicated to advance and protect the integrity of any field, extremes of caution have been observed repeatedly when the established paradigm is "challenged" by unexplainable anomalous facts. In the areas of physics and astronomy, for example, a similar crisis emerged with respect to planetary orbits. Specifically, Mercury's orbit does not conform to Newton's predictions — that is, Newton's laws of motion. Physicists at the turn of the previous century were busily developing mathematical formulas to "prove" that Newton was correct, accounting for deviations in Mercury's orbit with respect to various factors, such as a hidden moon, asteroid, or comet. However, rather than being blinded by the dictates of authority, Einstein offered a radically new theory that accounted for the apparent discrepancies. He proposed that instead of thinking of gravity in the ways of Newton, alternatively we might see gravity as a function of matter warping the nearly "nothingness" in which it resides. Orbital calculations based on this distinct metaphor nicely explained the deviations and thus enabled accurate predictions. Advances in science and practice demand not only that we develop the field in concert with accepted findings but also that we be open to the fact that because our models are not equivalent to the truth, ultimately they break down.

SOME HOMEOPATHIC REMEDIES

A few of the homeopathic remedies and some of their recommended uses follow. For more detailed information on this topic, see Lockie and Geddes (1995) and Gerber (1988).

Allium (red onion): Neuralgia or burning pain, colds, hay fever
Arnica (leopard's bane): Physical and emotional shock after a trauma
Aurum metallicum (gold): Depression, suicidal thoughts, headache, heart
   disease
Hamamelis virginiana (witch hazel): Hemorrhoids, varicose veins
Hypericum perforatum (St. John's wort): Depression, drowsiness, shooting pain

BACH FLOWER REMEDIES

Similar to homeopathy, in that it is believed to operate by way of subtle energy, are treatments based on flower essences. This approach to treatment was begun by Dr. Edward Bach (1880–1936), a pioneering pathologist and bacteriologist during the early 1900s, who developed a number of vaccines for treating intestinal bacteria associated with chronic arthritis and rheumatic disorders. He entered the field of homeopathy after reading Hahnemann's treatise, *The Organon of Medicine*, and finding himself in agreement with the homeopathic practice of giving minute doses of medicine. He eventually administered his own vaccines in homeopathic oral doses, rather than by injection. He had been looking for an alternative method of administration, because injections frequently resulted in unwanted side effects at the injection site.

Significantly predating psychoneuroimmunology, Bach came to recognize an integral relationship between personality temperaments, stress, emotions, and illness. In his search for ways to assist patients in overcoming disease, he observed that the mind evidences alterations prior to disease manifesting in the body. He came to believe that disease was an indication of disharmony between the physical and spiritual aspects of the person and that treating the spiritual aspect would be providing treatment at the most fundamental level.

Bach was not comfortable with administering noxious substances and intestinal bacteria to patients, even though they were given in low doses. He felt that there must be a better alternative in nature, and this brought him to a study of the beneficial effects of flower tinctures. As a highly sensitive, intuitive type, it is reported that by sampling the sunbathed morning dew drops on the flowers, Bach was able to experience the negative emotional states alleviated by various flowers. He developed 38 primary flower remedies in addition to a *rescue remedy,** an all-purpose stress reducer made from five flowers (Bach, 1933). These remedies are similar to homeo-

---

* Rescue remedy is a mixture of five flower remedies: cherry plum, clematis, impatiens, rose rock, and star of Bethlehem. It is often used to deal with stressful situations, trauma, anxiety reactions, etc. It has been used also to treat psychological reversal, a self-sabotaging state that is consistent with psychological problems that are highly resistant to treatment (Callahan, 1985; Durlacher, 1995).

pathic remedies in that they contain a minuscule amount of the flower stock in a mixture of 50% water and 50% brandy for preservation.

A few of the Bach flower remedies and some of their recommended uses follow. For more detailed information on this topic see Walther (1988) and Gerber (1988).

Aspen: Free-floating vague fears and anxieties
Cerato: Strong dependency needs, lacking confidence in one's own decisions
Impatiens: Impatience, easily frustrated
Rock rose: Panic and nightmares
Star of Bethlehem: Trauma, loss, grief
White chestnut: Obsession

CONCLUSIONS

Energy is a fundamental constituent of our reality, if not the most singularly fundamental aspect. It shows up throughout the universe in the makeup of galaxies, stars, planets, and life itself. It appears that our bodies possess an energy system with a constitution that is, at the very least, electrical and electromagnetic. It is self-evident that the body operates according to the same principles that pervade the universe and that have been discerned by the field of physics. In view of the research reviewed, this energy system cannot be considered to be simply an epiphenomenon of biochemistry, since it operates at a causal level. In this regard, the energy system is instrumental in regeneration, healing, and pain perception and may really serve to maintain the integrity of health. Additionally, while the bioenergy system interacts with the nervous system, it also appears to possess some uniquely independent features with its own "anatomical" structures, with the latter suggested in view of the fact that there is observed consistency of bioenergy pathways and functions. Further, it is suggested, as this book aims to demonstrate, that the utilization of this bioenergy system and biofields represents a highly efficient way to treat a variety of psychological conditions.

We turn our attention now to a brief history of applied kinesiology, which has paved the way from chiropractic medicine to diagnostic and therapeutic applications in the fields of psychiatry and clinical psychology. The applied kinesiology methods of manual muscle testing and therapy localization have provided empirical tools that have been necessary in the advancement of energy psychology.

4 Origins of Energy Psychology (Or Adding Muscle to Therapy)

Applied kinesiology is based on the fact that body language never lies.... The opportunity to use the body as a laboratory instrument of analysis is unparalleled in modern therapeutics, because the response of the body is unerring.

— George J. Goodheart, Jr.

Besides attending specifically to the subtle bioenergy systems harnessed by the meridian therapies, energy psychology's diagnostic and treatment methods also have roots in chiropractic medicine, specifically applied kinesiology (AK). This chapter traces the roots and offshoots of applied kinesiology and introduces applications in the areas of psychotherapy and prevention.

APPLIED KINESIOLOGY

In the mid-1960s, Detroit chiropractor George J. Goodheart, Jr., D.C., began the process of carving out an entirely new field, what is referred to as applied kinesiology. Specifically, applied kinesiology is a unique method of evaluating bodily functions by means of manual muscle testing. The procedures involve a comparison of the relative "strength" in the examined muscles as they relate to the muscles themselves in addition to associated neurologic, lymphatic, vascular, respiratory, energetic, mental, and other functions. "The examination procedures ... appear to be such that they can be used in all branches of the healing arts" (Walther, 1988, p. 2).

Muscle Testing and the Origin-Insertion Technique

Concerning his initial serendipitous discovery, Goodheart reports having evaluated a patient who was unable to get a factory job because he could not pass the physical due to a weakness in one of his arms that made it impossible for him to apply pressure in a forward direction. Observation revealed that there was a notable protrusion of the shoulder blade out from the chest wall. Although radiographs could not locate the cause of the problem and Goodheart felt that he had nothing to offer, often, to Goodheart's embarrassment, the man persisted in his request for assistance.

He would come into the office, and quite often in a crowded waiting room would ask me in a loud voice, "When are you going to fix my shoulder?" This embarrassed me somewhat, and I motioned him to come into the inner office quickly, away from the sight and scene of my embarrassment, and I would tell him that there wasn't much I could do about it. (Goodheart, 1987, p. 2)

Goodheart recalled that there is a muscle that holds the scapula in place against the chest wall, but he could not remember specifics about it. Therefore, he resurrected a book that a colleague had given him as a Christmas present, *Muscle Testing* by Kendall and Kendall (1949). This book revealed not only the muscle in question, the *anterior serratus anticus*, but also provided a method for testing it (Goodheart, 1987).

After studying this text, Goodheart reexamined the persistent patient. To his interest he observed that the muscle was not atrophied, regardless of extensive disuse and a 15- to 20-year history of the problem. He further discovered that there were tender nodules located at the origin of the muscle. After he massaged them deeply, the nodules disappeared, muscle strength immediately returned, and the patient's condition permanently improved:

Upon palpating the muscle I felt an unusual nodulation at the attachment of the muscle to the anterior and lateral aspects of the rib cage, which I didn't feel on the other side. The small nodulations were quite apparent to the palpating finger, and in an effort to identify their nature I pressed on them. They were not painful other than minimally so, and they seemed to disappear as I pressed on them with my palpating pressing finger.

Encouraged by the apparent disappearance of the first one or two, I continued to press on all of the small areas which we later learned to be avulsive in character, a tearing away of the muscle from the periosteum. The attachment of the muscle to the covering of the bone, the periosteum, was producing a nodulation which is characteristic in these cases of micro avulsion. They are small tearings away of muscles from their attachment.

Having palpated and pressed on all the small nodulations which coincided with the attachments of the muscle to the rib cage, I then surveyed the muscle. It felt the same, but this time I noticed that the scapula ... was lying in a normal position on the posterior chest wall.

Surprised but pleased, I repeated the test, having him place his hands in front of him against a plywood panel that separated one section of the office from another, and I pressed on his spine. The shoulder blade did not pop out, and he looked at me with an inquiring glance and said, "Why did you not do that before?" I looked at him serious of face and direct of eye and said, "Well, you have to build up to a thing like this. You didn't get sick over night." It was an automatic response, but all I could think of at the time.

He was pleased, I was delighted. It was an unusual thing to see this quick a response. (Goodheart, 1987, p. 2)

For more than 20 years, Goodheart had an opportunity to reexamine this patient, and the muscle remained strong after that single treatment. Goodheart continued to utilize this method of diagnosis and the discovered treatment technique with a variety of patients and found that many were aided in this manner. "This led to the original applied kinesiology technique of *origin and insertion treatment* [emphasis mine]. Goodheart presented this technique at the charter meeting of the American Chiropractic Association held in Denver, Colorado in 1964" (Walther, 1988, p. 2).

NEUROLYMPHATIC REFLEXES

Goodheart's next, most significant serendipitous discovery came about while he was treating a patient who suffered from an anomalous sciatic neuritis. The patient experienced pain in his lower right limb when standing, sitting, or lying down although the discomfort was not present while walking. This problem was also associated with weakness of the *fascia lata muscle*, a thigh muscle that makes it possible to move the legs outward. Goodheart reasoned that the problem, in view of the odd history, was related to the lymphatic system, the toxin-removing system that operates fundamentally through skeletal muscle movement.

> Because walking relieved [the pain], indicating [the] possibility [of lymphatic involvement], I palpated the lymph glands on the lateral aspect of the thigh and felt nothing unusual in comparison to the uninvolved left side. I palpated also for the potential of any sacroiliac disturbance, because occasionally we get lymph nodulation in the region of the sacroiliac joint if there is a sacroiliac disturbance. I found none of these, and the patient was in a great deal of distress while lying on his back. After palpating for diagnostic information, which I did not find, the patient looked up at me and said, "That's the first relief I've ever gotten." I looked at him and said, very bravely, "That's what you came here for," indicating that it was not the surprise to me that it was.
>
> Astonished by this rather quick success and yet not understanding the basis, I continued to initiate the palpation which I had accidentally used to relieve his pain. He remarked that the pain which he had experienced for many, many months was now completely absent, and subsequent investigation and diagnosis revealed a complete disappearance of the long-standing and chronic irritation of the sciatic nerve. (Goodheart, 1987, pp. 3–4)

In this instance Goodheart had correlated nerve and muscle dysfunction with another bodily system, namely, the lymphatic system, discovering that by massaging lymph glands he could restore function and alleviate pain. However, another clinical event clarified this relationship more precisely.

Goodheart's secretary at the time was troubled by a chronic sinus condition and an associated head tilt. He unsuccessfully attempted to alleviate the sinus condition and to correct the head tilt by application of the origin-insertion technique cited earlier. Next, he attempted to treat her in the same manner by which he had helped the patient with the sciatic problem: by palpating and treating the neck flexors. He found that rather than strengthening the muscles, his treatment weakened her further. "Then I thought, perhaps what I pressed on was something unassociated with the muscle itself, but associated with, possibly, some lymphatic circuit breakers which had been postulated by an osteopath named [Frank] Chapman" (Goodheart, 1987, p. 4). These cutaneous circuits are also referred to as "neurolymphatic reflexes" by another osteopathic physician, Charles Owens. Approximately the size of a shotgun pellet, these reflexes are located at intercostal spaces in the vicinity of the sternum and in the pelvic region.

Goodheart laboriously tested various muscles and eventually associated them with the neurolymphatic reflexes that Chapman and Owens had originally discussed. In time, he discovered not only which muscles were associated with these reflexes, but he also discovered additional neurolymphatic reflexes in other areas (Goodheart, 1987).

> By now I was becoming convinced that there was a relationship between muscles and particular viscera or organs. A moderately weak muscle on testing appeared to be associated with a weak viscera or organ, but every time I could see evidence of a weak pancreas, or a weak stomach, or a weak liver or a weak kidney dysfunction — of those organs which would be measured by x-ray or by biochemistry or by some other accepted biological test — I would find a correspondingly weakened muscle. This relationship, although rather tenuous at first, became more and more evident as time went on. (Goodheart, 1987, p. 5)

NEUROVASCULAR REFLEXES

Serendipity and persistent curiosity always on his side, while lecturing at a seminar in New York, Goodheart had the opportunity during the lunch break to treat a young boy who was having an acute asthmatic episode and was not responding to medication. The patient was referred to Goodheart by his doctor. While the boy was lying on his back, Goodheart noticed that while one foot was upright, the other was limp on its side. He unsuccessfully attempted to help the boy by a variety of approaches including massaging neurolymphatic reflexes, the origin-insertion technique, and the "lymphatic pump," which involves exerting pressure on the sternum to change the pressure in the chest. Next, he attempted a primitive cranial technique developed by Dr. James Alberts, which involves spreading cranial sutures.

> My index fingers were resting on the posterior fontanel area with the rest of my fingers spreading the sagittal suture which runs vertically along the top of the skull, separating the two halves of the skull and joining the parietal bones of the skull together. I felt that insistent pulsation, very faint at first, at the posterior fontanel; and despite the fact that the carotid arteries were beating at a rate of about 120 and his respirations were at 40, I noticed that the pulsations that I experienced with my fingertips were at the rate of 72 beats per minute.

> Thinking the beating was perhaps in my own fingers, I removed my fingers and placed them on a wall to identify if the 72 rate beating was in my own fingers. I noticed no change. I reapplied my fingers to the posterior fontanel and felt the continued pulsation, which became more insistent and more persistent and more evident in strength, until finally the young man gradually stopped his labored breathing, took a deep breath, began to breathe easily, and simultaneously his foot rotated up into a parallel position with its opposite member.

> The doctor attending the youngster, who had asked me to see the patient, looked at me and said, "Good gracious, Doctor, that's marvelous." And I looked at the doctor, very serious of face, and said, "That's what you came here for." (Goodheart, 1987, p. 8)

While attempting to treat the child with asthma with Alberts's cranial technique, Goodheart inadvertently stimulated neurovascular reflexes on the cranium.* A light, spreading touch with the fingertips on these receptors activated a primitive circulatory system germane to the capillary bed.† This, in turn, resulted in improved circulation to associated muscles, thus accounting for not only cessation of the asthmatic episode but also strengthening of the muscles associated with the foot lying loosely on its side.

Explaining the basis of this method further, Goodheart notes that "many muscles lack a 'thermostatic' configuration which allows them to function when under stress" (Goodheart, 1987, p. 9) and stimulating the neurovascular reflex is like adjusting a thermostat, which improves the circulation to the muscles and promotes the excretion of lactic acid and other waste products that can accumulate in muscles as a result of mechanical contraction. Activating the neurovascular reflexes causes a backup circulatory system to engage, taking over these functions, which are not being efficiently handled by the primary circulatory system.

CRANIAL-SACRAL PRIMARY RESPIRATORY MECHANISM

By now it should be evident that Goodheart possesses keen powers of observation, an ingenious capacity for detecting correlation, a willingness to work hard, and the luck of serendipity. These features were again revealed in his treatment of a 49-year-old patient who suffered from a 30-year headache. He also observed notable variations of muscle weakness and muscle strength on both sides of her body with detectable fluctuations while inhaling and exhaling. He additionally observed that her right ear was lower than the left and that this was not a congenital misplacement but rather evidence of deviations in the skull bones, which he confirmed by measurements.

Referring to the work of osteopath William Sutherland, who proposed that the cranial bones move in accordance with one's breathing, Goodheart attempted to adjust the mastoid process while having the patient breathe according to specific instructions. He pushed forward on the mastoid as she inhaled deeply and pushed in a backward direction as she exhaled. Within a few moments, the patient indicated that her previously intractable headache was relieved.

Goodheart then tested her muscles during various phases of respiration, finding interesting variations. Some tested strong in response to inhaling, some to exhaling, others to half breaths, and still others to breathing through the nostrils as compared

---

* These receptors were originally discovered by chiropractor Terence Bennett in the 1930s, who developed a training program to promote this work. After Bennett's retirement and eventual death, Floyd Slocum, D.C., took over this activity.

† Goodheart writes: "In the embryo there is no heart, and for the first three or four months the mother's placental circulation is augmented by a network of vascular circuits which, as the tissue grows, exert slight traction on the blood vessel which then causes the blood vessel's muscles themselves to pulsate in an augmented fashion, aiding the mother's placental circulation.... At about the fourth month the heart is formed, and many times the mother is delighted to hear the heart beat that the obstetrician allows her to listen to. At the advent of the heart beat, the heart takes over part of the burden of supplying circulation to the growing embryo, and the neurovascular circuit of supply and demand circuitry goes on a standby basis — something like a generator behind a hospital in case of power failure, which can be turned on for emergency use" (1987, p. 8)

to through the mouth. Some variations were even noted when the patient was breathing through one nostril as compared to the other.

> We then had the patient take a deep breath in and out. If the muscle was found to be weak and responded to inspiration, the mastoid process on the side of the skull that the muscle weakened was located and pressed forward at the temporal bone mastoid process with the thenar eminence of the hand, with about 4 or 5 pounds of pressure coincident with 4 or 5 deep inspirations.

> If the muscles found weak responded to expiration, the thenar eminence of the hand was placed anterior to the mastoid process of the temporal bone and ... pressed backward towards the occiput coincident with 4 or 5 deep expirations....

> This resulted in many, many cases improving from many, many conditions, and they postulated a concept of a cerebral spinal fluid flow rate something like a dual irrigation ditch — with someone turning the rheostat down on the pump, and the tomato vines withering somewhat, and then when someone turned the rheostat up on one side or the other, the tomato vines thriving due to an increased flow of the irrigation fluid. (Goodheart, 1987, p. 6)

Goodheart observed a holistic interplay of the cranial bones, respiration, and various muscles. He also found that the vertebrae and sacrum responded in a predetermined manner to respiration, moving forward with inspiration and backward with expiration.

> This new cranial finding coincident with a method of diagnosis aided greatly in the application of the cranial concept. The original Sutherland concept, as well as those that followed, used topographical, anatomical changes for cranial corrections; but the addition of respiration added a measure of diagnostic certainty and also safety to this relatively new science.... Time has shown that a respiratory relationship exists in the spinal fluid flow rates, and a critical factor in the production of routine cranial correction was to correlate muscle weakness to strengthen with respiration. (Goodheart, 1987, p. 7)

THE MERIDIAN CONNECTION

By this time, Goodheart had discovered four procedures for strengthening muscles that tested weak: origin-insertion, neurolymphatic reflexes, neurovascular reflexes, and cranial manipulation. He also observed a holistic connection between specific muscles and various organs and glands. For example, the hamstrings and tensor fascia lata muscles of the legs correlate with the large intestine, while the satorius and quadriceps muscles, also on the legs, are associated with the adrenals and the small intestine, respectively. It was becoming clearer that the whole is truly greater than the sum of its parts.

In 1966, Goodheart introduced acupuncture to applied kinesiology after studying a text by a British medical researcher, Felix Mann, *The Meridians of Acupuncture,* which discussed the *theory of the five elements.* Mann highlighted a relationship between acupuncture points and various organs and revealed multiple tonification or stimulation points to activate the organ and multiple sedation points for when the organ was overactive (Mann, 1964). This was right up Goodheart's alley.

> In an effort to relate these points to kinesiological parameters, we attempted stimulating the points for tonification and found occasional responses in muscles. We attempted to sedate other points and found occasional responses in muscles. Insertion of a needle at the so-called "first point" invariably would produce a strengthening of a muscle if found weak on testing, and insertion of a needle at the first point of sedation would invariably cause weakness of the muscle if the muscle was strong. We soon found that touching the first two points for tonification would result in strengthening of a weak muscle. The converse was also true. Touching the first two points for sedation and simultaneously the second two points for sedation would weaken the muscle. (Goodheart, 1987, p. 10)

As a substitute for needles, Goodheart explored and discovered the effectiveness of applying pressure to acupoints as well as percussing or tapping on the points. While the interconnection of glands, organs, and meridians was well known to acupuncture, by bringing his knowledge of muscle testing to the arena, Goodheart and his colleagues discovered a connection between the various muscles and meridian pathways. Referring to our previous example, it became clear that the hamstrings and tensor fascia lata muscles of the legs correlated not only with the large intestine itself but also with the large intestine meridian and that these muscles and organ could be effectively treated via stimulation of various potent acupoints along the large intestine meridian. In a similar manner, Goodheart was able to demonstrate that the quadriceps muscles are associated with the small intestine in addition to the small intestine meridian and that these muscles and this organ could be effectively treated via stimulation of various potent acupoints along the small intestine meridian.

FIVE FACTORS OF THE IVF

By this time Goodheart had five options available for diagnosing and strengthening weak muscles and various organs and glands throughout the body. A holistic system of health was emerging. In his words, "The healer within can be approached from without" (Goodheart, 1987, p. 11). While the method and related procedures did not cease in their evolution, at this point the essential foundation was laid.

The holistic applied kinesiology diagnostic and treatment procedures were now addressing what Goodheart referred to as the "five factors of the IVF," referring to the intervertebral foramen or spinal column (the place where the nerves exit the spine). The five factors "relate to the nervous, lymphatic, and vascular systems, along with the relationship of cerebrospinal fluid and the cranial-sacral primary respiratory motion, and with the meridian system" (Walther, 1988, p. 13).

Now, applied kinesiology clearly entailed a unique set of diagnostic and treatment procedures that could be applied in addition to standard procedures employed by many physicians. In addition to observation of the patient's posture and gait as well as gathering detailed history, elaborate manual muscle testing could be employed to assess relative muscle strength as it related to bodily functions. It should be apparent that muscle testing is not conducted to simply evaluate muscle strength *per se,* but rather to assess the functioning of the nervous system via muscle response. In this regard, it has been referred to as "functional neurology" (Walther, 1988, p. 2).

THE TRIAD OF HEALTH

As a holistic endeavor, applied kinesiology is consistent with the stated philosophy of chiropractic medicine that goes back to its origins with D. D. Palmer. This position attends to the "triad of health," which includes structural, chemical, and mental components. Thus, while many health fields emphasize one aspect of the triangle, applied kinesiology endeavors to enlist all three components.

For example, the allopathic physician may be inclined to use chemical treatments to address both the structural and mental aspects of the triangle, possibly prescribing muscle relaxants, anti-inflammatory drugs, and analgesics in an effort to correct structural deficits. When addressing the mental-emotional component, antidepressants, tranquilizers, mood stabilizers, and neuroleptics may be employed.

The traditional chiropractor, on the other hand, tends to utilize structurally-based treatments, such as adjustments to the spine, in an attempt to treat the structural imbalance directly. The chiropractor may also attempt to rectify mental and chemical aspects of the triad in this fashion.

Finally, the traditional psychologist may utilize various psychological treatments to alleviate mental-emotional distress. In that the psychologist attends to only one leg of the triangle, the mental aspect, he or she may also attempt to treat a structurally related problem such as pain via hypnosis, relaxation training, biofeedback, cognitive restructuring, and so on. As far as chemically based or partially chemically based conditions are concerned, such as allergies and depression, the traditional psychologist would again employ mental means toward amelioration.

Again, the emphasis in applied kinesiology is toward examination of all three aspects of the triangle to discover the primary factor(s)

Often a health problem starts on one side of the triad, and eventually involves all three aspects. It is important to recognize that any one side of the triad can affect the other sides, both as causative factors of health problems and as therapeutic approaches.

Applied kinesiology examination helps determine the basic underlying cause of the health problems. Structural balance is readily evaluated in the static and dynamic body. The neuromuscular reaction of the body to chemicals helps to evaluate the effects of nutrition and adverse chemicals. Insight into the patient's emotional status can be obtained by evaluating the nervous system, using applied kinesiology manual muscle testing. Mental health problems can sometimes be improved by nutritional and structural corrections, determined by manual muscle testing. (Walther, 1988, p. 11)

TOUCH FOR HEALTH

While developing applied kinesiology, Goodheart worked closely with a number of colleagues. In 1974, upon the recommendation of John Thie, D.C., one of his closest colleagues, Goodheart established the International College of Applied Kinesiology (ICAK) to regulate the field by standardizing curricula and establishing certification.

The basic applied kinesiology training entails 100 hours of approved material, and there is an extensive procedure in place for evaluating research projects.

However, the International College of Applied Kinesiology is for the professional and admits only licensed doctors who have the authority to diagnose in their respective fields. John Thie, on the other hand, wanted to see much of applied kinesiology available to a wider audience. He thereupon developed a synthesis of early material from applied kinesiology into what is referred to as touch for health (TFH). Thie's vision of touch for health was to make it possible for others without medical training or manipulative skills to apply kinesiological methods to enhance self-health and the health of family members. As it turns out, while the lay public has been receptive to touch for health, many professionals have also taken this training. Touch for health became the initial offshoot of applied kinesiology.

In addition to elaborating basic manual muscle testing to determine relative strength and weakness in a wide array of muscles, touch for health includes a number of procedures to strengthen and thus balance muscles. It should be emphasized that touch for health is not applied kinesiology. It is not a therapeutic approach that attends specifically to illness but rather a system of balancing. As Thie points out:

> A muscle which tests weak indicates some blockage or constriction in the energy flow. The process we use to unblock the energy and restore balance to the system is called balancing. There is no such thing as a touch for health treatment. Instead, no matter what the person has in the way of symptoms, we balance the body energies, and strengthen all of the weak muscles we find; this brings the posture into better balance. (Thie, 1973, p. 20)

At the most basic level, the touch for health entails testing at least one muscle (most bilaterally) associated with each of 14 meridians. When a weakened muscle is found, various strengthening techniques are employed until the muscle tests strong and remains strong to a challenge. There are several touch for health methods of strengthening weakened muscles. Several of these techniques are discussed briefly in the following subsections.

Spinal Vertebrae Reflex Technique

This procedure is used only when bilateral muscle weakness is found. It involves subcutaneous reflexes over various vertebrae that "can be activated by moving the skin over the spinal vertebrae tips in a head to foot motion stretching the skin rapidly but gently for 10–30 seconds" (Thie, 1973, p. 22).

Neurolymphatic Massage Points

These are identical to the neurolymphatic reflexes discussed by Chapman. They are massaged deeply in a circular motion for approximately 20 to 30 seconds. Each muscle is associated with specific reflex points. For example, the latissimus dorsi muscles, which hold the shoulders in place and the back straight, are associated with the neurolymphatic point on the front of the body in the depression on the left side between the seventh and eighth ribs. These muscles are also associated with neuro-lymphatic points on the back, 1 in. on either side of the spine between T-7 and T-8.

NEUROVASCULAR HOLDING POINTS

These are identical to the neurovascular reflexes discovered by Bennett. They are primarily located on the head and are activated with a light fingertip touch, while subtly stretching the skin over the area. In each instance, there are two points, and the person doing the procedure holds both reflexes, one with each hand, until the pulses at the points are synchronized for a period from 20 seconds to 10 min. Again referencing the latissimus dorsi muscles, the associated neurovascular holding points are located on the parietal bone, above and behind each ear.

MERIDIAN TRACING

Another means of strengthening involves tracing the meridian pathway. "The flow of energy through a meridian may be stimulated by using the hands to trace the meridian line in the proper direction on the surface of the body…. Using the flat of the hand … it is only necessary to come within 2 inches of the meridian, either off to the side or even above the skin and over clothing, for it to be effective" (Thie, 1973, p. 26).

ACUPRESSURE HOLDING POINTS

Various acupressure points throughout the body are associated with various muscles. Touch for health method involves holding specified points on the side of the body that tests weak for approximately 30 seconds. In the case of the latissimus dorsi muscles, associated with the spleen meridian, the acupoints used for strengthening are liver-1, spleen-1, spleen-2 on the feet, and heart-8 on the palm beneath the little finger.

ORIGIN-INSERTION TECHNIQUE

This procedure involves stimulating the weakened muscle at both its origin and insertion. This is accomplished by placing one's fingers at each of these ends of the muscle and moving the muscle back and forth. Again, with respect to the latissimus dorsi muscles, the origin is from T-6, down along the spine, between the lower portion of the scapulas, and down to hip level. The insertion is below the shoulder and inside the arm (Thie, 1973).

OTHER APPLIED KINESIOLOGY OFFSHOOTS

Since the initial developments of applied kinesiology and touch for health, a wide array of offshoots has emerged. Some are highly reputable and some are of questionable reputability. This appears to be partly the result of limited regulation of the field, where practically any designing person can hang a shingle and call himself or herself a kinesiologist. This gives kinesiology a bad name and is unfortunately all too common with emerging fields.

David Walther, D.C. (1997), one of the principal proponents of applied kinesiology, reported that recently legal action was being taken against a "kinesiologist" who "muscle tested" a child with cancer and informed the parents that other treatments were not necessary, merely the supplements the "kinesiologist" could provide. Obviously, this does not represent kinesiology at its best.

John Diamond, M.D. (1997b), noted that he gave a seminar where an attending "kinesiologist" discussed his "cancer practice," which he had for less than a year. When Diamond asked what the man did prior to his current practice, he stated that he had been a baker and had never had medical training. Appalled, Diamond expressed the perhaps too strong opinion that kinesiology should be outlawed.

Certainly regulation of the field is necessary. Professionals who utilize kinesiological approaches within their practices should be well trained and expected to utilize these skills only within the scope of their respective fields. With respect to psychotherapy, for example, kinesiological techniques practiced by well-trained, licensed psychotherapists and counselors is entirely distinct from that attempted by those not conversant in assessment, psychopathology, human development, psychotherapeutic approaches, and practice standards. Likewise, the psychotherapist has no business proclaiming proficiency in areas for which he or she is untrained, regardless of the level of kinesiological skills. This is discussed further in the final chapter. Now, we focus on some applied kinesiology offsprings.

CLINICAL KINESIOLOGY

A protégé of Goodheart, the late Alan Beardall, D.C., studied applied kinesiology and eventually made a large number of innovative discoveries that culminated in what is referred to as clinical kinesiology (CK), also called human biodynamics (HBD). This is a complex methodology employed by health professionals with expertise in manipulative skills. It is predicated on the assumption that the body functions biphasically, much like a computer, a biocomputer, and that health is a function of good communication among the body's various systems (Beardall, 1982, 1995; La Tourelle and Courtenay, 1992).

While Goodheart correlated more than 50 muscle tests with various reflexes, Beardall expanded on this by developing 576 muscle tests. He also developed more than 300 handmodes or mudras, which represent a uniquely advanced method of therapy localization. For example, by utilizing a handmode while testing an indicator muscle, the etiology of the problem in question can be traced to structural, chemical, psychological, neurovascular, or other causes. Additionally, Beardall developed 70 therapeutic procedures germane to clinical kinesiology, including Nutri-West® Core-Level™ nutrients (Levy and Lehr, 1996). He also pioneered the leg lock or pause lock, which facilitates diagnosis and treatment by locking in information ascertained through muscle testing so as to relate this data to other associated aspects of a problem. Using this method, he developed cumulative two-pointing, three-pointing, and four-pointing to determine priorities among associated symptoms, meridians, neurolymphatic reflexes, and other bodily systems.

Beardall postulated that illness symptoms represent a request for change from the human biocomputer. If the communication is appropriately responded to, health is restored; otherwise, the body becomes adapted to the illness and overall health and functioning are further compromised.

EDUCATIONAL KINESIOLOGY

Whereas applied kinesiology and clinical kinesiology are primarily directed at the diagnosis and treatment of health problems, educational kinesiology (Edu-K) is essentially applicable to learning, concentration, thinking, memory, academic skills, etc. Developed by Paul Dennison, Ph.D., in 1980 after studying touch for health in 1979, educational kinesiology entails a number of techniques to enhance hemispheric communication and functioning.

One of the educational kinesiology methods, lateral repatterning, involves improvements on homolateral crawl and cross-crawl exercises (Figure 4.1) originally derived from the work of Doman and Delacato (Delacato, 1966). In this regard, Dennison found that incorporating humming, counting, and specific eye movement patterns into the routine enhanced results in terms of improved attention and learning.

Another educational kinesiology method, Brain Gym®, entails a series of easily performed activities to prepare children (and adults) for learning and coordination skills. In addition to lateral repatterning, the activities include educational anchoring (associating a kinesthetic experience such as a movement with a new learning), Cook's hook-ups (specific postures to connect various energy centers in the body to restore balance), positive points (neurovascular reflexes at the frontal eminence on the forehead), and many more (Dennison and Dennison, 1989). Educational

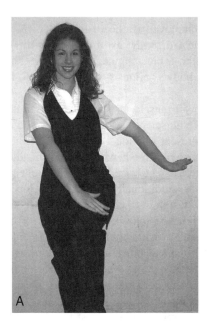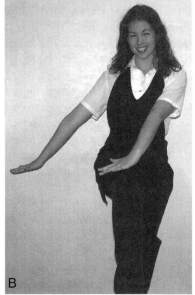

FIGURE 4.1 Basic cross-crawl exercises.

kinesiology also places emphasis on assisting the learner in establishing clear and positive goals.

THREE-IN-ONE CONCEPTS

Also referred to as *one brain, three-in-one concepts* is an approach to stress reduction developed by Gordon Stokes, D.C. and Daniel Whiteside, D.C. in 1972. It involves light touch, manual muscle testing to identify the client's stresses with their specific emotional characteristics (behavioral barometer) and pinpoint the origins of the stress through the process of age recession. This may entail having the client list various emotions that he or she may have repressed (e.g., anger, sadness, jealousy, etc.) and state specific time frames of the trauma's origin (e.g., 0–5, 5–10, etc.) while testing the indicator muscle. After tracking down the specifics of the stress by conducting this diagnostic procedure, choices from a wide array of stress diffusion techniques are employed.

PROFESSIONAL KINESIOLOGY PRACTITIONER

Since the development of touch for health, a new health profession of kinesiologists has emerged. To assist them in their development of skills beyond those contained in the touch for health course, Bruce Dewe, M.D., former faculty head of the Touch for Health Foundation, developed an extensive four-workshop program that leads to the designation of professional kinesiology practitioner (PKP). This program entails a synthesis of the most useful, recent, nonmanipulative findings from applied kinesiology, clinical kinesiology, and other branches of kinesiology (La Tourelle and Courtenay, 1992).

NEURO-EMOTIONAL TECHNIQUE

"There are two things in life: Money, which includes finances, career and job; and Love, which includes everyone you have ever loved and everyone who has ever loved you."

As you think of each one separately, we test an indicator muscle. "I see, It's Love! I can tell since your muscle strengthened on that one."

"Now the person in question is either male or female."

Again we test. "I see, again! It's a female."

"And there are two kinds of females, family and friends. So it's family."

"And there is immediate family (mother, sister, daughter) and extended family (grandmothers, aunts, nieces, cousins)."

Again we test the strength of the muscle. Is it on or off?

"So it's immediate family."

"Is it your mother? I see."

Thus proceeds the neuro-emotional technique (NET) originated by Scott Walker, D.C., in 1988, a method that helps to pinpoint the source of the patient's distress. After this is accomplished, the doctor locates the associated points on the Bladder Meridian on the spine that abolishes the weakness, and that spot is then tapped to relieve the trauma at the source of the problem.

Walker's neuro-emotional technique is available mostly to chiropractic and other physicians who seek to treat the mental leg of the triad of health effectively and efficiently.* It is Walker's contention, not a difficult one to accept, that many of the structural adjustments that do not hold are a function of this component. The neuro-emotional technique curricula also includes treatments for self-sabotage that block the standard neuro-emotional technique treatments from taking or holding, similar to what Callahan (1981) refers to as psychological reversal, as well as some other relevant applied kinesiology treatments. Besides the basic neuro-emotional technique training, advanced training is available.

BEHAVIORAL KINESIOLOGY

Australian psychiatrist John Diamond, M.D. began studying applied kinesiology in the 1970s and developed behavioral kinesiology (BK), which is an integration of psychiatry, psychosomatic medicine, kinesiology, preventative medicine, and humanities (Diamond, 1979). Early on, his approach came to be referred to as behavioral kinesiology and more recently, as life energy analysis. Diamond's work represents the first attempt to integrate applied kinesiology and psychotherapy, especially key elements of psychoanalysis.

Diamond's earlier approach involved the use of affirmations, the thymus thump, homing thoughts, imagery, and elements of the Alexander method to balance life energy or chi after a meridian imbalance was detected through kinesiological tests. He eventually expanded his approach to incorporate greater aspects of music and the humanities, as well as focusing on the individual's capacity for creative choice.

Diamond is a prolific writer and his publications include *Behavioural Kinesiology*; *Behavioral kinesiology and the Autonomic Nervous System*; *Your Body Doesn't Lie*; *Life Energy*; *Life Energy in Music,* Vols. I, II, and III; and *Life Energy Analysis: A Way to Cantillation*. Diamond's approach is discussed in greater detail in Chapter 5.

THOUGHT FIELD THERAPY

Clinical psychologist Roger J. Callahan, Ph.D., became interested in applied kinesiology in 1979, studying briefly with Diamond (Diamond, 1997b) and later becoming certified by the ICAK after attending the 100-hour applied kinesiology course given by Walther and Robert Blaich, D.C. He eventually developed a unique therapeutic approach based in part on applied kinesiology, what he referred to as the Callahan Techniques™, and more recently also as thought field therapy (TFT).

Thought field therapy entails diagnostic procedures to determine meridian imbalance combined with percussing at specific acupoints in a prescribed sequence in order to treat an array of psychological problems. Percussing along with affirmations is also used to treat what Callahan refers to as psychological reversal as well as some negative affects such as anger and guilt.

Callahan's major publications include *It Can Happen to You*; *Five Minute Phobia Cure*; *Why Do I Eat When I'm Not Hungry?*; *Thought Field Therapy and Trauma:*

---

* Since neuro-emotional technique can be taken by any health professional with a license to diagnose, many psychologists have also taken this training.

Treatment and Theory; and *Tapping the Healer Within*. Thought field therapy is discussed in detail in Chapters 6 and 7.

AND SO ON

There are a number of additional applied kinesiology offshoots. Some of the names in the roster include biokinesiology (BK), hypertonic muscle release (Hyperton-X), health kinesiology (HK), systematic kinesiology (SK), holographic repatterning (HR), and at least two approaches referred to as psychological kinesiology: William F. Whisenant (Whisenant, 1990) and Robert M. Williams (Psych-K Centre™, Denver, CO). To review all of these approaches would require a book in itself.* However, while many of these systems may have relevance to psychology and psychotherapy, others deviate so markedly from the norm that the field is not likely to seriously investigate them within the near future. Our present goal is to explore those approaches that are most clearly empirically based and are able to be tested.

The next few chapters focus on applications of the energy paradigm to the field of psychotherapy. We begin with a more detailed discussion of John Diamond's behavioral kinesiology, after which we explore Roger J. Callahan's thought field therapy. The following chapters include a detailed manual covering thought field therapy and related algorithms, various energy psychotherapy methods, and methodological considerations. It is hoped and intended that this coverage will provide the clinician and researcher alike with useful information to advance the field and the cause of promoting psychological health.

---

* I have developed energy diagnostic and treatment methods (ED×TM), which is a comprehensive energy psychology approach that includes elements of applied kinesiology, various applied kinesiology offshoots, and many clinical findings. ED×TM is covered in depth in *Energy Diagnostic and Treatment Methods* (Gallo, 2000) and high-quality certification training is available for professional psychotherapists and physicians (see www.energypsych.com for details).

5 The Diamond Method to Cantillation

We should like to show here that the ego is neither formally nor materially in consciousness: it is outside, in the world. It is a being of the world, like the ego of another.

— **Jean Paul Sartre**, *La Transcendance de L'Ego* **(1936/1957)**

When you come to a fork in the road, take it.

— **Yogi Berra**

This chapter reviews some of the psychotherapeutic methods developed by John Diamond, M.D., which have been variably referred to as behavioral kinesiology (BK), the Diamond method, and life energy analysis. His work represents an integration of psychiatry, preventative and psychosomatic medicine, psychoanalysis, music, and the humanities. While Goodheart (1987) has attended somewhat to the mental aspect of the triad of health by employing the emotional neurovascular reflexes,* Diamond's is the first comprehensive effort to utilize applied kinesiology principles in the diagnosis and treatment of psychological problems. Although we have space for only little more than a cursory exploration of his approach, it nonetheless lays some of the groundwork for that which follows. The inquisitive reader will want to explore Diamond's approach in greater depth.†

BACKGROUND

John Diamond, M.D., graduated from Sydney University Medical School in 1957 and obtained his diploma of psychiatric medicine in 1962. He is currently a Fellow of the Royal Australian and New Zealand College of Psychiatry and a Member of the Royal College of Psychiatrists of Great Britain. After practicing psychiatry in Australia, he came to the United States where he expanded into complementary medicine, becoming president of the International Academy of Preventative Medicine (IAPM).

---

* Stimulating the emotional neurovascular reflexes on the frontal eminence of the forehead, also referred to as the *emotional stress release* procedure, has been found to be highly effective in alleviating negative emotional states associated with a variety of stressors. See Chapter 7 for details.

† Several years ago, several colleagues and I had the occasion to spend more than a week with Dr. Diamond, exploring some of his most recent developments. Since that time, he has published a number of additional works that focus on his most current thinking.

In spite of his initial skepticism as well as his entrenchment in the psychoanalytic tradition, especially the approach proffered by Melanie Klein, he eventually undertook a detailed study of applied kinesiology with founder George Goodheart. Coming to appreciate the effectiveness of this method, he adapted it to his own work. In time, he began writing and lecturing on the subject prolifically, developing a newsletter called the Diamond Reports and publishing *Behavioral Kinesiology and the Autonomic Nervous System* in 1978 and *Behavioral Kinesiology: How to Activate Your Thymus and Increase Your Life Energy* in 1979. His work became more widely visible after the publication of *Your Body Doesn't Lie* in 1980(b), and especially after *Life Energy* in 1985. (See references and recommended reading sections for a detailed list of Diamond's works.)

Initially, membership in the International College of Applied Kinesiology (ICAK) was open only to chiropractic physicians. Dissatisfied with this policy, Goodheart convinced the members to alter the bylaws to open membership to any doctor with a license to diagnose. As a result of this change in policy, Diamond was able to attend training through the International College of Applied Kinesiology and to become a full member. As he was an officer of the International Academy of Preventative Medicine, which at the time excluded chiropractic physicians, Diamond, in the same manner, persuaded his board of directors to change the by-laws to allow chiropractic physicians to become members. Goodheart was subsequently admitted as a full member (Durlacher, 1995).

What greatly interested Diamond about applied kinesiology was Goodheart's discoveries concerning manual muscle testing. Of specific interest was the fact that a previously strong muscle would weaken after a patient entertained a distressing thought. Here was an apparent bridge between psyche and soma, dramatically negating any true separation between them. Diamond employed manual muscle testing and felt, to his satisfaction, that he was able to verify many psychoanalytic principles and to unravel the root causes of patients' issues much more efficiently than he could by free association and other analytic processes (Durlacher, 1995; Diamond, 1997b).

Diamond reported that after years of practicing traditional psychiatry, he came to realize that he and his colleagues had been doing little to truly benefit patients. He noted that the entire psychiatric process focused on the negative, steeped in the problem, and that this very activity was detrimental to both patient and doctor alike. Using manual muscle testing, he found that the majority of his colleagues tested "weak" while thinking about their professional activities. In essence, "their work takes away from their life energy and devitalizes them" (Diamond, 1985, p. viii). Given this realization and equipped with the tools of applied kinesiology, Diamond set forth on a different course, which led him away from the medical model and into the realm of life energy, ethics, and spirituality. In 1988, he wrote:

> Thirty years after graduating into medicine, I am at last graduating out of it…. I never really wanted to cure diseases, not even to diagnose them, just to transmute the patient's hatred into love. Increasingly I realized that this was all that mattered. But love is not in the textbooks, nor is it in the treatment manuals. (Diamond, 1988, p. 2)

LIFE ENERGY

Diamond's term *life energy* is synonymous with the *chi* of China, *prana* of India, Paracelsus's *archaeus*, Hippocrates's *vis medicatrix naturae*. In his view, life energy is also spirit.

According to Diamond as well as traditional Chinese medicine (TCM), life energy enters the body through the breath, travels through the acupuncture meridians beginning with the Lung Meridian, and vitalizes the bodily organs. After an imbalance in life energy occurs, which can be caused by any number of physical and/or psychological factors, in time disease will ensue. "When we are diseased, there will be an imbalance of chi, of life energy, of spirit, affecting a specific acupuncture meridian, leading to particular psychological and physical problems and ultimately to disease" (Diamond, 1985, p. 5). However, the imbalance can be corrected in a number of ways, including a shift in mental attitude, and the energy-initiated disease process can be deterred or even possibly reversed.

Diamond utilizes the applied kinesiology therapy localization procedures to evaluate the effects of various stimuli on life energy. Essentially, this approach involves testing the relative strength of an indicator muscle, generally the middle section of the deltoid group of muscles in the shoulder, while having the subject attend to the stimuli in question. He describes this standard deltoid test as "basically a test of life energy, and [it] can be used to gauge the relative functioning of the acupuncture meridians" (Diamond, 1985, p. 5) (Figure 5.1).

On the basis of conducting numerous manual muscle tests on a variety of subjects, Diamond has concluded that each acupuncture meridian is associated with a specific facial expression, gesture, vocalization, and "a specific negative and a specific positive emotional state" (Diamond, 1985, p. 5). For example, he finds that the heart meridian is associated with the positive states of forgiveness and love when energies are balanced and with anger when the meridian is not balanced. The large intestine meridian, on the other hand, is positively associated with feelings of self-worth and negatively associated with guilt.

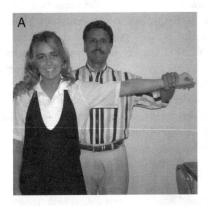 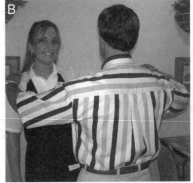

FIGURE 5.1 Standard deltoid "straight arm" test.

Utilizing this manual muscle testing procedure, Diamond has also been able to evaluate the effects of a variety of environmental stimuli on one's life energy.* For example, he has generally found that fluorescent lights, artificial fibers, refined sugar, quartz watches, and a variety of electronic devices result in weakening the test muscle and therefore, one's life energy. So, too, certain types of music (perhaps some types of Rock 'n' Roll in addition to alternative and industrial varieties) weaken or block the flow of life energy, whereas other modes (e.g., classical Bach and Beethoven) strengthen it. Diamond also reports that the effects of the individual conductor are relevant, such that whereas one conductor's rendition of a composer's work raises life energy, another's rendition of the same composition may lower life energy (Diamond, 1980b, 1985).

LIFE ENERGY ANALYSIS AND TREATMENT BY AFFIRMATIONS

To define the Diamond method more precisely, the following highlights some of the essential procedures involved in life energy analysis:

1. The tester stands opposite and to the left side of the subject. The subject extends the left arm perpendicular to the left side while the right arm is relaxed at the right side. The arm is straight, parallel to the floor, and the elbow is not bent. The tester may place his or her left hand on the subject's right shoulder to steady the subject, while placing his or her right hand on the subject's left wrist. The subject is asked to "hold" while the evaluator presses on the subject's wrist with a force of no more than 5 to 8 lb in an effort to move the arm downward. Assuming that the subject is not touching any location on his or her body or holding a particular issue in mind, emotionally charged or otherwise, this phase of the method is referred to as testing "in the clear."

2. Next, the subject is directed to place the fingertips of the free right hand "on the skin over the point where the second rib joins the breastbone (the sternomanubrial joint). This point ... is directly over the thymus gland. Now, with your subject touching the thymus point, test the indicator muscle again" (Diamond, 1985, p. 18). This is the thymus test point (Figure 5.2). If the indicator muscle tests strong, the subject's life energy is balanced, and the cerebral hemispheres will also show balance. If the indicator muscle tests weak, the subject's life energy is said to be in a state of imbalance. To further test the cerebral hemispheres, proceed as follows. Have the subject place the palm of the right hand opposite the right ear and approximately 3 to 4 in. away from the head. If testing the

---

* Diamond has expressed chagrin about the ways in which muscle testing often has been employed. He observes that some power-seeking persons have employed it to deleteriously undermine the person being tested. In other instances he feels that the testing is an unnecessary redundancy, that the desired information is simply obtainable via simple observation.

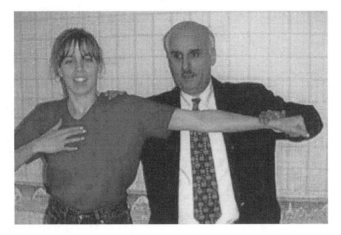

FIGURE 5.2 The subject therapy localizes the thymus test point with fingertips of the right hand while the tester conducts a deltoid "straight arm" test.

indicator muscle reveals a weakening of the muscle, the subject is said to be right-hemisphere dominant (Figure 5.3A). If the muscle remains strong, the opposite hemisphere is tested by having the subject place the right palm off the left side of the head by moving the right arm and hand across the front of the body and this time positioning the right hand opposite the left ear while testing the muscle (Figure 5.3B). If the muscle now tests weak, the subject is said to be left-hemisphere dominant.

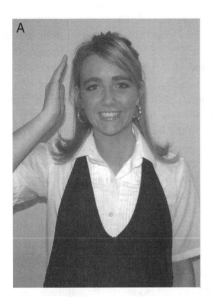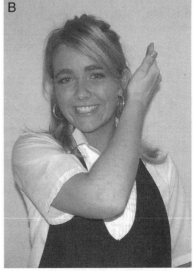

FIGURE 5.3 Test for cerebral dominance for the right hemisphere (A) and the left hemisphere (B).

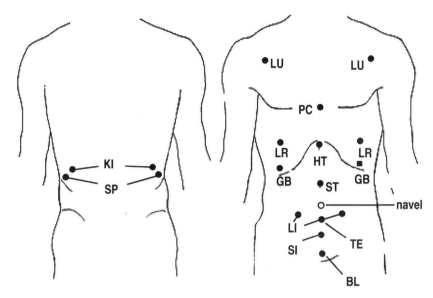

FIGURE 5.4 Alarm points for the 12 primary meridians.

3. If the right hemisphere tests dominant, this suggests that an imbalance exists in at least one of the following bilateral acupuncture meridians: lung, liver, gallbladder, spleen (also pancreas), kidney, or large intestine.
4. If the left hemisphere tests dominant, this suggests that an imbalance exists in at least one of the following midline meridians: circulation-sex (also pericardium), heart, stomach, thyroid,* small intestine, or bladder.
5. After conducting the *test for cerebral dominance* to determine which meridian is out of balance, the tester has the subject therapy localize the alarm points with respect to each meridian (Figure 5.4). For example, if the left hemisphere tests dominant, meaning that the indicator muscle tests weak while the right hand is positioned opposite the left ear, after securing a strong indicator muscle once again and having the subject touch the lower portion of his sternum between the breasts with his right fingertips will therapy localize the circulation-sex meridian. If the strong indicator muscle weakens, an imbalance in that meridian is present. Issues such as regret, remorse, and jealousy, specifically related to the circulation-sex meridian, can then be addressed psychotherapeutically.
6. While there are a variety of ways to alleviate the meridian imbalance, one way defined by Diamond is through the use of affirmations specific to the involved meridian. In the case of an imbalance in the circulation-sex meridian, having the patient congruently state one or more of the following affirmations will often alleviate the imbalance: "I renounce the past." "I am relaxed. My body is relaxed." "I am generous." If the imbalance were

---

* The term *thyroid meridian* appears to be specific to the Diamond method. Elsewhere, this meridian is referred to variably as the triple warmer, triple heater, tri-heater, and triple energizer.

in the heart meridian, the meridian of anger, the following affirmations will often prove of therapeutic value: "I love." "I forgive." "There is forgiveness in my heart."

7. After having the subject say the relevant affirmation several times, conducting the thymus test and the *test for cerebral dominance* will generally reveal that the imbalance has been alleviated.

8. Frequently, after one meridian-emotional issue has been transmuted, another layer of the problem will be revealed. For example, after conducting the thymus, *cerebral dominance*, and alarm point tests and locating, say, a heart meridian imbalance (i.e., anger), after transmuting the anger by using the appropriate affirmation (e.g., "There's forgiveness in my heart"), the thymus may yet test weak, although the heart meridian alarm point will not be active. This indicates that there is still an imbalance in the system, although it is no longer related to the heart meridian. Continuation of the basic procedure may next reveal a large intestine meridian imbalance (i.e., guilt), which can be treated with an affirmation such as, "I am essentially clean and good." Perhaps now the thymus will test strong, indicating that the imbalance is alleviated. Otherwise, we continue with the process until we arrive at the proverbial bottom of the barrel.

9. Diamond says that the last meridian imbalance revealed is the Achilles' heel. This is the person's most vulnerable issue. Given repeated use of the affirmation, in time the tendency for the meridian to go out may become less likely. When the meridian energy is balanced, the individual has better access to positive emotions and creativity.

MERIDIANS AND EMOTIONS

Just as Goodheart correlated the various muscles with specific meridians, Diamond has outlined an association between meridians and emotions (Table 5.1). While acupuncture lore has also connected meridians and emotions (i.e., liver meridian with anger, heart meridian with joy, etc.), Diamond's correlation is distinct in that he employed kinesiological tests to arrive at his findings (Diamond, 1997b). Additionally, he has lent greater specificity to the meanings of the various emotions by referring to their etymology and current usage.

For example, the positive emotion of the liver meridian is happiness and cheerfulness, while the negative emotion is unhappiness. On the other hand, the thyroid meridian, generally referred to as the tri-heater meridian or triple warmer meridian, is the seat of lightness, buoyancy, and hope at the positive pole and depression at the negative pole.

Diamond says that while depression and unhappiness have frequently been used synonymously in psychiatric literature, they are not equivalent. Depression includes sensations of heaviness and low energy, of being pushed down or depressed. The opposite of depression is lightness, feeling uplifted, feeling buoyed up with hope. In contrast to depression, unhappiness has to do with feeling unfortunate, of not feeling lucky. "The unhappy person feels that the fault always lies with someone else.... With the state of unhappiness there is always the feeling that if only the

TABLE 5.1
Meridians and Associated Emotions

Meridian	Negative Emotion	Positive Emotion
Lung	Disdain, scorn, contempt, intolerance, prejudice	Humility, tolerance, modesty
Liver	Unhappiness	Happiness, cheer
Gallbladder	Rage, fury, wrath	Love, forgiveness, adoration
Spleen	Anxiety	Security, faith/confidence
Kidney	Sexual indecision	Calm, sexual assuredness
Large intestine	Guilt	Self-worth
Circulation-sex/Pericardium	Regret, remorse, jealousy, sexual tension, stubbornness	Renunciation of the past, relaxation, generosity
Heart	Anger	Love, forgiveness
Stomach	Disgust, bitterness, disappointment, greed, hunger, deprivation	Contentment, tranquility
Tri-heater	Depression, despair, grief, hopelessness, loneliness, solitude, despondency	Hope, lightness, elation, buoyancy
Small intestine	Sadness, sorrow	Joy
Bladder	Restlessness, impatience, frustration	Harmony, peace
Governing	Embarrassment	Healthy pride
Central	Shame	Healthy pride

Source: Adapted from information contained in *Life Energy* (Diamond, 1985)

powers that be (which in our psyche always comes down to our parents) had given me more, I would now be perfect, I would now be happy" (Diamond, 1985, p. 114). The happy person, on the other hand, feels lucky and cheerful.

The stomach meridian is positively associated with contentment, which is from the Latin *continere*, meaning to contain, as the stomach contains food. Among the negative emotions of this meridian are disgust, dis + *gustare*, from Latin meaning to eat, and old French *desgouster*, meaning "to lose one's appetite." Other related associations include bitterness, greed, emptiness, deprivation, nausea, and hunger, all of which pertain to the negative aspects of the stomach meridian.

Table 5.1 lists a number of Diamond's findings on the connection between meridians and their emotions. Determining the specific meridian and associated emotion provides the therapist and client with the means to apply relevant affirmations and other therapeutic procedures and to diagnose their effectiveness. The interested reader should refer to *Life Energy* (1985) for in-depth treatment of this topic.

THE THYMUS GLAND

Diamond maintains that the thymus gland, which is the immune system's source of T cells (*T* stands for thymus), is also the principal gland or "master switch, the master controller, of the acupuncture energy system of the body" (1985, p. 20). He concludes this on the basis of manual muscle testing combined with therapy local-izing the thymus test point on the sternum. He observes that if the subject's indicator muscle tests weak while therapy localizing the thymus, having the subject test touch other areas on the skin will generally not produce the same results. He reports that when the thymus tests weak, having the subject chew a thymus extract tablet, in contrast to other glandular extracts, will reestablish strength in the indicator muscle while therapy localizing the thymus. Additionally, he finds that negative and positive thoughts have a significant bearing on the test, such that if the subject's thymus tests weak, a highly positive thought will activate the thymus, resulting in the indicator muscle testing strong. A strong thymus test, on the other hand, will be abolished when the subject accesses a highly negative thought.

Diamond emphasizes that the strength of the thymus is indicative of our will to health and that activating the thymus and the will is a primary ingredient in effective treatment.

> The thymus also reflects our will to be well. Whenever the thymus tests weak, it means we don't have sufficient will to be well. Our life energy is not high enough to carry out the healing processes. This finding has been of great value in clinical practice. The doctor's first goal must be to activate the patient's will to be well. (Diamond, 1985, p. 20)

Contrasting the level of functioning in the thymus gland, Diamond describes high-thymus and low-thymus types. The high-thymus type accentuates the positive and responds with strength in the face of tragedy. The primary positive thymus attributes are faith, trust, gratitude, and courage. The low-thymus type, by contrast, dwells in the negative, passively accepts a low level of functioning, and does not respond with strength to tragedy. The primary negative thymus attributes are fear, hate, and envy.

THE THYMUS THUMP

One way to activate the thymus and therefore one's life energy is by a simple procedure called the thymus thump (Figure 5.5). Diamond notes that the thymus gland used to be considered of little relevance with passing age, since medical studies concluded that the thymus shrunk with age. The only problem with this conclusion was that it was based on observations of cadavers in which the thymus has invariably shriveled. Diamond relates this to a dearth of life energy for which the cadaver is well known.

If the thymus tests weak, having the person thump on the sternum above the thymus can activate the thymus, increasing the availability of life energy. Diamond recommends that the thymus thump be done in a Waltz beat rhythm, since he has reportedly found this pattern to be most beneficial.

HOMING THOUGHTS

Another way of enhancing one's life energy and thymus functioning is by using a homing thought (Diamond, 1985). Stressful circumstances and even stressful

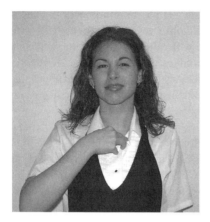 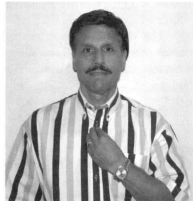

FIGURE 5.5 The thymus thump is used to activate the thymus by having the person thump on the sternum above the thymus.

thoughts can deplete life energy. This is evident when we ask the subject to think of something negative and then test his or her indicator muscle. The muscle will almost always weaken, indicating that the life energy has been compromised. However, if we have the subject think of something positive, the muscle will remain strong, and thus the life energy as well. The homing thought is based on this simple principle.

The difference between a homing thought and any other positive thought is that the homing thought involves a highly positive sense of self, a pervasively strong thought, an image, a feeling of what one is aiming to become. The homing thought is fashioned in the positive (e.g., being healthy) rather than in the negative (e.g., absence of illness or not ill). It is also developed without comparison to someone else. In many respects it is a meditation, a kind of prayer.

> Thinking about your homing thought, your thymus will test strong and you will be centered, your vulnerability to stress will be reduced, your life energy will be raised so much that factors that earlier might have stressed you now will not. When you are in touch with your true self through your homing thought, you are above being affected by most of the environmental factors that stress us from day to day. Your life energy has been dramatically raised. Furthermore, your own life goals will be clearer to you and you will have new confidence in your decisions. (Diamond, 1985, p. 77)

An appropriate homing thought can be ascertained by initially listing a variety of life goals. These can relate to any number of areas: profession, health, relationships, hobbies, musical and artistic activities, etc. Any one or a combination of these thoughts or aspirations can then be subjected to the indicator muscle test without touch testing the thymus. Those thoughts that test strong can be further tested by exposing the subject to a stressor that previously caused the indicator muscle to weaken. These might include loud noises, looking at a disconcerting picture, looking at a fluorescent light, yelling "Boo," etc. The thoughts that hold strong are effective homing thoughts.

Diamond points out that the homing thought is not constant and will evolve in time as one regularly contemplates it. Additionally, the homing thought, as it becomes thoroughly assimilated, will guide our actions in a positive direction. For example, a homing thought of oneself being healthy and upright in posture will influence one's diet, exercise, activities, choice of chairs and shoes, etc.

REVERSAL OF THE BODY MORALITY

In addition to the thymus testing weak when the will to be well is low, Diamond describes an even more insidious problem, which he refers to as "reversal of the body morality" (Diamond, 1988, p. 15). In this instance, the indicator muscle will test reversed, such that good tests as bad and bad tests as good; love tests as bad and hate tests as good; etc. When the body morality is reversed, healing cannot occur. Life energy is directed away from where it is needed. This is reminiscent of Becker's research on nonunion fractures (Becker and Selden, 1985) and Langman's research on electrical polarity with cervical cancer (1972). Freud's concept of *thanatos* is also called to mind.

With regard to manual muscle testing for this reversal, the method involves establishing a strong indicator muscle and then determining the variable responses to statements such as the following: "I want to be well." vs. "I want to be ill." or "I want to live." vs. "I want to die." Absent a reversal of the body morality, the subject will test strong for wanting to be well and to live, and weak for desiring illness and death.

Alleviation of this reversal is a complex problem. While Diamond reports that the condition can be corrected by having the patient regularly take brain RNA with choline, it is yet another matter to convince the reversed patient to take the supplement. By definition, the patient with a reversed body morality would be adverse to taking anything to improve his or her health, since health and illness are reversed.*

THE FORK IN THE ROAD: THE UPSILON (Y) FACTOR

Although a variety of therapeutic procedures may prove temporarily beneficial, in Diamond's view profound change often comes about only by returning to the fork in the road when the patient made the negative choice or attachment, perhaps unconsciously, that resulted in the reversal of the body morality. Referred to as the *upsilon* (Y) *factor*, this approach involves energetically attuning the moment of inception of the psychoenergetic problem and redeciding or reconcluding. It is applicable to a variety of other meridian problems. The therapist skilled in manual muscle testing will be able to employ Diamond's therapy localization method to determine which meridian and which specific meridian point is involved. Thereupon, the treatment point can be stimulated in some manner, such as by percussing or tapping, pressure, an acupuncture needle, with sound, cold laser light, and so forth.

---

* Diamond has extended this concept further with the notion of *illness diathesis*, which addresses the specific disease that the patient develops. This is related not only to a reversal of the body morality but also to an unconscious choice to develop a particular illness condition (Diamond, 1997b).

But even so, Diamond is of the opinion that although these methods may result in a noticeable change, a profound philosophical shift or indeed a spiritual shift is generally needed for endurance. Like Edward Bach, homeopath developer of the Bach flower remedies, he believes that every disease is fundamentally a spiritual problem (Diamond, 1997a,b).

> I would like to consider my profession as being what Freud called "a new profession of secular minister of the soul."
>
> But instead of just minister, which can also have religious connotations, rather a healer. A healer of the soul suffering, a healer of the spirit. Not a spiritual healer, for I don't think of myself as healing by spirit, but instead helping the sufferer overcome his pain by encouraging the workings of the Healing Power of his own Spirit, which I refer to as Life Energy. (Diamond, 1997a, p. 5)

For example, let us say that a man's mother died when he was 12 years old. In the face of such a trauma, the boy might make the decision that having a relationship with a woman is far too painful and will eventually result in profound loss. At this fork in the road, where he might have chosen acceptance and love, instead he "unconsciously" chose the low road, and at that moment a meridian problem was established. Clearly, this is a problem of the ego, but additionally, it is an acupuncture meridian energy problem. If we were to conduct an applied kinesiology therapy localization test with him, we might find that the heart meridian is involved, and in this instance the meridian problem would involve anger (from middle English, old Norse *angr*, meaning sorrow*). Or perhaps the circulation-sex meridian would be involved, given a perpetual state of regret (from the Germanic, *greter*, meaning to weep). Additionally, the energy block could be more precisely located at a specific point on the heart meridian, such as at heart-7 or heart-9, or on the circulation-sex meridian, such as at circulation-sex-8.

How can such a condition be effectively alleviated? With the Diamond method we have a measure of the condition in that we can muscle test in order to precisely locate the bioenergy block. We can also test to discern the moment when the choice was made that produced the meridian problem. Concerning the latter, after establishing that there is a disruption in a specific meridian, the patient is directed to think back to various time frames to precisely locate the moment of origin. For example, the man who lost his mother might be asked to think back to an innocuous event when he was 25 years old. Testing reveals that the meridian problem is already present. It is also present at ages 20, 19, 15 and 12. However, when he thinks back to an event at age 11, the meridian problem is no longer detectable. He is then asked about events within the 11- to 12-year-old time frame until the precise decisive moment is located. Perhaps it is the moment his father returned from the hospital, painfully announcing the loss. Or perhaps it was earlier if his mother suffered an extended illness. Or possibly the decision did not occur until a specific moment at the funeral home. Nonetheless, at that moment the problem began, since at that

---

* Interestingly, anger has frequently been understood as a secondary or cover-up emotion, a response to feeling afraid or hurt. This understanding apparently has an etymological basis.

moment a negative choice was made, creating an ongoing meridian problem. He decided, perhaps unconsciously, not to love, possibly to avoid the inevitable pains of love. The long road of suffering was paved.

The choices at this point are many. The man might be asked to direct his attention to that specific point in time while various points along the involved meridian are therapy localized to find that point that makes the indicator muscle strong. Then that point can be tapped or stimulated in some other effective manner. While this frequently results in a change in muscle response and alleviation of the energy block, Diamond is quick to point out that this is merely a temporary correction. More is needed.

A deeper level therapeutic choice would direct the man's attention to that point in time and redecision the moment. With each redecision attempt, the therapist can again challenge the indicator muscle. When a change has occurred at the energy level, it will show in the muscle test with the muscle testing strong. However, even when a change has been facilitated in this way, Diamond advises "eternal vigilance" (Diamond, 1997a,b). In most instances, it will be necessary to reaffirm the new choice frequently over time until it is resolutely established.

IDENTITY AND CONTROL

Returning to the fork in the road, often it is apparent that the person has lost a sense of personal identity and control to another, and this accounts for the meridian problem. The person is controlled by the introjected other, and thus his or her life energy might be zapped. Personal power is only available when one's actions come from one's self. In the theater, this might be similar to the distinction made between the Stanislavsky method and method acting.

> With every meridian problem, a control factor will always be found to be operant. Control is a specific instance of introjection and occurs when we have lost, or perhaps never attained, a sense of our own identity in a specific area of personality. In a desperate search for identity we hungrily take in that aspect of the personality of another which is missing in ourselves, and then act as if it were us. (Diamond, 1988, p. 37)

Diamond observes that the loss of identity is often to another that one perceives as more capable. Otherwise, introjected identity is also the plight of the one who controls, who specifically defines himself or herself in the context of the relationship as the one who controls the other. It is therefore imperative, for the freedom and growth of both therapist and patient, that the therapist's sense of self be solid as to not wish to control the patient or to be controlled in return.

With regard to method, when a specific problem has been located, manual muscle testing can be used to identify the introjected identity. Stating the name of the introject will generally reveal a distinction in muscle response. For example, if a patient has a phobia of dogs, thinking about the phobia will typically result in a weak indicator muscle response. If the patient is not "in" his or her own identity with the problem, the patient's indicator muscle will remain weak when saying, "I am [myself] with this fear of dogs." On the other hand, the indicator muscle will test strong when the introjected identity is stated: for example, "I am [Gloria] with this problem." From here, the therapist can continue to employ muscle testing creatively to determine when the problem originated. It is simply a matter of phrasing relevant questions in a yes–no format. Once the precise moment and context has been located, the patient may be able to make a positive creative choice. Again, the patient (or student, as Diamond would prefer) is assigned "eternal vigilance."

SURROUNDING THE ENEMY

Another therapeutic option is what Diamond refers to as "surrounding the enemy" (Diamond, 1997b). In *War and Peace*, Tolstoy describes the defeat of Napoleon's army by the Russians simply by surrounding the enemy, cutting off supplies, and allowing the Russian winter to defeat the enemy. In a similar manner, if a meridian problem is actually originated and maintained within the ego, assisting the patient in transcending ego would be akin to the Russian strategy and would not necessitate a head-on attack with the "enemy." That is, it may not be necessary to more specifically direct the therapy. In this regard, Diamond posits that at essence a human being has soul or in actuality is most fundamentally soul. Recall that Diamond sees life energy as spirit. By having the patient engage in creative activities in such a way as to "step out" of the ego, the meridian problem is transcended. Reading high-energy, cantillating poetry; singing; free-form dancing; and playing percussion instruments can prove of therapeutic benefit if done in a love- and healing-giving, self-*un*conscious manner. The therapist assists the patient in letting go of self-consciousness as the creative activity is entered in a life energy-enhancing manner.

CANTILLATION

The choice of the therapeutic creative activity is imperative in the same way that the homing thought is unique and relevant to the individual. One seeks that creative activity that is consistent with cantillation. This is a matter of discovering the "song" in one's heart. Diamond refers to this as "singing the song of love for the Love" (Diamond, 1997b). One method of ascertaining the "cantillating" activity is to have the person think about varieties of creative activities while testing the strength in the indicator muscle. The activities might include swimming, running, dancing, singing, teaching, carpentry, and so on. Each time we determine the degree of strength in the muscle. The muscle strength indicates one's cantillation.

> A life of Cantillation is one of love, of gratitude. A perpetual reaffirmation of the Love, the Tao, the Buddha nature. With increasing Cantillation there is the ever-increasing state of lovedness, of oneness, of beauty. On and on, higher and higher, beyond and beyond. (Diamond, 1988, p. 56)

Consistent with his Kleinian roots and on the basis of years of life energy analysis, Diamond concludes that:

[U]nderneath all the problems arising out of the various negative desires … there is always one basic problem: hatred of one's mother. When this is overcome through the specific act of creativity, all the more superficial problems disappear. But one, even deeper, remains: the absence of the belief in the love of the mother. Cantillation commences when we find The Mother in our mothers. (Diamond, 1988, pp. 4–5)

Diamond's work has led him from a precision analysis of chi, life energy, to a deep appreciation for creativity and spirituality. His current mission, which has indeed been his ongoing homing aspiration, is to assist others in transcending the distortions and the hypocrisy of the ego and arriving at their souls. He sees the soul as perfect, innocent, and good. The more one is in touch with one's soul, the more profoundly balanced one's life energy becomes. His is a philosophy, a realization of the God within.

Buddhist-like in sentiment, Diamond holds to the *four nobel truths* and sees cantillation as a means to enlightenment and the alleviation of human suffering. He posits that although life is suffering through the accumulation of our negative decisions, life can be the greatest joy. A way to achieve this is through life energy analysis and cantillation.

ADDENDUM

This has been only a rudimentary overview of the work of Dr. John Diamond. There is much more to tell about this approach that can be incorporated into what we do therapeutically and proactively with ourselves and others. But that will be covered in more detail in a future work. For now, we turn our focus to how this work has been instrumental in the development of one of the most efficient therapies to cross our paths in recent years, thought field therapy.

6 Thought Field Therapy

Therapy as a process is an advance into a higher state of freedom, maturity, and development in a similar way that mature development brings about a growth advance into increased personal freedom.

— **Roger J. Callahan (1994b)**

Thought field therapy (TFT) is among the most efficient of psychological therapies. Similar to other approaches based on applied kinesiology, thought field therapy addresses the acupuncture meridians and employs therapy localization to determine effective treatments. Thought field therapy is distinct from other approaches, however after a specific sequence of energy meridians is diagnosed, treatment entails having the patient tap on or near beginning or ending acupoints respective to the involved meridians while continuing to attune or think about the psychological problem (e.g., trauma, phobia, or depression). This is consistent with Goodheart's finding that tapping or percussing on specific tonification and sedation acupoints is effective in the treatment of physical pain conditions (Walther, 1988). Additionally, the thought field therapy procedures involve assessing subjective units of distress (SUD) periodically during treatment so as to have an ongoing measure of the effects of the treatments.

Originated by Roger J. Callahan, Ph.D., thought field therapy appears rather esoteric when compared to traditional approaches to psychotherapy. Even the theoretical position, like all energy approaches to medical and psychological treatment, significantly deviates from the "currently" accepted zeitgeist. That is, the fundamental causal factors according to thought field therapy are hypothesized to be the perturbations (disturbances) located within a subtle energy field rather than a function of disturbances in cognition, environmental contingencies, conditioning, chemical imbalances, or other seemingly more substantive factors. Because Callahan's method is indeed so contrary to standard contemporary approaches in psychiatry and psychology, it has, to some extent, aroused hostility and ridicule on the part of some traditionally trained professionals. While Callahan's method does not fit these traditional molds, he nonetheless appears to have tapped into something quite remarkable.

Callahan maintains a practice in Indian Wells, CA, where he and wife Joanne provide training and telephone therapy services to people from all parts of the globe, addressing a wide variety of psychological problems. When treating over the phone, the procedure involves testing the patient's voice to determine the specific meridian imbalances involved in the patient's psychological problem. Callahan refers to this proprietary methodology as the voice technology™ (VT™). He describes the voice

83

technology as an "exclusive … technology which allows for the rapid and precise diagnosis of [*perturbations*] by telephone through an objective and unique voice analysis technology" and notes that "the relevant information can be demonstrated to be contained in holographic form within the voice by means of Fourier transforms" (Callahan and Callahan, 1996, p. 110).

While similar diagnostic approaches have been available in many guises throughout the kinesiology industry, Callahan's entails some distinct innovations. Therefore, he also considers his basic diagnostic approach to be proprietary.*

Callahan sees the causes of psychological problems as involving distinct disruptions in the individual's thought field, what he refers to as *perturbations in the thought field*. In this respect, thought itself is assumed to exist bound in energy fields, likely electromagnetic in nature, similar to some other fields. A perturbed thought field is viewed as a configuration that contains information that in turn causes specific disruptive effects in the energy system and in turn within other bodily systems.

More specifically, the thought field therapy approach entails having the patient think about or attune the problem while the energy system is assessed either by therapy localization via muscle testing when the patient is seen in the office or by assessing certain qualities in the individual's voice over the telephone. These methods provide information regarding the precise sequence of energy disruptions and the structure in which the disruptions are encoded. Clients are then asked to numerically rate the level of distress on a 10-point scale while continuing to attune the psychological issue, after which the client is directed to stimulate the respective energy meridian points or acupoints on the body by tapping with the fingertips. Generally, within a matter of a few minutes, the anxiety, anger, depressed mood, or other negative affect associated with the condition is significantly or completely relieved. While many patients require repeated treatments over time to realize a permanent cure, an appreciable number find their problem permanently resolved after one brief treatment.

Callahan used to practice traditional approaches to psychotherapy. He describes himself as having been a practitioner of cognitive therapy at one point, and he even conducted seminars in rational emotive behavior therapy (REBT). He also developed expertise in client-centered therapy, systematic desensitization, biofeedback, and other contemporary methods of therapy. As an accomplished hypnotherapist, for a time he was even a fellow of the American Society of Clinical Hypnosis.

However, in his search for increasingly better and faster ways of doing treatment, he came upon applied kinesiology. Callahan reports that he initially learned of this method from a psychiatrist friend, Harvey Ross, M.D., who demonstrated an interesting muscle phenomenon that he had learned from Goodheart. As Callahan describes it:

> He asked me to hold my arm out straight to my side, and he pushed down upon it while asking me to resist. My arm felt quite strong. He then asked me to think of something upsetting and this time I could not hold my arm up. I was amazed and asked

---

* Callahan has two diagnostic approaches: one that is conducted by direct contact in person with clients via specialized manual muscle testing and the voice technology, which is conducted over the phone via voice analysis.

him to repeat this a number of times. It worked the same each time. (Callahan, 1990, p. 7)

Although Callahan did not immediately realize the full implications of this method, he did readily observe that negative states somehow disrupt the body's strength, while positive states were in some way consistent with balanced or increased strength. This demonstration so interested him that he went on to study applied kinesiology, completing the International College of Applied Kinesiology (ICAK) 100-hour certification program under the instruction of chiropractors David Walther, D.C., and Robert Blaich, D.C. For a brief time he was also associated with John Diamond, M.D. (1997b), incorporating Diamond's specific therapy localization methods to evaluate psychological problems (Callahan, 1985). He eventually made some of his own contributions to applied kinesiology, conducting clinical research and presenting at various International College of Applied Kinesiology conferences. In the course of his practice, he arrived at his own unique integrative approach. He reports that he initially tested his approach with a client with phobia in 1980.

THE CASE OF MARY

Mary had a severe water phobia and had been in treatment with Callahan for approximately 18 months, realizing little progress — a sad but true testimonial to the lack of curative power in the psychological therapies available at the time. After this period of client-centered therapy, rational emotive behavioral therapy, systematic desensitization, hypnosis, and other therapies, she was only able to sit near the shallow end of a swimming pool, dangling her feet in the water. "However, she had a splitting headache after each meeting, she couldn't look at the water, and it was difficult each time for her to go to the pool; it took real courage" (Callahan, 1990, p. 9). Additionally, Mary continued to have difficulty taking a bath, only using a small amount of water each time, and she could not even go out of the house when it was raining. She also suffered weekly nightmares about water consuming her. As Mary had had this severe phobia all her life, and there was no evidence of a trauma that led to its development, it certainly appeared to be a hereditary condition.*

Given such minimal progress, Callahan decided to evaluate Mary via a variation of the applied kinesiology diagnostic testing methods that he was studying. He had her think about water while assessing energy "flow" through the various meridians. He thereupon discovered that only her stomach energy system was out of balance.†
Given this "diagnosis," he simply had Mary continue to tune into the thought of water while he gently tapped on the bony orbits under her eyes with his fingertips.

---

* It is Callahan's position that most, if not all, specific phobias are hereditary conditions, albeit not necessarily in the genetic sense. In this regard, he references the work of biologist Rupert Sheldrake and experimental psychologist William McDougall.
† According to the ancient acupuncture maps, the stomach energy system begins under the eyes and travels downward toward the sides of the chin, thereupon changing course upward to the sides of the forehead, through the head, down the sides of the neck, through the chest and stomach, and down the legs, ending on the second toe of each foot. For a more precise description of this and other meridians, see *Applied Kinesiology: Synopsis* by David S. Walther (1988).

Within a minute or so Mary said that the problem was gone, that she no longer got "that sick feeling" in her stomach while she thought about water. Callahan thereupon decided to test out the results *in vivo* by inviting Mary to go outside to the swimming pool, as he was treating her in his home office at the time. Here is how Callahan reports the event:

> I fully expected her to resist as usual but, to my surprise, I had to hurry to keep up with her on the way to the pool. For the first time, she looked at the water, put her head near it and splashed water in her face, from the shallow end. I watched in amazement as she joyfully shouted, "It's gone, it's gone!"
>
> Mary's next move frightened me. She suddenly ran toward the deep end of the pool, and this sudden total absence of fear around the pool was so unusual for her that I shouted, "Mary, be careful!" I was afraid that she might jump in the pool and drown. She laughed when she saw my alarm and reassured me, "Don't worry Doctor Callahan, I know I can't swim." [Fourteen] years experience with the treatment has since taught me that the treatment does not cause sudden stupidity. Respect for reality, I have learned, is not diminished by successful treatment. (Callahan, 1990, pp. 10–11)

That was more than 18 years ago, and Mary remains cured of her previous debilitating fear of water. Such a seemingly absurd treatment actually cured Mary of a condition that none of the other therapies could even touch.

This therapy apparently had nothing to do with cognition, other than the fact that it required Mary to think about water while she was being treated. However, there was no attempt made to directly challenge or alter her ways of thinking about water, even though one can be sure, judging by the enthusiasm of her actions, that her beliefs about water and herself shifted automatically with the change brought about by tapping. The cognitive therapy that she had previously received attempted to directly effect a change in her beliefs to little or no avail.

Also, this was not a hypnotic procedure, nor was it an obvious desensitization method. Recall that Mary had previously been ineffectively treated with hypnosis and systematic desensitization, methods that emphasize relaxation, desensitization, and suggestion.

And surely this change could not simply be accounted for as the result of a placebo. A placebo seems to require at least some degree of positive expectations on the part of the client and/or therapist. One would certainly not be inclined to anticipate such a dramatic change as a result of simply tapping under one's eyes. Besides, if a placebo was to hold the answer, one would definitely have expected the previous 18 months of various treatments to have delivered on that count, as they are much more complex, attentive, ritualistic, and scientific in appearance.

It would also be incorrect to conclude that the treatment simply worked as a result of distraction because the other techniques used would certainly have produced some level of distraction as well. To the contrary, there appears to have been something more to this treatment, something that cannot be simply minimized, explained away, or interpreted in terms of the generally accepted paradigms in the field.

As far as chemical effects are concerned, most psychopharmacologists and allo-pathic physicians would agree that while depressions and many anxiety disorders often respond favorably to certain psychotropic medications, phobias are an entirely different matter.* According to Callahan, many experts even go so far as to assert that phobias cannot be successfully eliminated. Besides, as far as thought field therapy is concerned, there was no ingestion of any chemical compound involved. Tapping under Mary's eyes may have resulted in various chemical changes at some level, such as by elevating the level of neurotransmitters or endorphins, although that aspect of the treatment effect has not been substantiated at this time.† Rather, Callahan believes that the ancient meridian maps are correct and that the tapping facilitated a fundamental balancing of the stomach energy system while Mary's thought field entailed awareness of water. Perhaps another explanation could hold more water, but at this point, the energy system appears to be the most promising receptacle.‡

THERAPEUTIC SEQUENCES

Although the successful treatment of Mary was fairly simple in that it merely involved single bilateral treatment points, there is much more to this therapy than meets the eye. When one really thinks about it, knowing to tap under the eyes to cure a phobia is akin to finding a needle in the galactic haystack. How would one ever come to select that specific procedure among the infinity of possibilities that must exist? Again, the answer lies in a major shift in how one thinks about psychological problems. This shift is on the same order as that which led Copernicus to perceive that the heliocentric view of the universe was in error, or that which made it possible for Newton to conclude that the same force that makes an apple fall to the ground also holds the moon in orbit, or that which led Einstein to conceptualize gravity as a manifestation of matter-warped space. In a similar manner, Callahan shifted his focus away from cognition, psychodynamics, learning, chemicals, and development as the principal causes of psychological problems and instead, came to view the role of energy as the central, pivotal component.

Callahan discovered that he could successfully treat only about 20% of his phobic patients by using the same treatment he used with Mary. The other 80% needed something more. Within a short period of time, however, he was able to double his success rate as he discovered that phobias, as well as many other psychological problems, could be further differentiated in accordance with the specific energy meridians involved. For example, while some phobias involve disruption of the stomach meridian, others affect the spleen meridian. Still others

---

* Certain cardiac medications such as beta blockers (e.g., Tenormin and Inderal) have often been effective in temporarily reducing the symptoms associated with some phobic conditions. Anxiety is also frequently blocked with certain benzodiazepines such as Xanax and Ativan, although drug dependency and other side effects often pose a problem. Antidepressant medications including some tricyclics — Tofranil, Elavil, Pamelor, etc. — and selective serotonin reuptake inhibitors (SSRIs) — Prozac, Zoloft, Paxil, etc. — are also employed by some healthcare professionals in an attempt to contain the symptoms.

† Although acupuncture and thought field therapy are distinct, Pomeranz (1996) has proposed an acupuncture-endorphin theory that suggests that "acupuncture stimulates peripheral nerves that send messages to the brain to release endorphins ... [which] block pain pathways in the brain" (p. 86).

‡ Actually, chemical involvement is not excluded here. The thought field therapy theory proposes that perturbations in the thought field produce a disruption in the energy system, which in turn activates disruptive changes in the neurology, neurotransmitters, hormones, and cognition.

require treatment of the stomach meridian followed by treatment of the spleen meridian (also called the pancreas meridian), while still other phobias require the reverse of this sequence or sequences involving yet other meridians. Callahan became convinced that the sequence in which the meridians are treated is relevant, indeed critical to successful treatment.

Callahan came to refer to this phenomenon as a kind of combination lock that necessitates a specific order of turns if it is to be unlocked. For example, he concluded that the sequence for treating most specific phobias involved tapping directly on the bony orbits directly under the eyes (stomach meridian), 6 in. under the armpits (spleen meridian), and then under the collarbones at the acupuncture K-27 point (kidney meridian). In many cases, however, he found that to successfully treat claustrophobia, flight turbulence, or a spider phobia, the same meridian points are utilized, albeit with a variation in sequence as follows:

spleen (under arm) stomach (under eye) kidney (under collarbone)

Callahan concludes that the disruptions that exist with each condition often reveal a pattern unique to the condition itself, a specific sequence, and thus treatment needs to be conducted in the same specific order. This is partially consistent with Diamond's observation:

> One of the most incredible findings … is that meridians that tested strong will later be revealed as weak after the meridian which is currently testing weak is corrected.… It is only after you uncover and correct that first layer of meridian energy imbalance that the second meridian problem reveals itself. There is a definite order in which these layers reveal themselves. (Diamond, 1985, pp. 203–204)

Another way of conceptualizing this distinction of order in meridian stimulation is in terms of syntax and meaning. With regard to words, the sequence of letters is of obvious importance in the conveyance of meaning. Thus, the letters n, o, and w can spell now or won, depending on the ordering of the letters. The meaning is contingent on the order or sequence. This same relationship applies to the arrangement of words in a sentence. For example, the following arrangement does not convey the same meaning as the sentence you have just finished reading: *Reading finished just have you sentence the as meaning same the convey not does arrangement following the example for.* The sequence of meridians carries the same kind of relationship that we observe with sequences of letters and words. While the thought field therapy alphabet has only 14 primary symbols, as is discussed in the following section, taking the factorial of 14, over 87 billion possible treatment sequences are theoretically possible.

Recently, Callahan has proposed the term *healing data* for the therapeutic input to the energy system (Callahan, 2001). In this regard, he suggests that the sequence of meridians involved in a problem is similar to a DNA code and that the stimulation of the respective acupoints inputs healing information into the system. Since he has observed an improvement in heart rate variability (HRV) after such treatments, he concludes that the treatment not only resolves psychological problems but improves aspects of physical health as well.

DIAGNOSIS AND DIAGNOSTIC PROCEDURE

Thought field therapy diagnosis is a far cry from traditional diagnostic approaches. While the official diagnostic manual of the American Psychiatric Association, DSM-IV, may yet remain relevant with regard to syndromes and statistical considerations (as well as for the purpose of filling out insurance forms*), this standard psychiatric nomenclature as well as psychodynamic, cognitive, and many other theoretical formulations are not viewed by Callahan as hitting the most fundamental causal mark. Additionally, any diagnosis that could be based on neurotransmitter depletion would be a little closer to some aspects of the mark but would still miss the bull's-eye by a considerable distance. According to Callahan, these developmental, cognitive, and chemical aspects are tertiary or secondary rather than primary. It is his claim that the fundamental causal factor is the interaction of the energy system and perturbations in associated thought fields.

As noted, the energy system in thought field therapy is the same as that attended to by therapeutic approaches such as acupuncture, acupressure, and related meridian methods. This energy system comprises specific pathways or meridians through which the energy flows.† Many of the meridians are designated by the name of a bodily organ through which the meridian is routed. While a number of connecting meridians exist, the 12 primary and 2 collector meridians employed in thought field therapy are as follows:

1. Bladder (Bl)
2. Gallbladder (Gb)
3. Stomach (St)
4. Kidney (Ki or K)
5. Spleen (Sp)
6. Lung (Lu)
7. Small intestine (SI)
8. Large intestine (LI)
9. Circulation-sex (CX) also called pericardium (PC)
10. Tri-heater (TH) also called triple-warmer (TW)
11. Heart (Ht)
12. Liver (Lv)
13. Central or conception vessel (CV)
14. Governing vessel (GV)

---

* Possibly the accuracy of the DSM statistics is affected by the reality of third-party payers that will reimburse for some diagnoses and not others.

† This energy has been referred to as qi, chi, ki, prana, universal life force, and a number of other terms. This energy is subtle, and many believe that it is largely electromagnetic.

Concerning thought fields, Callahan hypothesizes that they contain subtle energy features, perturbations, when a psychological problem or other disruptive condition exists. If a client has an elevator phobia, for example, the awareness about elevators occurs within the context of a thought field that entails perturbations — disruptions within the energy system that are the fundamental cause of all negative emotions. When the perturbations are removed, the psychological discomfort or distress is likewise alleviated. The perturbations manifest in precise complexes or gestalt — holons — that can be diagnosed and treated via any of at least four increasingly precise assessment methods discussed in the following sections.

THERAPEUTIC ALGORITHMS

The most basic treatment approach entails the utilization of a therapeutic recipe or algorithm that has generally been found to be effective in the treatment of specific conditions. These algorithms have been arrived at via other procedures as a result of effectively diagnosing and treating a large number of individuals having similar problems, and distilling the common pattern of their thought fields' perturbations. For example, many traumatic conditions such as acute stress disorder (ASD) and post-traumatic stress disorder are often effectively treated by utilizing a specific sequence of acupuncture meridian energy points. In this regard, the algorithm entails treatment of the bladder meridian and kidney meridian, although other meridians are sometimes addressed as well, depending on the emotional complexity of the trauma (e.g., anger, guilt, rage, depression).*

From the standpoint of thought field therapy, it should be noted that the algorithm approach to treatment does not entail diagnosis in the strictest sense. That is, diagnosis at this level simply involves matching a packaged sequence of treatments, a recipe, to alleviate problems that have already been diagnosed or categorized by observation or interviewing. In this regard, algorithms exist for specific phobias, generalized anxiety, anticipatory anxiety, panic, addictive urges, depression, anger, guilt, and so forth. These and other algorithms are detailed later in this chapter and the next.

ALGORITHMS AND INTUITIVE UNDERSTANDING

A more advanced level of "diagnosis" and treatment entails an understanding of the emotional and contextual aspects of a condition in terms of its relationship to respective meridians. For example, a person who suffers from depression is likely to have a disruption associated with the tri-heater meridian, while one who evidences chronic anger problems may reveal disruptions in the heart, liver, or gallbladder meridians. The practitioner who understands these and other relationships has a greater chance of clinically estimating the therapeutic needs of the client in terms of energy balancing and is therefore prepared to develop effective algorithms or energy meridian sequences.

Additionally, it appears that the experienced therapist tends to synchronize with the client while working on a specific issue and thus develops an intuitive sense of

---

* This algorithm is detailed in the section on trauma cases.

what is needed at the moment. This is really no different from what occurs with mastery across any number of fields, in that the expert is in touch with "something" that transcends mere conscious processing or technique. In the field of psychotherapy, we often refer to clinical intuition in this regard.

MANUAL MUSCLE TESTING

While the previously noted "diagnostic" approaches appear to equip the energy practitioner with the means of more successfully treating a wider array of clients than many other psychotherapeutic approaches, a significant level of precision is often lost with these methods. A much more precise level is purportedly attained when diagnosis is arrived at through a specific form of muscle testing. In this way, disruptions in the body's energy system can be detected by assessing relative muscle strength while the client is tuning-in to the condition to be treated. Similar to other applied kinesiology offshoot methods such as the Diamond method* and neuro-emotional technique (NET),† thought field therapy offers a muscle testing/therapy localization procedure that yields highly specific information for treating psychological problems. The diagnostic method provides the means for delineating sequences of energy meridian–thought field disruptions (i.e., perturbations), which are effective in treating the particular problem in question. Thus, even though many traumas may be treated successfully with the basic trauma algorithm of eyebrow, collarbone 9 gamut treatments eyebrow, collarbone (notationally specified as eb, cb 9G Sq) (see the trauma cases section for further details), a small percentage of others suffering from trauma may require diverse sequences due to different complexes of perturbations, referred to as holons. Often, these variations can be effectively delineated via this more precise diagnostic method.

VOICE TECHNOLOGY

According to Callahan, the most advanced level of diagnosis is achieved by way of voice technology (VT). This method affords the luxury of diagnosing or decoding the condition by assessing the client's voice. In this regard, the voice, which also involves muscles, carries the information about the structure of the problem (i.e., the perturbations in the thought field) while the client speaks or is directed to count while attuning the problem. Callahan reports that this information is obtained in an instant, as it is holographically represented, rather than by having to proceed through the linear process necessitated when doing muscle testing. Additionally, at times there are confounding variables with muscle testing in that the tester may inadvertently influence the results due to physical contact with the client and the necessity of making judgments regarding the quality of muscle strength in response to the

---

* The Diamond method was developed by psychiatrist John Diamond, M.D. He has also referred to his approach as behavioral kinesiology and, more recently, has discussed his work in terms of life energy analysis (see Chapter 5).
† Neuro-emotional technique (NET) was developed by Scott Walker, D.C. Similar to thought field therapy, this method may also involve some stimulation of meridian points, although the points selected are the associated points off the bladder meridian along the spine.

condition being assessed. Further, if both the tester and the subject are in states of psychological reversal at the time (see the following section), the testing procedure becomes even more complicated. According to Callahan, these factors do not pose a problem with voice technology. The advantages of voice technology would appear to be rather far reaching when one considers that most people can be effectively treated over the telephone, which is how Callahan and others who employ voice technology conduct their practices. This would appear to entail advantages in treating disorders such as panic and other conditions that often require immediate, on-the-spot attention.

As noted earlier, voice technology is considered by Callahan to be proprietary, and therefore he does not disclose its specifics except to those who purchase and obtain specific training in the technology. While there are some advantages to such a technology, the scope of its effectiveness must at present remain in question, since it has not been experimentally validated. While Callahan has done some preliminary research and also reports that his clinical work with the technology has verified its effectiveness (see Callahan, 1987; Leonoff, 1995), at least two practitioners who have worked with voice technology have concluded that it provides no advantage over a comprehensive algorithm (Craig, 1993, 1997) or even over random sequences of treatment points (Pignotti, 2004).

PSYCHOLOGICAL REVERSAL

Callahan considers psychological reversal (PR) and effective ways of treating it to be among his most important contributions, increasing success rates with many psychological problems upward of 95%. This phenomenon is related to *Tibetan energy*, figure "8" energy, and over-energy (Rochlitz, 1995), as well as Diamond's independent discoveries of *reversal of the body morality* and the *umbilicus problem* (Diamond, 1980a).

Psychological reversal is a negativistic condition whereby one's "motivation operates in a way that is directly opposed to the way it should work" (Callahan and Perry, 1991, p. 41). This situation is apparent among the pathologic as well as the normal. It accounts for a wide array of conditions such as the inability to maintain resolve to quit drugs, lose weight, relate better to one's in-laws, or golf consistently better. Highly negativistic orientations are also manifestations of psychological reversal. In Callahan's words, psychological reversal is described as follows:

At times we all become aware that we are behaving in a destructive and hurtful way toward people we love, and yet we seem helpless to stop behaving that way. It is almost as if our willpower is suspended and we seem unable to do anything about it. At such times we are what I call psychologically reversed.

When you are psychologically reversed, your actions are contrary to what you say you want to do. You might say that you want to quit eating when you aren't hungry, and in your heart of hearts you really do want to quit overeating. But in reality you are continuing to overeat. You are sabotaging your own efforts, you feel helpless and you don't know why. (Callahan and Perry, 1991, pp. 40–41)

Callahan reports observing psychological reversal with an overweight person who had been unsuccessfully attempting to lose weight for a number of years. He employed the applied kinesiology muscle testing procedure, having her extend her left arm horizontally while he tested the strength in the middle deltoid muscle of her shoulder by pressing down on her arm while she attempted to resist his force. He then had her picture herself as thin as she said she wanted to be. Rather than testing strong, as would be expected if this image deeply appealed to her, she tested weak instead. Similar results were obtained when she stated that she wanted to be thin, in that her arm again tested weak. What's more, when Callahan had her picture herself even heavier and state that she wanted to gain weight, her arm tested strong (Callahan and Perry, 1991). Consistent with Goodheart's dictum that "the body never lies," this woman's body was apparently announcing the truth of the matter. This should not be interpreted to mean that the patient is lying, however, but rather that there is a conflict or stress in the system, such that the idea of achieving the stated goal arouses notable stress, whereas not achieving it produces quite the opposite effect in the tested muscle.

Obviously, something is awry when psychological reversal is present. This polarized energy reversal prevents the patient from achieving results consistent with his or her consciously expressed intention. Also, as long as one is psychologically reversed on a specific condition (i.e., depression, phobia, traumatic memory, etc.), clinically significant therapeutic results cannot be achieved. However, this situation is not the same as secondary gains — the patient being unwilling to improve due to his or her perception (perhaps unconscious) of somehow benefiting from the "undesirable" state of affairs.

Psychological reversal, to be certain, manifests as a form of self-rejection to various degrees. However, it is not entirely correct to simply conceptualize reversal in such a traditional manner, which is consistent with psychodynamic and cognitive models. Rather, psychological reversal is best thought of in terms of electrical or electromagnetic poles, such that the therapeutics or the individual's expressed intentions cannot be metabolized or assimilated by the system when the energy flow is in the "wrong" direction. Additionally, it is hypothesized that when a patient is psychologically reversed, this reversal of energy flow accounts for the self-sabotaging behaviors, which are seen as epiphenomena of the electromagnetic substrate.

One possible mechanism underlying the phenomenon appears to operate at the perceptual level whereby sensory data are misinterpreted, yielding an opposite or incongruent affect or emotion to that normally experienced. Thus, that which is negative for one feels positive when experienced in a state of psychological reversal, and is therefore engaged in despite one's conscious, cognitive understanding of its detrimental effects.

SPECIFIC AND MASSIVE PSYCHOLOGICAL REVERSAL

Psychological reversal can be quite specific, limited to clearly defined contexts, or it can be so extensive that it manifests globally, what Callahan has referred to as *massive psychological reversal* (MPR), extending across contexts and generally infesting many or most aspects of the person's life. Concerning the latter, this is quite apparent among people with highly negativistic elements in their personality, such as with patients diagnosed as having personality disorders including the proposed self-defeating personality disorder.* The person who is massively reversed might be deemed his own worst enemy. Additionally, it seems possible that chronic psychological and even medical conditions entail psychological reversal at some level, either delimited to the specific condition or pervasively present.

PSYCHOLOGICAL REVERSAL TREATMENTS

While psychological reversal has been known by other terms and treated by various means, Callahan eventually developed his own unique treatment for this barrier to treatment effectiveness. Initially, Callahan began in a traditional manner, focusing on assisting the patient toward achieving self-acceptance. He found that simply having the patient make a self-accepting statement would often temporarily interrupt the reversal. For example, an affirmation, such as "I profoundly and deeply accept myself with all my problems and all my shortcomings," (Callahan, 1985, pp. 59–60) would often correct the reversal long enough for other needed treatments to work (e.g., sequences of major treatments). This is equivalent to Diamond's finding that meridian imbalance can be corrected by utilizing affirmations (Diamond, 1985). Eventually, Callahan learned that the therapeutic effects of the affirmation could be enhanced by physically addressing certain aspects of the energy system at the same time. In this regard he discovered that it was especially useful to have the patient stimulate the small intestine meridian by tapping on the little finger side of a hand at small intestine-3, while simultaneously stating or thinking about the self-acceptance statement three times† (Figure 6.1).

Callahan further discovered that having the patient vigorously massage a tender intercostal neurolymphatic reflex on the left side of the chest while stating the affirmation worked particularly well, especially in cases of recurring reversal and massive psychological reversal (Figure 6.2). The latter has already been highlighted, while the former entails a tendency for the client to reverse again fairly quickly after the psychological reversal has been corrected. Callahan hypothesizes that the neurolymphatic reflex approach to treating reversal works by draining toxins from the person's system and that certain levels of toxins are generally if not invariably associated with psychological reversal. This may also be the major factor involved in correcting reversal by treating the small intestine meridian in view of the fact that the small intestine is a major source of absorption in the body.

---

* The hallmark of all personality disorders must entail psychological reversal to a large extent, especially because such conditions are deeply ingrained and relatively more difficult to treat than other psychological problems, such as anxiety disorders.

† Callahan eventually discontinued using affirmations in favor of simply having the client tap at the relevant acupoint or stimulate (rub) the neurolymphatic reflex (i.e., "sore spot"). In addition to the finding that the affirmations are not essential, possibly this change in position also helps to distinguish thought field therapy from cognitive therapies. Many other treatment approaches that stem from thought field therapy continue to employ affirmations with percussion or other stimulation of acupoints.

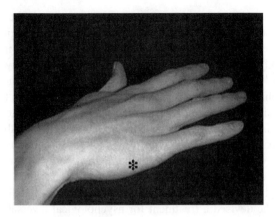

FIGURE 6.1 PR treatment at small intestine-3 (SI-3), little finger side of hand.

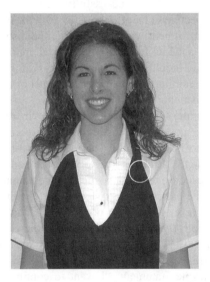

FIGURE 6.2 Neurolymphatic reflex (NLR) on the left side of the chest for treating psychological reversal. In thought field therapy, this reflex is also referred to as the "sore spot," since most people report a sore or tender sensation at the location. The neurolymphatic reflex is stimulated with rotating finger pressure.

MINI PSYCHOLOGICAL REVERSAL

Callahan has also described a type of psychological reversal that often interrupts effective treatment, what he refers to as mini psychological reversal (mPR). In the instance of mini psychological reversal, the patient level of distress or subjective units of distress (SUD) steadily decrease with a specific sequence of tapping on the involved meridian points after which a standstill is reached whereby the subjective units of distress remains at a specific level. For example, the patient may report subjective units of distress of 10 that descend to and remain at a 6 after a series of treatments, with continuing attempts at treatment having no effect. Thus, progress has been interrupted or halted, likely indicating a mini psychological reversal.

In this instance, treatment for psychological reversal is again introduced in one of the aforementioned ways, albeit with a different, appropriately specific verbalization, such as "I deeply and profoundly accept myself even though I *still* have *some* of this problem." Note that the altered statement recognizes that progress has occurred to a point. It would not be as precise for the patient to state, "... even though I have this problem." The latter does not convey the fact that some level of progress has already been achieved. This may seem to be quibbling with words, but the unconscious, which is consistent with the bodily energy system, seems to function at a specific and concrete level in this regard.

Concerning the discovery of mini psychological reversal, Callahan reports that some time after he devised a treatment for psychological reversal, he encountered a number of patients who continued to experience some degree of their psychological problem, even though it was treated successfully for the most part. For example, if the patient reported subjective units of distress of 10 prior to the onset of treatment for a phobia or trauma, treatment was able to lower the distress to 5 but no further. While he notes that the patients frequently expressed appreciation, Callahan wondered why his treatments could eliminate all traces of the problem with many patients, whereas others continued to experience a level of discomfort. What would it take to resolve those patients' problems completely?

Callahan reports that the solution occurred to him "in a flash" one day while he was working with a patient. After the distress level lowered but would not descend all the way to a 1 on the 1-to-10-point scale, he tested for psychological reversal. The strength in the patient's arm was strong while he had him say, "I want to be over this problem." In response to the opposite statement, that is, "I want to continue to have this problem," the patient's arm tested weak. Therefore, the patient did not evidence psychological reversal. Then it occurred to Callahan that there might be resistance to being completely over the problem. He thereupon tested the patient's arm while having him say, "I want to be completely over this problem." Lo and behold, the patient's arm tested weak. As would be expected, the arm tested strong in response to the opposite statement, "I want to continue to have some of this problem." The correction simply entailed having the patient tap on the little finger side of the hand (small intestine-3) while stating three times, "I deeply accept myself even though I *still* have *some* of this problem." This aspect of psychological reversal is similar to understandings arrived at through hypnosis. The unconscious mind can be quite linguistically concrete and literal.

OTHER LEVELS OF PSYCHOLOGICAL REVERSAL

In addition to specific, massive, and mini psychological reversal, Callahan and others have explored a number of levels or degrees of psychological reversal. In this regard, Callahan reports what he refers to as deep level psychological reversal; the treatment entails having the patient tap under the nose at a point on the governing vessel while repeating several times, "I deeply accept myself even if I *never* get over this problem."

James Durlacher, D.C. (1995) and Gallo (1994b, 1997b) have independently elaborated other levels of reversal that entail relationships to various criteria. One type of reversal in this category may be referred to as deservedness reversal. This block is treated by having the patient tap under the bottom lip (i.e., central vessel) or on the little finger side of the hand (small intestine meridian) while repeating the following affirmation three times: "I deeply accept myself even if I don't *deserve* to get over this problem." These and other criteria-related reversals* are discussed further in Chapter 7.

ANCILLARY TREATMENTS

Callahan refers to the primary energy meridian treatment points as major treatments and differentiates these from psychological reversal treatments. He has also developed a variety of other odd sequences that are utilized alone or in conjunction with the major treatments to achieve therapeutic results. Included among these procedures are the nine gamut treatments (9G), floor-to-ceiling eye roll (er), and collarbone breathing exercise (CBB). The essentials of each of these treatments are discussed in the following sections.

THE NINE GAMUT TREATMENTS

The nine gamut treatments (9G) are a series of fine-tuning procedures that likely activate various areas of the brain to enhance the effects of the major treatments. Thus, after a patient with a phobia has been directed to tap under his or her eye, arm, and collarbone (i.e., major treatments), the nine gamut treatments are inserted, followed by a repeat of the major treatments (i.e., eye, arm, collarbone). The nine gamut treatments are done by continuously tapping on the gamut spot between the little and ring fingers on the back of either hand (the tri-heater meridian at TH-3) while participating in a variety of tasks including opening and closing the eyes, moving and placing the eyes in different positions, humming a tune, and counting (Figure 6.3).

After the nine gamut treatments are completed, usually the subjective units of distress lower. However, often it seems that the nine gamut treatments primarily serve to attune other relevant aspects of the problem or thought field for treatment. In such instances, a lowering of the distress may not be evident. Callahan comments:

> The theory behind the gamut treatments is that we are balancing various functions of the brain with each treatment in regard to the particular problem we are treating. Each problem needs to be treated separately. It is as if the brain must be tuned to the right frequency for each problem for the treatment to work. (Callahan, 1990, p. 15)

Familiarity with neurology and neuropsychology suggests the possible relevance of this procedure in terms of stimulating varied brain functions and areas. For

---

* A number of criteria-related reversals (a term I coined) were originally developed by Dr. James Durlacher and me. This approach has not been incorporated into Callahan's approach to thought field therapy.

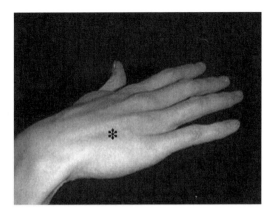

FIGURE 6.3 Thought field therapy gamut spot at triple-heater-3.

example, humming a tune may be consistent with activation of the right or nondominant hemisphere, while counting coincides with activation of the left or dominant hemisphere. It is further assumed that the various eye positions serve to stimulate other specific areas and functions of the brain; this is similar to Bandler and Grinder's (1979) observations that various lateral eye movements correlate with functions such as kinesthetic sensations (lower right), internal dialogue (lower left), and internal eidetic and constructive imagery (upper left and upper right, respectively). However, according to Callahan, the important issue here is not the ultimate truth of why this treatment works but rather that it does work. The procedure was developed empirically and is therefore utilized because of its effectiveness alone.

THE FLOOR-TO-CEILING EYE ROLL

The floor-to-ceiling eye roll (er) is a rapid relaxation procedure, reminiscent of the work of Moshe Feldenkrais (1972, 1981) and also similar in some respects to a test of hypnotic susceptibility. This technique entails slowly rolling one's eyes upward from the floor to the ceiling while steadily tapping the gamut spot.

After a patient has been treated on a particular issue by utilizing an appropriate series of major treatments, this technique is employed to further lower the level of discomfort if any still remains. On a 1 to 10 scale, if the patient is down to a 2 or 3 after being treated with a particular sequence, the er can then be used to lower the subjective units of distress to 1. Even if the distress is down to a 1 after the patient has completed the *majors* 9G *majors*, frequently practitioners find it beneficial to introduce the er for good measure.

This procedure can also be used alone or in combination with the nine gamut treatments for rapid relaxation purposes.* When used with the nine gamut treatments, the overall treatment is as follows:

---

* See *Why Do I Eat When I'm Not Hungry* by R. J. Callahan and P. Perry (1991).

$$er \rightarrow 9G \rightarrow er$$

I have frequently applied this method to facilitate hypnotic induction.

NEUROLOGIC DISORGANIZATION AND COLLARBONE BREATHING

The collarbone breathing exercise (CBB) is Callahan's answer to neurologic disorganization, a condition that kinesiologists refer to as polarity switching or simply switching.* In applied kinesiology, switching is assumed to entail left-brain/right-brain disorganization, in addition to other features. Some of the signs that are frequently indicative of switching include reversals of letters and numbers, confusing left and right, and saying the opposite of what one means. Neural disorganization is also evident when an individual is significantly awkward or clumsy. When this condition exists, the client's psychological problem is generally slow to respond or recalcitrant to treatment sequences that should otherwise work to alleviate the problem.

The collarbone breathing exercises are designed to rectify this situation, at least long enough for the correct thought field therapy treatments to work. Some clients are instructed to practice this procedure daily, sometimes several times a day, while other treatment procedures are being employed. In other instances, however, the need for the collarbone breathing exercises is realized within a set of major treatments. This latter phenomenon appears to be at variance with traditional applied kinesiology lore in that certain conditions apparently have switching nested within them such that switching can be activated at various levels of the disturbance. This suggests that switching is more a function of energy disruption rather than a strictly hemispheric event.

This procedure entails simultaneous stimulation of the tri-heater meridian at the gamut spot (tri-heater meridian-3) and the kidney meridian at the collarbone points (kidney-27) while proceeding through an extensive breathing routine, which is described in the following chapter. While this procedure appears to be very odd and some may find it difficult to subscribe to, it is nonetheless highly effective. Oftentimes the value in correcting neurologic disorganization is found simply in that treatment proceeds more quickly and efficiently afterward. In other instances, the collarbone breathing exercise is necessary in and of itself or as an aspect of the overall treatment in order to rectify conditions such as attention deficits and extreme awkwardness and clumsiness. At other times, treatment cannot proceed at all unless the switching is corrected. Frequently, this condition cannot be corrected at all, such as when an energy toxin or a structural imbalance is affecting the energy system. In such instances, correcting the primary cause of the energy disruption will simultaneously rectify the neurologic disorganization. (See Chapter 7 for specific instructions on the collarbone breathing exercises.)

---

* A typical applied kinesiology approach to treating switching involves cranial manipulation, a rather complex procedure employed by some osteopathic and chiropractic physicians. There are also a number of other methods available for correct switching (see Chapter 7).

ENERGY TOXINS

While most people can be assisted in overcoming a wide array of psychological problems by treating the various psychological reversals; utilizing sequences of major treatments; and employing other odd sequences/treatments such as the nine gamut treatments, floor-to-ceiling eye roll, and the collarbone breathing exercises, recalcitrance to therapeutic results is often seen by Callahan as indicating the presence of a kind of toxicity. In this case a substance such as alcohol, caffeine, nicotine, aftershave, perfume, laundry detergent, or even corn or wheat may profoundly disrupt the energy system so that therapeutic results cannot be realized or otherwise the positive effects of treatment will degrade after the substances have been consumed. In the latter instances, it becomes necessary to track the individual's exposure to substances and eliminate those that account for the difficulty. This is accomplished by treating the individual and then recording when the target symptom returns, noting the various substances that the individual was exposed to prior to or concurrent with the return of symptoms. Given this information, a thorough analysis is conducted by employing a specific muscle testing or voice analysis procedure to pinpoint the substance(s) causing the difficulty. Once this or these substances are eliminated, sustained therapeutic results often follow easily and swiftly.

It should be noted that sensitivity to substances is not the same as an allergy. An allergy involves the inappropriate activation of the immune system in response to an allergen. Substance sensitivity or energy toxin, however, refers to the effects of the substance on a person's energy system. It may be that the substance in question also causes an allergic reaction; however, this is not necessarily the case. In the instance of a substance causing a toxic effect on the energy system, the substance causes the energy system to go out of balance in such a way that the needed sequence of treatments cannot rectify the specific psychological problem. In a sense, the toxic substance causes effects similar to PR or neurologic disorganization, albeit at a more pervasive level. The individual must eliminate exposure to the substance for a period of time before the energy balancing treatments can work. Once the condition being treated has been eliminated for a sufficient period of time, the person may be able to resume exposure to the specific substance without a relapse. However, this is often not advisable, as the substance may produce other undesirable effects.

Callahan reports an interesting case in which a female client had a highway phobia that did not improve for any duration with the diagnosed sequences. It was later discovered that she experienced an energy-toxic effect from corn. After corn was eliminated from her diet for a considerable period of time, the phobia resolved when the appropriate sequence was employed. Given a considerable length of time without the phobic response, she resumed eating corn and the driving phobia did not return. However, later she developed a severe public speaking phobia, and corn again had to be eliminated from her diet in order for this phobia to be resolved as well.

While Callahan posits that energy toxicity poses a significant problem in the alleviation of psychological problems, one must be careful not to utilize this concept as a "garbage pail" for instances in which the thought field therapy treatments prove ineffective for a specific patient. Of necessity, most models contain within them an explanation of when a proposed effect does not occur, assuming that the procedures emanating from the model would surely produce results if it were not for the assumedly "identified" culprit. Such mechanisms promote the survival of the model and also deter forfeiting the model prematurely. Surely, every model has its actual limits, and this model is no different. At the risk of being pedantic, no model is the truth; otherwise, it would be preferable to simply refer to it as the truth.

With this caution firmly in mind, it should be noted that other environmental factors can be involved in neurologic disorganization and interference with treatment effects. If the body really does have an energy system that has electromagnetic characteristics, and we submit that it does, it is feasible that other energy sources such as power lines and microwaves can exert a negative influence (Becker, 1990). Additionally, according to Douglas P. Hetrick, D.C., neurologic disorganization "can be caused by many things including poor nutrition, allergic reaction, environmental pollution, stress or trauma" as well as structural problems such as foot subluxations (Valentine and Valentine, 1985). It has also been proposed by Diamond (1980a) that neurologic disorganization as well as other serious conditions can occur as a result of exposure to certain kinds of music, especially certain brands of rock music. Instances of switching have also been observed as a result of extended exposure to computer monitors.

COMPLEX TRAUMA ALGORITHM

Given the application of thought field therapy by a large number of practitioners over the course of several years with varieties of clinical conditions, the quality and rapidity of therapeutic results have generally been highly impressive. The opportunity to also compare thought field therapy with other methods, such as eye movement desensitization and reprocessing (EMDR), neurolinguistic programming (NLP), hypnosis, flooding, and cognitive therapies, has created a basis for empirical evaluation short of controlled experimental studies. In a majority of cases, thought field therapy has been found to be superior in many respects, although the other approaches noted have also proved effective. Given the efficacy of their effects, thought field therapy, eye movement desensitization and reprocessing, neurolinguistic programming's visual/kinesthetic dissociation (V/KD), and traumatic incident reduction (TIR) have been referred to as "power therapies" in the treatment of post-traumatic stress disorder by Charles Figley, Ph.D., chairman of the Psychosocial Stress Department at Florida State University in Tallahassee.

One of the most effective areas in which thought field therapy shines is with regard to the rapid resolution of trauma and various trauma-based conditions such as post-traumatic stress disorder. The essential algorithm or sequence for the treatment of relatively complex trauma is as follows:

$$PR \rightarrow eb, ue, ua, cb \rightarrow 9G \rightarrow Sq$$

where PR = psychological reversal treatment (where needed)
      eb = either eyebrow immediately above bridge of nose
      ue = under an eye on the bony orbit

ua = approximately 4 in. below either armpit
cb = between the clavicle and first rib, on either side of sternum
9G = nine gamut treatments
Sq = repeat sequence of major treatments (i.e., eb, ue, ua, cb)

To describe this treatment procedure in more concrete terms, the therapist begins by having the client attune to the painful memory and rate the level of discomfort or subjective units of distress on a 10-point scale. If psychological reversal is detected via muscle testing, then the client is instructed to either repeatedly tap the little finger side of either hand (i.e., karate chop) or vigorously rub the neurolymphatic reflex "sore spot" on the left side of the chest while saying three times, "I deeply accept myself even though I'm upset." Next, the client is directed to tap approximately five times at each of the following meridian energy treatment points in sequence: either eyebrow point immediately above the bridge of the nose (eb), immediately under an eye on the cheek bone (ue), approximately 6 in. under either armpit (ua), and between the clavicle and first rib on either side next to the sternum (cb). An evaluation of treatment effectiveness may be made at this point by asking the client to once again rate the subjective units of distress 1 to 10. Generally, the distress will be lower from the initial rating by at least two points. (If it has not lowered, all of the preceding treatments, including the psychological reversal treatment, are repeated before proceeding.)

Next, the client is guided through the nine gamut treatments. While simultaneously and repeatedly tapping between the little finger and ring finger on the back of either hand, which is on the tri-heater meridian, the client is guided through the following treatments: close eyes, open eyes, look lower left, look lower right, whirl eyes in a circle left, whirl eyes right, hum a few notes, count to three, hum again. An evaluation can be taken once again at this stage of treatment, and usually the rating is lower yet.

Next, the sequence of major treatments is repeated: eyebrow (eb), under eye (ue), under arm (ua), and under the collarbone (cb). Again, a reevaluation should reveal progress. If the rating reveals some level of distress, the treatments are repeated. One or two go-rounds frequently settle the matter with the memory no longer bothering or causing emotional distress to the client. The individual is still able to recall the event, as this method does not eliminate the memory itself. Rather, it is simply the negative emotionality that is eliminated.

If some level of distress should return, however, this does not present a major concern, since the trauma can be successfully treated again within moments with the client returning to a state of quiescence. Given repeated treatments, the individual comes to realize an enduring positive change. Even after a successful treatment, the therapist alerts the client to the remote possibility that the trauma could return to bother him or her. If this should happen, the client is advised to contact the therapist immediately so that appropriate treatments can be provided. This support is important also since many traumas are complex, with many aspects requiring treatment. (The specifics of the trauma algorithm are delineated in even greater detail in Chapter 7. Also see Gallo, 1994a, 1997a.)

TRAUMA CASES

Here are some of my cases that illustrate the effectiveness of this treatment modality. Certainly there have been instances where the basic trauma algorithm and its extensions for more complex trauma have not achieved sufficient results; however, it appears that this is an exceptionally rare occurrence.

RAPE TRAUMA

Barbara was raped by an 18-year-old boy when she was 13. The trauma she suffered haunted her well into her early 30s, creating extreme devastation in her life. She had an extensive drug and alcohol problem and evidenced a notably depressive lifestyle in most respects. This entailed frequent bouts of deep depression with suicidal thoughts and attempts, insomnia, appetite disturbance, loss of pleasure, feelings of hopelessness and worthlessness, guilty feelings, and periods of excessive energy or hypomania. She was variably diagnosed as having major depression, bipolar disorder, borderline personality disorder, alcohol dependence, and polysubstance dependence. She had received treatment at a number of inpatient and outpatient facilities by a variety of psychiatrists, psychologists, and therapists. At the time of treatment she was also taking a regimen of psychotropic medications, including lithium, Prozac, and trazadone. Even with this and years of counseling, she was not doing very well at all.

After gathering some basic history, the details of the rape were discussed. As she elaborated about the event, it was vividly evident that she was traumatized. She cried deeply about what happened and, in many ways, seemed to be reliving the memory. She exclaimed that she was to blame, that she should have known better, that she should have listened to her mother, that she was terribly rebellious, etc. While it was doubtful that all of her psychological disturbance could be traced simply to the rape, there was no question that this was a significantly painful memory that required intensive intervention.

Initially, she was assisted in altering her mood by being asked to shift her focus. She was asked to describe various objects in the office, such as the end table lamp, knickknacks on the bookshelves, the texture of the material on the chair, sounds coming from outside the office, and so on. In this way she moved her attention away from distressing internal sensory data and toward the external environment.* She was then offered the possible benefits of the aforementioned trauma algorithm. This treatment took less than 10 min, and it completely resolved Barbara's painful memory. All she had to do was briefly attend to the memory and then tap on the specified points in sequence a number of times. Not only did she no longer experience painful

---

* In neurolinguistic programming (NLP), this is referred to as an uptime strategy. Neurolinguistic programming attends to how we organize experiences via our senses. Thus, experience at any point in time is a combination of internal and external sensory factors. In this example, Barbara's experience was primarily organized internally. That is, she was internally reexperiencing the past event visually, auditorily, kinesthetically, and possibly olfactorily as well. I assisted her in shifting her attention to the external environment along the same sensory dimensions and thus interrupted the flashback.

emotionality while reviewing the memory, but her belief about the situation and herself changed in a radically positive direction as well.

Right after the treatment was completed in that incredibly brief time, she was able to tell me with obvious conviction that it was "just something that happened" in her past and that she was "not to blame." To say the least, this was completely and utterly amazing. Astonishment might be a better description. Her conviction was also tested by reminding her of the self-incriminating statements that she made earlier, but her confidence and conviction remained unshaken. The meaning of the event was transformed completely and profoundly without directly attempting cognitive techniques such as reframing.*

Follow-ups were conducted for more than 5 years, and the trauma remained resolved. She was able to recall the event in detail; however, it no longer caused her emotional pain. As therapy progressed, she improved easily in other aspects of her life in that her drug and alcohol problem resolved and her overall mood and self-concept improved. Barbara was well on her way to total recovery. Should one be so bold as to use the term "cure"?

The reader should not get the mistaken idea that Barbara was instantly and completely cured of all her problems as a result of this brief treatment. However, the painful memory was absolutely and completely resolved within a few minutes. That change, in turn, made it easier for her to realize change in other areas of her life as well. It should also be pointed out that as therapy progressed, other thought field therapy procedures as well as other psychotherapeutic methods were employed to help her in other ways. As far as thought field therapy is concerned, however, specific algorithms were utilized to help her overcome addictive urges whenever they emerged. Algorithms to help her transcend depressive moods and anxiety were also provided. To say the least, Barbara was pleased. (These treatment algorithms are covered in detail in Chapter 7.)

One might think that resolving the traumatic memory would then resolve all of the pathology. While this might prove true in some situations, this is obviously not always the case. Perpetual disruption of one's energy system as a result of a trauma tends to infest other aspects of the individual's functioning. This was especially true in Barbara's case, where she had plenty of years to approach life from a self-hatred stance. In time, she developed severe anxiety problems as she consistently numbed her feelings by using alcohol and drugs. Thus, this became an independent issue. Probably the heavy use of sedating chemicals in combination with persistent guilty feelings and other aspects of irresponsible living culminated in clinical depression as well. More than likely, toxic effects were also contributing to Barbara's condition.†

---

* Reframing is a linguistic technique directed at changing the interpretation or meaning that one attributes to an event or situation in an attempt to eliminate the negative emotionality associated with the event and the original meaning prescribed. For example, perhaps depression may be positively reframed as slowing down to reevaluate one's life; jealousy might be reframed as an indication of deeply loving; and stubbornness might be reframed as tenacity.

† There is little doubt that hereditary factors often play a role in depression, alcohol dependence, certain phobias, and many other conditions.

Vehicular Trauma

Thought field therapy treatment was provided to a 52-year-old man who had suffered a severe accident with his tractor trailer, a five-vehicle pile-up in which one person died and several others were seriously injured, including the client. He reported that he was in psychiatric treatment, which included antidepressant and antianxiety medications, for approximately a year because of the trauma. Although he felt the treatment was somewhat beneficial, he continued to experience nightmares of the accident as well as anxiety while driving. Utilizing thought field therapy, he was relieved of all symptoms associated with the trauma within a matter of minutes. Several weeks of follow-up revealed no return of the symptoms. He has been able to consistently drive without any discomfort, and the nightmares also ceased.

War Trauma

A Vietnam vet presented with an alcohol problem and depression that had plagued him since the war. While he received metals of honor for his valor, he also bore emotional and physical evidence of his presence there. The physical condition included shrapnel scars, the aftermath of Agent Orange exposure, a severe gastrointestinal condition, and a host of other problems. As one would guess, he suffered from post-traumatic stress disorder. For him, this entailed frequent reminders of the war visited upon him as nightmares, flashbacks, and otherwise traumatic memories. Essentially, this hero's life was in shambles. He was unable to keep a job, his relationships were suffering, and he remained on many medications, psychiatric and otherwise, in order to cope with life.

During the second therapy session, he related an incident in which he had to kill an enemy soldier. As he described the event, he became pale, began to shake, and looked like he was about to vomit. While he seemed to be reliving the trauma in his mind, he gasped that he could never be forgiven for what he did, not by God, not by himself. He was in the throes of great distress.

Rather than attempting to assure him that he was not to blame, that he did the best he could at the time, that his actions were required by the fact that he was fighting a war for the sake of his country, that it was either him or the other guy, and other such rational comments, which he must have heard a thousand times over, the thought field therapy procedure was offered to him as an alternative. Within minutes he was amazed to find that the distress had greatly diminished. On a 10-point scale the upset had decreased from a 10 to a 5 after the first few seconds of treatment. With repeated tapping, the distress was eliminated altogether within the span of approximately 3 to 5 min. By the close of that session he was unable to feel distressed about that awful memory, that horrible scene. Not only was the emotional distress relieved, but he also instantaneously changed his beliefs about the event as well as himself. His comments revealed that he no longer considered this to be an unforgivable sin. When he was seen 2 weeks later, he reported that he was feeling rather peaceful, actually quite joyful, still unable to feel bothered about the event. A follow-up approximately 2 years later revealed that the level of relief remained without having to repeat the treatment for this trauma. He had obviously benefited from that brief, ludicrous-appearing treatment. Again, it should be noted that thorough treatment generally requires more than simple alleviation of a trauma, although trauma resolution would certainly seem to be an important aspect of treatment if sufficient recovery is to occur.

RESEARCH

Five studies supporting the effectiveness of thought field therapy have been reported for the treatment of phobias and other anxieties (Callahan, 1987; Leonoff, 1995), phobias and self-concept (Wade, 1990), post-traumatic stress disorder symptoms (Carbonell and Figley, 1995), and acrophobia (Carbonell, 1997). While the studies by Callahan (1987) and Leonoff (1995) revealed significant decreases in subjective units of distress ratings, given the fact that these studies involved treating call-in subjects on radio talk shows, they could not include control groups, double-blinds, placebo treatments, follow-up evaluations, or other evaluative measures. The Carbonell and Figley study was a systematic clinical demonstration study conducted at Florida State University, evaluating the effectiveness of thought field therapy a number of other approaches, including visual/kinesthetic dissociation (V/KD),* eye movement desensitization and reprocessing (EMDR),† and traumatic incident reduction (TIR)‡ in the treatment of post-traumatic stress disorder symptoms. This study was more sophisticated and detailed in evaluative measures and also included follow-along and follow-up assessments. The Wade (1990) and Carbonell (1997) studies are the only ones that included a control group, paper–pencil measures, and SUD ratings. The latter also included placebo control, double-blind, and behavioral measures. (These and other energy psychology studies are discussed in greater depth in Chapter 8.)

While the number and quality of thought field therapy studies are limited, there are an increasingly respectable number of anecdotal reports from clinicians trained in thought field therapy. This is not unusual in the fields of clinical psychology and psychotherapy, especially during the early phases of a method's development. However, anecdotal studies are not controlled experiments, and this leaves something to be desired from a traditional experimental viewpoint. Since case studies do not generally entail randomization, control groups, and other methodological necessities, an obvious criticism is that one cannot be certain about the source of the therapeutic

---

* Visual/kinesthetic dissociation is one of a multitude of neurolinguistic programming techniques. Neurolinguistic programming is a method based on linguistics, sensory processing, and cybernetic notions. This approach was developed by computer scientist and gestalt therapist Richard Bandler and linguist John Grinder.

† Eye movement desensitization and reprocessing initially involved the utilization of bilateral eye movements while the patient tuned in the traumatic memory, phobia, etc. Other forms of stimulation, such as sounds and even simply focusing on a single spot, have been found to be effective as well. This method was initially theorized as entailing desensitization; however, currently an information processing model is believed to be more appropriate according to developer Francine Shapiro.

‡ Traumatic incident reduction is a metapsychology procedure developed by Frank Gerbode, M.D. This approach requires the client, referred to as the "viewer," to repeatedly view and report about the traumatic incident until the memory no longer causes distress. While this method appears to entail flooding to a large extent, the methodology is actually much more sophisticated.

effect. Obviously, case studies can be called into question due to plausible factors such as therapist enthusiasm, placebo effect, demand characteristics, suggestion, simple exposure, etc.

SCOPE OF EFFECTIVENESS

Thought field therapy appears to be effective in the treatment of a wide array of psychological conditions. The methodology has been successfully applied in the treatment of specific and complex phobias, generalized anxiety, panic disorders, clinical depression, addictive urges, anger and rage disorders, trauma, grief, eating disorders, and physical pain conditions, to mention a few. Callahan believes that this approach to the treatment is applicable to most, if not all, conditions. However, on the basis of the experience of many practitioners trained in the method, thought field therapy is most profoundly effective with anxiety-based conditions. Psychotic symptoms, such as hallucinations and delusions, do not appear to consistently respond to these treatments. In general, other conditions that respond to psychotherapy also respond to thought field therapy, albeit at a much more accelerated rate. Conditions such as post-traumatic stress disorder, which do not respond efficiently to most psychotherapeutic approaches, generally respond quickly and profoundly to "the tapping therapy."

In an effort to make many aspects of thought field therapy and other effective energy psychotherapy methods more widely available, we now turn to Chapter 7, The Energy Therapist's Manual.

7 The Energy Therapist's Manual

The benevolence of Natural law lies in assuring us that ... miracles are open to us, but it does not tell us how to accomplish them; it is for us to discover the keys, the encodings and decodings, by which they can be brought to pass.

— **Robert Rosen**, *Life Itself* (**1991**)

KNOWING WHERE TO TAP

The first time I heard this story was when I was an adolescent. My father had just returned from a meeting of the Wolves Club, an Italian service organization that owes its name to the myth of Romulus and Remus, the legendary founders of Rome. Among other activities, this organization is noted for supporting disadvantaged youths in their pursuit of higher education. Similar to other organizations, a noted professional in the area would be invited to present a brief talk. The speaker that evening told this rather amusing and poignant story as an introduction to his talk. My brothers, sister, and I listened as our father laughed incessantly along the way to the punch line.

It seems that a factory was experiencing difficulty with its boiler, and a number of experts had attempted in vain to repair it. The manager then heard about a master technician who was known far and wide for his expertise. And so he requested his assistance.

On the day that the technician arrived, the manager was somewhat taken aback, since the technician was dressed in a shirt and tie, not the typical garb that one would don before doing greasy boiler work. Also, the man carried with him only a very small toolbox, which could not have weighed more than a few pounds.

After the technician was escorted to the boiler room, he casually surveyed the monstrosity, looking at the gauges and tilting his head as he listened. He thereupon set his toolbox on a nearby table, opened it, and removed a tape measure and a pencil.

At this point, the technician did a bit of measuring and made three distinct marks with his pencil on the wall of the boiler. He then replaced the pencil and measure in the box, removed a small ball-peen hammer, and proceeded to tap lightly on the boiler at the precise locations he had marked. Immediately everything "fell into place," and the boiler worked perfectly from then on.

A month or so later, the manager received a bill for $1000 from the technician. This appalled the manager greatly because the technician was only at the factory for about 10 minutes. The manager hurriedly scribbled a note, requesting an itemized statement and expressing displeasure for being charged so dearly for, as he said, "simply tapping the boiler with a hammer!"

Several weeks later the manager received a note from the technician, indicating that he "absolutely" agreed that it would be unconscionable for him to charge so much for "simply tapping the boiler with a hammer." As requested, the technician also enclosed an itemized statement as follows:

Tapping boiler with hammer	$5.00
Knowing where to tap	$995.00
Total	$1000.00

INTRODUCTION

This chapter provides the "nuts and bolts" of applying a number of energy therapy or energy psychotherapy procedures, including thought field therapy algorithms, also referred to as therapeutic sequences or therapeutic recipes, for treating a variety of clinical problems. The algorithms *per se* are applicable to an even greater number of clinical conditions than those discussed here. Nonetheless, to introduce the reader to thought field therapy, algorithms are provided for specific phobias, anticipatory and performance anxiety, addictive urges and addiction, generalized anxiety, panic and agoraphobia, trauma and post-traumatic stress disorder, obsession and obsessive-compulsive disorder (OCD), depression, physical pain, anger and rage, guilt feelings, jealousy, frustration, impatience and restlessness, fatigue, embarrassment, shame, and stress reduction. Where the thought field therapy recipes leave off in the present context, other methods and procedures are introduced that have proved of clinical value and that have some research support.

Additionally, an overall treatment methodology is provided. Effective utilization of these algorithms and other energy techniques must frequently be nested within an overall treatment approach. Further, although various detailed diagnostic procedures are available for discerning specific treatment sequences, that aspect of the methodology is not covered in this book.* Because thousands of professionals have been trained by me (and others) in thought field therapy and other energy psychology algorithms and reports of clinically significant results with such an approach continue to emerge, it seems that algorithms represent an effective and efficient means of conducting treatment and introducing the professional to this technology. Furthermore, regular utilization of algorithms, as discussed in Chapter 6, assists the practitioner in developing an intuitive sense of this work, thus precluding the necessity of meridian diagnosis in many instances.

Nonetheless, the reader is provided with instruction in a method of diagnosing psychological reversal, neurologic disorganization or polarity switching, and what is referred to as criteria-related reversals, since identification of these aspects is

---

* Callahan offers training in his thought field therapy diagnostic procedure, including what he refers to as the voice technology (VT™). His basic training provides procedures for discerning specific therapeutic sequences, specifically tailored to the individual. In essence, the sequences discerned are often idiosyncratic to the individual patient.

frequently essential to providing effective treatment, even when the therapist primarily relies on algorithms and intuition to achieve therapeutic results. It should be emphasized, however, that the "diagnostic" methodology presented here is not equivalent to Callahan's thought field therapy diagnostic procedure or my diagnostic methods,* which involve ways of precisely determining effective treatments for treating various psychological problems via direct assessment of the bioenergy aspects of the condition.

Before presenting this methodology and varieties of algorithms and methods, it should be pointed out, especially with regard to thought field therapy, that while much of what is discussed in this chapter is consistent with what has been referred to as "orthodox" or "pure" thought field therapy, many aspects of this presentation deviate from such a path.

As much as possible, the reader is alerted to the differences. Any distinctions or omissions are not intended to misrepresent thought field therapy.

PRELIMINARIES

RAPPORT AND THE THERAPIST–CLIENT RELATIONSHIP

Rapport and a positive relationship between the therapist and client are often considered to be among the primary active ingredients in effective psychotherapy. Certainly, this has been the position of a number of practitioner-theorists and researchers, including Rogers (1942, 1957), Sullivan (1954), Truax (1963), and others. If the therapist is accepting of the client, which is an aspect of rapport, it is assumed that the client will come to accept himself or herself and this will promote positive change.

While rapport can be studied externally, observing the behavioral and verbal interactions between persons in a state of rapport (Condon, 1970), it would be a mistake to assume that the mere mimicking of such behaviors alone (e.g., synchrony of specific verbal characteristics and gestures) constitutes a genuine relationship. The methods of the con artist are well known. Rather, true rapport is consistent with a positive feeling between the people who are in a state of rapport. Nonetheless, the process of mirroring a client's verbal and nonverbal outputs may serve to facilitate the therapist entering the client's model of the world and could then lead the way to authentic rapport.

Although rapport and positive relationships are valuable in and of themselves, it would appear that this has little to do with the effectiveness of the therapeutic procedures covered in this chapter. Whether or not one is in a state of rapport with the client, these treatments appear to work in and of themselves. That is, rapport and an otherwise positive relationship between therapist and client do not appear to be the necessary and sufficient condition for therapeutic effectiveness.

---

* I have developed a series of diagnostic and treatment procedures nested under the rubric of energy diagnostic and treatment methods (EDxTM). This methodology includes a variety of protocols for evaluating bioenergy features with respect to affect, core beliefs, peak performance issues, energy toxins, etc. Not all of the methods covered in this approach are meridian based.

Given that it is healthy and pleasurable for both therapist and client, maintaining rapport is highly desirable. Rapport brings additional benefits to the therapeutic context that are independent of the therapeutic procedures themselves. Further, since rapport appears to be an active ingredient with many therapies, it may also enhance the therapeutic effects of these methods as well. There is also little doubt that clients tend to be more compliant when the therapist relates in such a manner; this is especially important because the procedures are odd and because, in many cases, the client is called upon to practice some of the procedures between sessions.

Pacing

Pacing is related to rapport. Here, the therapist meets the client where he is before moving on to perhaps bigger and better places. The client generally needs to feel understood and accepted by the therapist before he or she is willing to follow therapeutic directives. Of course, an opposite means of gaining compliance is through playing on opposition, although this is not necessarily antithetical to rapport.

All too frequently, some therapists forget about this obvious, commonsense principle after learning a new technique. At such times, the exuberant therapist rushes in to apply the "magic" that is thought to be the "real" therapy. While the technique may be truly powerful and therapeutically beneficial, to attempt to force it on the client violates therapeutic etiquette and may serve to alienate. This is when the therapist encounters resistance, and this is often when the client does not return. And so everyone loses out.

While pacing may not be absolutely essential to the success of the methods described here, it is an example of poor planning not to take it into account. Pacing paves the way for the treatment.

One final important note on pacing: It should be obvious that some clients enter therapy simply to have an understanding professional to talk to, someone who will help them resolve an important issue in their lives. They do not want to tap on their bodies, whirl their eyes in circles, hum tunes, and extend their arms to be pushed on. This is not consistent with their expectations. Also, they will not readily "buy into" the view that it is best to neutralize or otherwise let go of negative emotions. Rather, they believe that the negative feelings are important and that tapping them away is not the way to resolve something. This is where the client is at the moment, and conceivably, this is where he or she will remain. They are not seeking energy means to therapeutic ends. At such times, the therapist and client will be best served by the therapist's choosing to stretch his or her paradigm a bit further by assisting the seeker in other creative ways. Otherwise, perhaps a period of rapport, pacing, and attending to expectations will lead the client to become receptive to such a shift.

Belief in the Treatment

It is commonly held that the therapist's and client's belief in a psychotherapeutic method is essential to its effectiveness. Similar to the issue of rapport, it is suggested that belief in the method may enhance the effectiveness of the procedures. It is well known that the effectiveness of medication is improved as a result of the prescriber's belief in and enthusiasm for the medication. Thus, it would appear to follow that the same factor applies to certain therapeutic procedures. As the therapist's and patient's belief in the method increases, so should the effectiveness of the procedure, regardless of the independent power of the method.

This is the issue of Pygmalion and the placebo effect, which is really the power of belief and influence. This issue, however, is actually independent of the effectiveness of a medication or psychotherapeutic procedure itself. Rather, the claim is being made here that these procedures are effective, independent of placebo. In other words, while placebo may account for some of the therapeutic result, like most placebos we would assume that at best, placebo can account for approximately 30%.* The other 70% then would be attributed to the procedure itself, independent of the therapist's and patient's belief in the procedure. Of course, empirical research is needed to test the accuracy of this claim, but on the basis of the clinical experience of a considerable number of thought field therapy practitioners as well as practitioners of other energy approaches, this hypothesis is offered for evaluation with considerable confidence.

ATTUNEMENT

Tuning or what is also referred to as attunement is essentially a process whereby the therapist directs the patient to access the appropriate thought field or psychological problem for treatment. In most cases, all that is necessary is to ask the individual to "think about" the problem. This does not require visualization, although if the patient is visualizing while thinking about the problem (e.g., snakes, if patient is phobic of snakes; a memory of a trauma, if the patient has post-traumatic stress disorder; etc.), one can be certain that the attunement condition has been fulfilled.

In other cases, the patient may access the negative emotion as it is associated with an auditory component, such as the tone of voice of a person with whom distress is experienced, the exploding sounds that occurred when the person suffered an automobile accident, etc. Of course, any other stimuli may be relevant toward stimulating the targeted emotional response, including tactile, olfactory, and gustatory stimuli.

Many problems do not include a primary visual or auditory component, and therefore, attuning in this manner will not be relevant. For example, depressed or generally anxious patients experience noteworthy feelings, but there may not be an attached or associated visual or auditory representation. In such cases, it is the feeling of emptiness or dread that the patient may attend to in order to attune the thought field. Nonetheless, in most cases, there is a feeling of discomfort experienced either independently or in concert with an image or auditory component.

---

* The accuracy of this percentage has been debated inasmuch as the placebo effect must preclude all factors except for that of the patient's belief. Many of the studies that conclude that approximately 30% can be accounted for by placebo may entail methodological problems that magnify the magnitude of the placebo effect.

Repression of Affect

Some patients are unable to access the negative emotion unless they are in the real-life situation. They may be repressed or dissociated from their feelings when merely thinking about the circumstance. An example would be patients who are fearful of flying but cannot feel any fear when merely thinking about flying. In such instances, they may state that they cannot feel the fear because they know that thinking about flying is not the same thing as actually flying. They may report that they know that they are not in an unsafe situation as they sit comfortably in the office discussing the "fear." Some of these people have learned this process as a way of generally coping with distressing life situations.

This situation need not pose a problem from the standpoint of attunement or therapeutic effectiveness. In many instances, simply asking the client to think about the situation will be enough to ensure adequate attunement of and successful treatment of the problem or perturbed thought field. Often, the presence of the thought field can be assessed by manual muscle testing: testing the strength in the isolated muscle while having the patient think about the "distressing" situation. Once the problem has been adequately treated by whatever means, testing the muscle again while the patient thinks about the "problem" area should result in a different muscular response. When the problem has been resolved, disruption within the body's energy system will no longer be evident, as the indicator muscle will now test "strong" (see the manual muscle testing section later in this chapter).

However, when this approach does not work to alleviate the psychological problem, meaning that the problem field or biofield has not been adequately engaged, sometimes it will be desirable to treat the patient in the context in which the problem presents itself. In such an event, this should be done in a gentle and gradual manner, similar to *in vivo* systematic desensitization, albeit utilizing the appropriate algorithm or other procedure, rather than employing progressive relaxation or related relaxation and desensitization processes.

Alternatively, one might attempt other procedures designed to produce the affect. A number of patients have been assisted in accessing the affect related to the phobia, trauma, etc. by having them think about the problem sequentially and in as much detail as possible. For example, a patient who has difficulty getting in touch with the discomfort associated with needles can be asked to recall a specific event in which he or she received an injection from beginning to end silently and then to report it aloud. One or a few go-rounds of this process will frequently produce sufficient subjective units of distress to be able to be certain of attunement and to assess the effects of one's treatment procedures.

Attunement vs. Exposure

An important distinction worth noting is that between exposure and attunement. The psychotherapy field is replete with exposure therapies, including flooding, implosive therapy, primal scream therapy, emotional reliving, etc. Characteristically and intentionally, these methods result in rather prominent, painful emoting or abreaction, as it is assumed and apparently also proved to be therapeutically effective in many cases. However, while behavioral flooding is reported to be effective in relieving anxiety (Cooper and Clum, 1989; Keane et al., 1989; Pitman et al., 1991), it also produces untoward side effects including panic episodes, exacerbation of depression, and alcoholic relapse (Pitman et al., 1991).

While some level of exposure occurs when the patient is asked to attune a thought field, such as the memory of a trauma or a phobic situation, the purpose of the attunement is not for exposure per se. Rather, in this regard the therapist's goals are twofold: (1) to obtain a measure of the distress associated with the thought field (i.e., subjective units of distress) and (2) to lock in the thought field (i.e., resonance locking or entrainment) so that it can be treated. It is necessary that this aspect of the method be conducted briefly so that the patient does not suffer needless emotional distress or abreaction.

Obviously, if the psychological problem is to be treated, it must be available for treatment, and that is what attunement accomplishes. However, it is not necessary for the patient to become wholly involved in recalling the trauma, accessing the phobia, delving the depths of the depression, and the like. The purpose of attunement is not to promote painful emoting toward the goal of extinguishing the stimulus–response bond. This is not considered to be therapeutic from the standpoint of energy psychology or several other approaches. To the contrary, after the relevant thought field is attuned, it is not necessary for the patient to continue to think about the psychological problem while the treatment process is being conducted, except for brief intermittent reevaluations of subjective units of distress. It is assumed that once the thought field is attuned, it is locked in for a sufficient period of time and therefore can be treated.

EXPLAINING THE METHOD

Given the strangeness of thought field therapy and energy psychotherapy in general, as compared to traditional psychotherapy, in many cases the client may desire an explanation. This is not only an aspect of informed consent, but it also helps to maintain rapport and to promote compliance. It is therefore suggested that the therapist explain the method in as much detail as is appropriate, given the client's age, level of intellectual functioning, scholastic attainment, academic orientation, etc.

The scholastically or scientifically sophisticated may prefer a detailed explanation. Thus, the therapist may wish to offer discussion concerning the theoretical underpinnings and to direct the client to research and anecdotal reports about energy psychology as well as acupuncture. Information presented in earlier chapters should prove of value in this regard. Additionally, the work of orthopedist Robert O. Becker (1976, 1990; Becker and Selden, 1985) should prove beneficial toward documenting the relevance of meridian acupoints and establishing that the body has an electrical system. The work of radiologist Bjorn Nordenstrom (1983) and acupuncture researchers Stux and Pomeranz (1995) should also prove relevant in this regard. Further, the theoretical notions of Rupert Sheldrake (1981), David Bohm (1980), and Arthur Young (1976a,b) can be explored in some depth with the interested client. Callahan's self-published monograph entitled *Thought Field Therapy and Trauma: Treatment and Theory* (Callahan and Callahan, 1996) and *Energy Tapping* (Gallo and Vincenzi, 2000) should also prove valuable when discussing Callahan's theoretical position. There are also several articles that the therapist may like to offer to the client (see Gallo, 1996a,b,c, 1997a).

The therapist should allow the client to ask questions as needed and not bother the client with a barrage of unwanted information. Too much detail could prove boring and not in pace with the client. As much as possible, one should follow the adage to keep it simple.

The less academically oriented may be content with no explanation at all ("That's OK, I trust you, Doc") or simply being told that many consider this method to balance electrical flow in the body, thus eliminating the basic or fundamental cause of negative emotions. Often, we like to offer concrete examples or to show pictures of the acupuncture meridians. There are many books and charts available that are beneficial in this regard.

Young children seldom require detailed explanations. They often experience these procedures as an enjoyable game. The therapist should readily pace the child's brand of understanding creatively. Obviously, the younger the child, the less relevant explanations will be. However, the parents or guardians will require adequate information so that the requirements of informed consent can be fulfilled.

As a general adult explanation when specifically introducing thought field therapy, consider the following, which can be abbreviated or embellished as needed. Other energy psychotherapy methods can be similarly introduced with appropriate modifications.

> I'd like to offer you a therapy that could eliminate the negative emotions that you feel with regard to this trauma (phobia, relationship, etc.). This therapy is really different from any other you've likely heard of or have been treated with. It simply involves having you think about the problem while tapping at specific places on your body, making certain statements, moving your eyes in different directions, humming, counting, and doing various other activities as I guide you through them. The places you will tap are at specific points on your face, under a collarbone, under your arm, and on your hands. Other than if you were to tap too hard, which you really shouldn't do, there is no danger with this therapy. It either helps or does nothing at all.

> This therapy has been around since 1964, in various forms. But it is based on knowledge that has been in existence for more than 5000 years. You've probably heard of acupuncture and acupressure, which involve using tiny needles or pressure on potent points on the body in order to relieve pain and other problems. This therapy is similar in that it is also working with an energy system in the body in order to treat psychological problems and even some physical conditions such as pain. It seems that when you have a psychological problem, there is an imbalance in this energy system, and the tapping procedure helps to restore the balance and eliminate the problem. It does this by stimulating the flow of the energy through what are referred to as meridians or pathways. Of course, this is only a theory at this point. Some scientists have other ideas as to how and why the treatments work. But there is little doubt that the method has helped many people. Do you have any questions about this?

The therapist should feel free to modify these introductory comments in any way seen fit in order to prepare the client for therapy. Clients will often ask questions about how much they should think about the problem or if it matters which hand they tap with or which side they tap on (e.g., under the eye, at the beginning of an eyebrow, etc.). In such instances, simply state that generally it does not appear to matter but recommend that the client tap with the tips of two fingers firmly and with enough pressure to feel it but not enough to cause discomfort.

SCALING 1 TO 10

The procedures covered in this manual are empirical methods that afford the therapist and client immediate feedback regarding the effectiveness of each therapeutic trial. Scaling is one way to obtain such feedback. After the client has been asked to think about the psychological problem, the therapist requests a measure of distress or what is referred to as subjective units of distress. A request such as the following is apropos in this regard: "When you think about the (trauma, phobia, etc.), how much does it bother you *now* on a 10-point scale, with 10 the worst level of distress and 1 representing no distress at all?"

The client will then provide a number such as 8, 9, or 10. It is important to ensure that the client is referring to how he or she is feeling at the present time, not how he or she felt when the event occurred, how he or she tends to feel when he or she is in the phobic situation, or how he or she thinks he or she should feel. With this in mind, the therapist might emphasize the distinction with a statement such as the following: "What I'm asking for is how you feel right *now* as you think about what happened, not how you felt at the time of the rape (accident, robbery, etc.)." Or "As you think about flying in a plane right *now*, where are you on the 10-point scale? I'm not talking about how you think you would feel if you were in a plane but rather how you feel *now* as you think about it."

Thus, a pretest is obtained, after which a therapeutic sequence is introduced. Upon completing the sequence, a post-test measure of the distress is requested: "Where are you *now*?" Or "Again, on a 10-point scale, how do you feel when you think about that situation?" Or "OK, tune in again. Where are you *now*, 1 to 10?"

By evaluating the distress level after each set of treatments, the therapist is readily informed about what is needed next. This informs both the therapist and client if all is on course or if perhaps an alteration is needed. While other measures of treatment effectiveness are useful in their own right, there is really no substitute for subjective units of distress, since they provide moment-to-moment feedback of the client's experience. Even if physiological measures such as heart rate, galvanic skin response (GSR), or electromyography (EMG) were obtained while treatment was being conducted, one would still want to know about the client's subjective experience. Subjective units of distress are an efficient method for obtaining this information.

Although some therapists prefer the 11-point scale (0 to 10) instead of the 1 to 10 scale, I have encountered a number of clients who are not inclined to provide a rating of "0," regardless of the fact that there does not appear to be any remaining distress. Perhaps these individuals do not believe that it is possible to experience an absence of distress or discomfort about the issue treated. In such instances, perhaps a more useful measure is obtainable by using the 10-point scale, as the subjective units of distress rating guide the therapist through the stages of treatment. In this respect, it is my tendency to continue to direct the client through the therapeutic sequences until there are no reported signs of distress. If a client becomes involved in "hair-splitting" (e.g., 0.75, 0.5, etc.), this could unnecessarily complicate the treatment process.

That said, many therapists may still prefer to use the 0 to 10 scale, since 1 does not as easily translate into "none" as 0 does. However, given such scaling, the therapist will be unable to emphatically commend the client by exclaiming, as Dr. Callahan has characteristically tended to do, "ONE-derful!" after a rating of 1 has been obtained.

ALTERNATIVE "SCALING"

There are many instances where standard scaling may be inappropriate or impossible, such as when treating a child or an intellectually challenged individual. In such instances, other methods of obtaining a measure of treatment effects should be considered. Children can be asked to measure out the degree of change by holding their palm-facing hands out in front of them: the closer together, the less distress. Another visual-kinesthetic measure would be to indicate the "height" of the distress: the lower the height, the lower the level of distress. Some therapists have reported the value in measuring out the change in affect as one proceeds along a line from far right (i.e., 10) to far left (i.e., 1), either noting the shift visually or by actually walking the line. A series of five "happy" faces transitioning from very unhappy to great distress is another option that may be useful with children as well as some adults.

While other methods of scaling can be creatively developed, in some instances a secondary measure may not be at all necessary, even though a "numerical" measure of the change is lost in the process. Simply asking the client how he or she feels after a treatment has been provided may prove sufficient. In this respect, statements such as the following are surely informative: "That's better." "I don't feel as fearful now." "That tightness in my stomach has lessened." "It's not gone but it's a lot less now." "It was decreasing, but now it's intensified." "It's gone!"

MANUAL MUSCLE TESTING

Another way of obtaining a measure of the stress level of a perturbed thought field is by conducting a simple applied kinesiology muscle test. The most detailed descriptions of this method are provided by Kendall and Kendall (1949), Kendall et al. (1971), and Walther (1981, 1988). Less complex approaches, more suited to our purposes, are outlined by Diamond (1977, 1980b, 1985), Callahan (1985), Levy and Lehr (1996), and Gallo (2000). Garten (1996) offers a summary of the various muscle qualities observed during manual muscle testing and attempts to explain the muscle test phenomenon. Manual muscle testing outcomes have been shown to be reflective of central nervous system changes (Leisman et al., 1989). Also, significant interexaminer reliability has been demonstrated when a single muscle is isolated for testing but not when muscle groups are tested (Lawson and Calderon, 1997). While there is some research that supports the usefulness of muscle testing for examining psychological issues (Monti et al., 1999), traditionally muscle testing has been used widely by physiatrists, physical therapists, osteopaths, chiropractors, etc. to evaluate muscular strength and weakness (Kendall et al., 1971). When evaluating psychological issues, the test is distinct from assessing the muscle itself. Rather, the application of muscle testing here is equivalent to the way it is used in applied kinesiology — to determine if the muscle tests "on" or "off" in response to a psychological issue or challenge. The muscle response is used as a gauge to evaluate something else.

When conducting manual muscle testing, it is necessary to isolate a muscle, referred to as the *indicator muscle* (IM), such as the triceps or biceps of the arm, a deltoid muscle in the shoulder area, etc. Generally, the latter is preferred, as long as the patient does not have a condition that prohibits such a test (e.g., a damaged rotator cuff or an arthritic condition affecting the shoulder region). First, the test is conducted "in the clear," which means that the subject is not touching or thinking of anything in particular, especially not something stressful, while the muscle is tested. The essential test proceeds as follows:

1. Initially, ascertain that it is safe to press on the client's extended arm if one is using the deltoid muscles. This may be referred to as qualifying the indicator muscle. That is, if the client has a physical problem that would prohibit pressing on the arm, that, of course, should not be done. In such an instance, another muscle or muscle group should be isolated. (The triceps of the upper arm can be isolated by having the client bend his or her elbow with the arm partially flexed. Testing is conducted by exerting some pressure against the back of the wrist, attempting to push the hand in the direction of the shoulder while the client resists the pressure. The opponens pollicis longus can be isolated by having the client make a ring with his or her fingers by touching the tip of the thumb to the little finger. Testing is conducted by attempting to separate the thumb and little finger. Some separation is normal; however, a "strong" muscle is expected to lock.)

2. When testing with the middle deltoid muscle, ask the client to stand erect, look down at the floor at a 45° angle or off to the side and away from the examiner, and extend the left or right arm directly out from the side and parallel to the floor. The elbow should not be bent, and the arm should not be rotated in either direction.

3. Face the client, avert your eyes, do not smile (since this appears to impair the test), and place one hand on the shoulder opposite the arm that is extended so as to steady the client (usually the right shoulder). At the same time, place the fingers of your other hand (usually right hand) on the client's wrist, directly above the hand. Alternatively, you may simply stand off to the client's side with your hand on the wrist and perhaps your other hand resting on the shoulder of the arm being tested. Frequently, the latter is preferred, as this seems to least interfere with testing the indicator muscle.

4. Tell the client that you are going to press on his or her arm, and ask the client to resist your force and attempt to hold the arm in the fixed position.

Alternatively, tell the client each time you test the muscle to "hold." However, the client should not attempt to raise the arm higher than the parallel position or to rotate the arm in either direction so as to further brace it. The palm should be relatively parallel to the floor.

5. Next, test the muscle in the clear by applying pressure slightly above the wrist away from the hand in an effort to push the client's arm down. This pressure should not be too great. A good rule of thumb is to apply approximately 2 to 5 lb of pressure for 2 seconds with two fingers. Some practitioners have developed skill with an even softer touch. The goal is not to attempt to overpower the client's arm but rather to get a feel for the strength or the spring in the arm. When the arm is strong in the clear, there is a "locking" at the shoulder with an associated springing sensation. The reason this is referred to as testing in the clear is because the client is simply being asked to concentrate on resisting the pressure and not to touch any part of his or her body or to simultaneously engage a thought field.*

6. At this point, ask the client to think about something positive and then press on the arm similarly to evaluate the relative strength. The arm should test strong, perhaps even stronger than when the test was conducted in the clear. Draw the client's attention to this by asking if he or she notices the strength in the arm.

7. Now ask the client to think about something stressful and rate the distress 1 to 10. While the client is thinking about this "issue," ask him or her to "hold" or "resist" and again press on the arm. In most cases, a "weakening" of the muscle will be evident. The shoulder may not lock or some other aspect of weakness will be detectable. It is important not to press any harder than when testing "in the clear." In this respect, the test is not only a test of the effects of the disturbing issue (i.e., the perturbed thought field) on the client's body, but it is also a test of your own integrity in conducting the test.

The specifics of muscle testing and its value are delineated in more detail throughout this chapter and in another publication (Gallo, 2000). However, for the moment, it should be apparent that if the muscle weakens while the client is thinking a distressing thought, then once the thought field has been treated effectively and alleviated of associated distress, the muscle will test strong. In this way the muscle test can serve as somewhat of a physiologic measure or biofeedback to supplement the subjective units of distress that the client reports before, during, and after treatment.

The face validity of muscle testing is evident in everyday life. When under stress, most people observe a feeling of weakness, which is consistent with the weakening of one's muscles. Many of us have also been asked or advised others to sit down or hold on to something sturdy prior to being presented with "bad news." It is apparent that muscles weaken when one is under stress. Accessing a stressful thought field

* *In the clear* has a wider meaning in applied kinesiology in that it relates to therapy localization in a variety of ways.

during muscle testing produces the same qualitative effect, albeit not as dramatically in most instances.

Another way to think of muscle testing is not so much in terms of "strong" and "weak" muscles, but rather in terms of biphasic communication, much in the same way that a computer operates. This is also similar to ideomotor signaling, which is frequently employed in hypnosis. In this respect, a signal is established with the patient's unconscious such that a specific finger twitches when communicating "yes" and another finger twitches to communicate "no." In this way, the operator can ask questions in a yes–no format to gain access to a large amount of information.

As displayed in Step 6 of the basic muscle testing procedure, it is often useful and informative after conducting the test in the clear to ask the client initially to entertain a pleasurable thought while conducting the muscle test, after which the test is again conducted while the client attunes a stressful thought. This helps to clearly establish the distinguishing effects on the muscle of a negative thought as compared to a positive thought. Furthermore, some clients are wont to protest that they cannot hold a thought in mind while their arm is being pressed on, and this objection can be easily avoided or otherwise addressed if it should arise when it becomes clear that the positive thought did not result in interfering distraction.

The "Apex Problem" (or Cognitive Dissonance)

When treated with energy psychology, or any rapidly effective psychotherapeutic procedure for that matter, oftentimes a patient will respond with an interesting brand of disbelief such that he or she will not attribute the change in affect to the procedure itself. Some patients will proclaim that they were "distracted" or "confused," and that this accounts for the lessening of distress even though they continue not to feel distress after the "distraction" or "confusion" has ceased. Others will apparently "forget" the level of distress that they reported prior to receiving the treatment (e.g., 8, 9, or 10), offering comments such as, "I don't think it bothered me much at all." Still others will recognize that although the distress has been alleviated, it must be due to some other "more plausible" factor such as thinking about it "differently" or "rationally" (e.g., in reference to a previously distressing trauma: "After all, Doc, that was something that happened long ago. It's over and done with now.").

Borrowing the term from Arthur Koestler (1967), Callahan has referred to this phenomenon as the *apex problem*, suggesting that the individual is not functioning at the apex of his or her intelligence or perceptual ability at the time. Callahan suggests that this phenomenon may be accounted for in the same vein by which Gazzaniga (1967, 1985) accounts for confabulation observed in split-brain research, namely, what he refers to as the *left brain interpreter*. Another parallel is evident with posthypnotic suggestions/amnesia such that the patient offers an explanation for his posthypnotic behavior that does not reference the hypnosis.

The apex problem, which in many instances appears to be a type of cognitive dissonance, does not pose much of a "problem" if the therapist takes sufficient time to prepare the client for the procedure prior to its being administered. Frequently, the apex phenomenon is a function of the therapist feeling awkward or possibly even skeptical about the therapeutic procedure. If the therapist feels comfortable with the method and takes care to explain to the client that it significantly differs from traditional forms of therapy, cognitive dissonance usually can be avoided. Often, an introduction such as the following will prove beneficial in this regard:

> The procedure we are going to do is rather odd in many respects in that it generally produces rapid results. Frequently, within a matter of moments one experiences the distress level significantly or completely relieved. This can be confusing, and some people mistakenly conclude that the distress has been relieved as a result of distraction, confusion, or something unrelated to the treatment procedure itself. I can assure you that that is not the case, and I believe you will also discover the truth of this shortly. However, if you would like, we can discuss this fact in more detail later.

The above preparatory instruction prepares the client for the objections that may be raised and thus implicitly discredits such objections. Surely this is not the only way to prepare the client. The therapist is encouraged to explore other options for addressing this issue creatively.

At this point some may question the relevance of being concerned about this issue. While it may not be of much relevance in many cases, if the client mistakenly receives the impression that the technique was merely a distraction or an attempt to manipulate him or her, repercussions for the client and therapist may result. For example, the client might cancel future sessions, thus discrediting the therapy and the therapist, as well as missing out on the opportunity of benefiting from a highly effective therapy. As much as possible, we should want the client not only to benefit from the therapy but also not to get the wrong idea. Taking the time to prepare the client will prove highly beneficial.

It should be noted that it is not absolutely imperative to offer a detailed explanation about the possibility of cognitive dissonance prior to conducting the treatment. With many clients, this issue can be easily addressed immediately after the treatment procedure has been provided. If the therapist has good rapport with the client, an explanation after the fact is generally well received.

One final note on this issue: Some patients treated with energy psychology methods will recognize that the distress or negative emotion has been relieved and will make a statement, such as "It doesn't bother me right now." In this respect, the patient is absolutely correct; however, the statement also generally implies a disbelief that the relief will persist. This disbelief also likely accounts for the fact that such patients do not respond with amazement or obvious gratitude. Instead, they respond seemingly unimpressed and unemotionally. While the patient's skepticism is understandable and logically valid in that one does not know that an effect will persist until it does so, there is an obvious fact that is often elusive at such times. This becomes apparent after asking the patient, "When have you been able to think about this trauma (phobia, etc.) and not feel discomfort?" Generally, the patient will respond in the negative. For example, "I've never been able to think about this and not feel bothered. It's always bothered me." The fact that the issue invariably bothered the patient prior to receiving the treatment is often overlooked at such times unless the therapist draws the patient's attention to it.

Assuredly, "the proof is in the pudding," and we have to await the persistence of relief over time. However, the fact that the treatment relieves negative emotion at the time is nevertheless highly relevant. For a more extensive discussion of this issue, see Callahan's "Cure and Time" chapter in his 1996 monograph, *Thought Field Therapy and Trauma: Treatment and Theory.*

CHALLENGING RESULTS

After a client has been successfully treated, with the subjective unit of distress (SUD) now at a "1," it is often useful to challenge the results. That is, we wish to test for stability. In this regard, we ask the patient to try to become distressed about the issue, to really think about it. Perhaps we assist the patient in visualizing or "reenacting" to determine if it is possible to experience a return of negative emotion. Alternatively, *in vivo* exposure may be utilized in this effort. If the patient is unable to experience a return of symptoms, probability is high that the patient will not be bothered again.

Client: "It doesn't bother me now" (after treatment has been provided).

Therapist: "Well let's be certain. Really think about it. See if you can get upset if you really think about it."

Client: "OK. Let me see" (long pause while the client thinks back on the incident of having been in a severe automobile accident). "I can see it and it doesn't bother me. I don't feel the fear now. It all seems more distant."

Therapist: "I see. It seems farther away. Is that right?"

Client: "Yes. And it's like it's way over there, away from me" (gesturing in direction across the room).

Therapist: "Is it like you're watching yourself 'over there' rather than being in the scene?"

Client: "Yes. That's it. It's far away and it's like I'm not in the car. I'm seeing myself, me at the time, in the car over there" (points again).

Therapist: "Well, if you don't mind, I'd like you to think about it differently. If you could think about it like it really happened. Like put yourself back in the car and go through the accident again in your mind. Like it's really happening again. Instead of it being 'over there' away from you. Could you do that?"

Client: "I think I understand. See it from inside again. Let me see" (long pause while client thinks back, apparently visualizing the event). "I can see it like it was. I'm in the car. And now I'm slamming on the brakes and crash! It doesn't bother me. I still don't feel any fear."

Therapist: "OK. Good. I just wanted to be sure that we got it all. I wanted to be sure that it doesn't bother you anymore. Can you think of any bit of it that bothers you? I mean is there any part that causes any upset?"

Client: "No. I don't think so. I'm a one."
Therapist: "Good. That should continue to be the case. Most of the time
             that's the way it works. If it bothers you again, we'll just have
             to repeat the treatment until it absolutely doesn't bother you.
             We'll check on this again next time. However, if you were to
             become distressed about this prior to the next scheduled session,
             please feel free to call. We could even do some treatment over
             the phone if needed."

DEBRIEFING

After a patient has been treated in this manner, a detailed debriefing is advisable.
The debriefing should involve a number of areas including cautions concerning the
possibility and implications of reemergence of symptoms, what to do in case of
reemergence, homework assignments, and standard clinical guidelines.

In a high percentage of cases, there will not be a reemergence of symptoms with
regard to the treated issue. For example, if a specific trauma or phobia is successfully
treated in the session, rarely does it bother the patient in the future. When symptoms
of distress do return, however, repeating the treatment procedure one or a couple
more times will generally alleviate the distress altogether. Other conditions such as
depression, panic, generalized anxiety, addictive urges, and physical pain frequently
require repeated treatments over time before sustained improvement is evident.
Additionally, it appears that exposure to noteworthy psychological stress and even
certain substances, such as specific foods and chemicals (in this context referred to
as energy toxins), can undo the treatment effects. It is certainly advisable to inform
the client of these possibilities at the end of the session to prevent the patient from
losing confidence in the treatment and to enlist the support of the client in ascertaining the effects of stress and substances with regard to symptom reemergence.
Toward this end, the therapist might include a statement such as the following in
the debriefing:

> Although you do not feel any distress concerning this matter at this time, and it is
> highly likely that this will not bother you in the future, we never really know that
> something is going to last until it does last. If this were to return to bother you, generally
> one or a couple follow-up treatments will get the results we want. If distress were to
> return, it could mean that we did not get all the aspects of the problem or that additional
> psychological stress affected the results. Also, some problems are more complicated
> than others and require more detailed attention. In some instances we find that certain
> substances* that we are exposed to can undo the treatment until we have had a chance
> to track them down. Here, I am referring to the effects of certain chemicals, allergic
> reactions, and such.

---

* Callahan maintains that certain substances, specific to the patient, can undo or prevent the treatment
from benefiting the client. These are referred to as "energy toxins" and are in some ways similar to
allergens, although an immune response is not necessarily present with the former. Energy toxins may
include the obvious such as alcohol, tobacco, and certain perfumes, as well as the not-so-obvious such
as corn, peas, herbs, etc.

Holons

With complex psychological problems, there are frequently many aspects or facets involved. Borrowing again from Arthur Koestler (1967), Callahan refers to these arrangements of perturbations as "holons." Essentially, a holon is a perturbation or cluster of perturbations that may be "independently" associated with or connected to another cluster of perturbations. A holon is a whole that in turn can be a part of a greater whole. For example, after a patient has been treated for feelings of depression with a specific sequence of perturbations (a holon), another holon may emerge that might entail related feelings of depression, anger, or guilt. This is another sequence of perturbations (a holon), which when subsumed or collapsed may or may not be connected to another holon. A holon is in some ways similar to the description Shapiro (1995) offers for the eye movement desensitization and reprocessing procedure of stimulating or activating a target/node, which then results in processing along various associative channels. These are the proverbial layers of the onion. Callahan defines a holon as follows:

> Holon refers to an architectural feature of TFT [thought field therapy] which refers to the therapy sequence: majors 9 gamut majors. Most problems require but one holon but some complex problems may require 40 or more holons before relief is experienced. Each gamut can define a holon. (Callahan and Callahan, 1996, p. 102)

Energy Toxins

The specifics of tracking toxins are a rather complex matter that will not be elaborated in detail in this book. However, it appears that practically any substance can trigger a return of symptoms if that substance is energy toxic to the individual. An apt phrase is "One man's meat is another man's poison."

While allergens are probably energy toxic to the individual who experiences allergic reactions to them, an energy toxin does not necessarily result in an allergic reaction. The essential feature of an allergen is that the immune system reacts to it as though the body has been invaded by a germ or virus. This is not necessarily the case with an energy toxin. Rather, energy toxins result in a disruption of the energy system such that there is a return of a successfully treated condition or the condition cannot otherwise be successfully treated.

When a patient has been successfully treated and later there is a return of the symptoms, determining the situation and time when the symptoms returned can be useful in preventing future relapse. Frequently, the symptoms return within an hour of the patient's consumption of or exposure to the energy toxin. Some typical examples of such toxins include perfumes, gasoline fumes, detergents, shampoo, makeup, herbs, corn, legumes, coffee, and tobacco. While there are diagnostic procedures available for tracking down the toxin, having the patient keep an "exposure diary" with notations concerning emotional reactions can prove quite informative and beneficial.

Once the relevant energy toxins have been identified, having the patient abstain from usage and avoid exposure will make it possible for the treatments to work and hold. After a period of time, depending on the severity of the patient's condition, exposure to the substances will not promote a relapse.

Even if the relevant energy toxins have not been identified, it has frequently been observed that there are often "windows of opportunity" in which the energy toxin is not predominant. At such times the treatment can bypass or break through the toxic barrier. In this regard, Gary Craig, a Stanford-trained engineer who worked with thought field therapy and Callahan's voice technology for a number of years, coaches his clients to regularly use a complex treatment algorithm, what he refers to as emotional freedom techniques (EFT), which reportedly eliminate the identified problem over time, even when energy toxins have interfered with treatment in the short run (Craig and Fowlie, 1995). It is feasible that treating the psychological problem regularly through many energy psychology approaches also serves to increase the body's tolerance to the energy toxin. It stands to reason that if the toxin is interfering with resolution of the psychological problem, it is also attuned while the psychological problem is being treated. Therefore, treatment may be simultaneously "balancing" the energy system in relationship to the toxin.

While there are reports of a variety of methods to alleviate the negative effects of allergies and energy toxins (Hallbom and Smith, 1988; Nambudripad, 1993; Fleming, 1996b), it has been Callahan's position that energy toxins are essentially irreversible in that the individual lacks a necessary enzyme to combat the toxin. While he recognizes that there are procedures that can alter the muscle test in response to a toxin (i.e., the muscle now responds as "strong" rather than "weak" after the treatment has been provided), at this writing he has maintained the stance that this is merely a means of overriding the muscle test, not truly altering the individual's systemic response to the substance.

ENERGY PSYCHOTHERAPY TREATMENTS

TREATMENT POINTS

As indicated in Chapters 3 and 6, there are 12 primary and 2 collector meridians that are addressed by the various forms of meridian therapy, including acupuncture, acupressure, moxibustion, etc. While there are other acupoints along the meridians that are used in various forms of meridian therapy, including sedation points (which reduce energy flow in the meridians) and tonification points (which increase meridian energy flow), the thought field therapy treatment points are specific acupoints at or near the beginning or end of each of the meridians, regardless of the type of acupoint involved (Figure 7.1). A description of each of these treatment points follows. In some instances, the abbreviations for the treatment points have been altered for ease of remembering.

1. The thumb point (abbreviated T) is the 11th or final acupoint on the lung meridian (LU-11), located at the radial nail point of either thumb (i.e., except for the central vessel and governing vessel, the meridians are bilateral). These points are easily located by holding the palm of either hand up to one's face. The side of the thumbnail farthest from the fingers

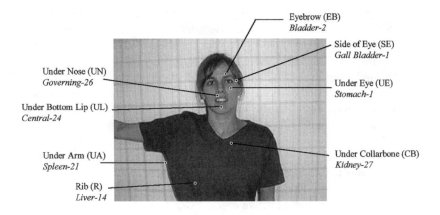

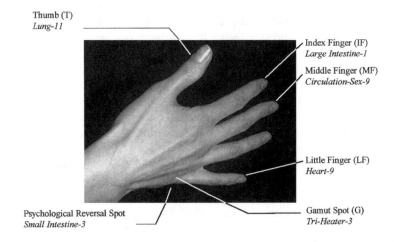

FIGURE 7.1 TFT meridian treatment points.

is the side where this point is located, approximately where the nail meets the end of the thumb. I have often found this treatment point relevant in the treatment of emotional issues such as disdain and intolerance, in addition to obsession and obsessive-compulsive disorder.

2. The index finger point (abbreviated IF) is the first acupoint on the large intestine meridian (LI-1), located at the radial nail point of either index finger. Again, facing the palm of the hand, the side of the index fingernail closest to the thumb is where the point is located, the corner of the nail where it meets the cuticle. This treatment point is often important to relieving guilt feelings and diagnostically often presents when an energy toxin is present.

3. The under the eye point (abbreviated UE or E) is the first acupoint on the stomach meridian (St-1), located on the intraorbital ridge or bony orbit

directly below the center of the pupil when the eyes are focused straight ahead. A slight notch is often detectable at this location. This point is important in the treatment of anxiety, addictive urges, and feelings of deprivation.

4. The under the arm point (abbreviated UA or A) is the 21st or last acupoint on what is referred to as the spleen or pancreas meridian (Sp-21), located on the lateral thorax at the level of the sixth intercostal (between ribs) space on the mid-axillary line, approximately 4 in. under either armpit. Men can easily locate this point by placing a hand on the breast nipple and sliding the hand toward the same level under the armpit. Women can locate this point since it is approximately where the under strap of a bra meets the side under the armpit. This treatment point is relevant when treating anxiety and addictive urges.

5. The little finger point (abbreviated LF) is the last or ninth acupoint on the heart meridian (Ht-9), located at the radial nail point of the fifth or little (pinkie) finger. These points are located by looking at the back of either hand, noting the inside aspect of the little finger nail, where the nail meets the cuticle on the side facing the fourth or ring finger. The LF point is frequently important in the treatment of anger.

6. The little finger side of the hand point (abbreviated SH) is the third acupoint on the small intestine meridian (SI-3), located on the ulnar edge of the hand at the crease from the palm when a fist is made. This acupoint is approximately 1 in. down from the crease where the little finger meets the hand. This point is relevant in the treatment of psychological reversal as well as feelings of sadness.

7. The eyebrow point (abbreviated EB) is the second acupoint on the bladder meridian (Bl-2), located at the beginning of either eyebrow at the bridge of the nose. Included among the conditions treated with this point are restlessness, impatience, frustration, and trauma.

8. The collarbone point (abbreviated CB or C) is the last or 27th acupoint on the kidney meridian (K-27), located at the juncture of the first rib, clavicle, and sternum. This point is easily located by placing one's finger in the notch above the sternum (i.e., supersternal notch), moving the finger down the sternum approximately 1 in. and then perpendicular to either the right or left 1 in., under the collarbone. The collarbone point is important in the treatment of a wide array of clinical conditions.

9. The middle finger point (abbreviated MF) is the last or ninth acupoint on the circulation-sex or pericardium meridian (CX-9 or PC-9), located at the radial nail point of the third or middle finger. This treatment point has often been important in treating jealousy, regret, sexually related problems, and inhalant-type allergies.

10. The gamut spot (abbreviated G) is the third acupoint on the tri-heater or triple warmer meridian (TH-3), located on the dorsal surface of the hand (back of hand) proximal to and on the ulnar side of the fourth metacarpal head. (For simplicity, I refer to this as the back of hand, or BH, point.) This point is easily located by making a fist with either hand and noting

the indentation between the little finger knuckle and ring finger knuckle on the back of the hand. This point is important in the treatment of depression, loneliness, despair, and physical pain and as an aspect of various thought field therapy treatment procedures, including the nine gamut treatments.

11. The side of the eye point (abbreviated SE) is the first acupoint on the gallbladder meridian (GB-1). It is located $\frac{1}{2}$ in. lateral to the lateral eye canthus. This point is located by placing a finger at the temple side of the bony orbit of the eye socket and sliding the finger $\frac{1}{2}$ in. in the direction of the temple. This treatment point is important in the treatment of rage.

12. The rib point (abbreviated R) is the last acupoint on the liver meridian (LV-14), located at the upper edge of the eighth rib inferior to the nipple. This point is located by moving one's hand down from the breast to approximately where the ribcage ends. This treatment point is rarely used in thought field therapy, although it may be relevant in the treatment of general unhappiness.

13. The under the nose point (abbreviated UN or N) is the 27th acupoint on the governing vessel (GV-27), at the juncture of the philtrum and upper lip, directly under the nose. This point is relevant in the correction of deep level psychological reversal and has often proved beneficial in the treatment of nasal congestion and embarrassment.

14. The under bottom lip point (abbreviated BL) is the 24th acupoint on the central or conception vessel (CV-24), at the depression between the lower lip and the chin. This point has often been beneficial in alleviation of feelings of shame.

STIMULATION OF TREATMENT POINTS

The thought field therapy treatment points are stimulated by tapping, or percussion, with the tips of the fingers, a procedure introduced by Goodheart. According to Callahan, tapping on the acupoints transduces kinetic energy into the meridian. It should be observed, however, that in all cases the tapping on these acupoints occurs on or in proximity to bone, and this probably creates a piezoelectric effect (i.e., mechanically generated electricity or electrical polarity in dielectric crystals that have been subjected to mechanical stress). That is, since bone is crystallized calcium, the tapping generates a small amount of electrical current that enters or otherwise stimulates the meridian.

The tips of the index and middle fingers are generally used with the therapist or patient tapping firmly enough to stimulate the respective meridian acupoint. In most cases, it is preferred that the patient performs the tapping on his or her own body. The patient may be instructed as follows:

> I am going to direct you to tap on various points on your body after we have gotten a measure of the distress level associated with this (trauma, phobia, depression, etc.). I will verbally indicate the location while simultaneously tapping on the same points on my own body to assist you in locating them. You'll need to tap firmly enough to feel it but not so hard as to hurt. Five taps at each point will be sufficient.

Frequently, it is beneficial for the therapist to model the tapping for the patient by simultaneously tapping the same points on oneself. Consider the following rationale:

1. It is visually instructive, helping to prevent confusion as to point location.
2. Some patients may find it embarrassing to do the tapping while the therapist is watching. If the therapist taps at the same time, this concern is reduced.
3. Synchronization of tapping, like any synchronization process, is consistent with and possibly helps to promote rapport between the therapist and client.
4. Many therapists have found the process of tapping on meridian points to be a great stress reducer, affording a soothing experience for the therapist as well as the client and also possibly aiding in the prevention of secondary traumatization or compassion fatigue for the therapist.
5. Finally, if it is true that energy from our bodies resonates, which is admittedly highly speculative, perhaps the therapist's tapping serves to affect the client's energy system, adding an extra therapeutic boost to the process.

In most instances, only five taps at a treatment point are needed before moving on to the next point in the sequence. The exceptions to this rule are when doing the nine gamut treatments (9G), floor-to-ceiling eye roll (er), collarbone breathing exercises (CBB), and when treating depression and physical pain conditions. In these instances, the client taps on the treatment point continuously throughout the procedure.

There are a number of other ways of stimulating the energy system. Some therapists have reported beneficial effects of treating patients with chronic pain by stimulating acupoints with a cold laser. This ingenious method makes it possible to treat patients without requiring them to tap on painful areas of their bodies.

Rubbing at the points as well as simply holding the acupoint with some pressure, both processes similar to acupressure, have been found effective at times. However, in most instances, percussion appears to more profoundly stimulate the acupoint and produce more rapid results. Nonetheless, if a client feels uncomfortable with tapping, alternative ways of stimulating the energy system should be considered.

Finally, some clients report the rather intriguing phenomenon that merely thinking about tapping on the treatment points can be effective. However, imaginary tapping is probably most effective after the client has initially had some exposure to tactile tapping.

Major Treatments

Callahan refers to the treatment points as *majors*. This distinguishes them from other treatment procedures such as the nine gamut treatments, floor-to-ceiling eye roll, and treatments to correct psychological reversal. The basic thought field therapy architecture is depicted by the following linear formula:

$$PR \rightarrow Majors \rightarrow 9G \rightarrow Majors \rightarrow er$$

This formula instructs the therapist and client to correct initially for psychological reversal, assuming that psychological reversal is present. Next, the major treatments are provided, generally entailing a sequence of treatment points such as ue, ua, cb. Then the nine gamut treatments are provided, after which the majors (e.g., ue, ua, cb) are repeated. Finally, the patient is taken through the eye roll after the subjective units of distress are within the range of 1 to 3.

NINE GAMUT TREATMENTS

As discussed in Chapter 6, the nine gamut treatments are a procedure that possibly stimulates or engages various aspects of the neurology to enhance the effects of the major treatments. Therefore, after a patient has been directed to tap on a series of major treatment points such as under his eye, arm, and collarbone, the thought field therapy architecture next involves the nine gamut treatments, followed by repetition of the major treatments (e.g., eye, arm, and collarbone).

The specifics of the nine gamut treatments entail having the patient tap continuously on the gamut spot between the little and ring fingers on the back of either hand (the tri-heater meridian at TH-3) while doing the following:

1. Keeping eyes closed
2. Keeping eyes open
3. Moving eyes down in one direction
4. Moving eyes down in opposite direction
5. Rotating eyes 360° in one direction
6. Rotating eyes 360° in opposite direction
7. Humming a few notes or a tune
8. Counting to three
9. Humming a few notes or a tune again

After the nine gamut treatments are completed, frequently the patient reports a lowering of the subjective units of distress. For example, if the distress level is a 10 prior to initiating treatment and lowers to an 8 after the majors are completed, the discomfort generally reduces even further after the nine gamut treatments are provided, perhaps down to a 6 or less. Repetition of the majors generally results in additional reduction in subjective units of distress.

It should be noted that the nine gamut treatments frequently seem to primarily tune in other relevant aspects of the problem or thought field for treatment. In such instances, a lowering of the subjective units of distress will not necessarily be evident. Callahan offers the theory that the nine gamut treatments serve to attune or access the problem and to balance various aspects of brain functioning with respect to the specific problem being treated:

> The theory behind the gamut treatments is that we are balancing various functions of the brain with each treatment in regard to the particular problem we are treating. Each problem needs to be treated separately. It is as if the brain must be tuned to the right frequency for each problem for the treatment to work. (Callahan, 1990, p. 1)

Neurological and neuropsychological research suggests the possible relevance of this procedure in terms of stimulating varied brain functions and areas. For example, humming a tune is consistent with activation of the right or nondominant hemisphere, while counting coincides with activation of the left or dominant hemisphere. It is further assumed that the various eye positions stimulate other areas and functions of the brain; this is similar to Bandler and Grinder's (1979) observation that various lateral eye movements correlate with functions such as kinesthetic sensations (i.e., lower right positioning of the eyes), internal dialogue (i.e., lower left positioning), internal eidetic (upper left), and constructive imagery (upper right). According to Callahan, the important issue here is not the ultimate truth of why this treatment works but rather that it does work. The procedure was developed empirically and is therefore utilized because of its effectiveness alone.

FLOOR-TO-CEILING EYE ROLL

The floor-to-ceiling eye roll is a rapid relaxation procedure, reminiscent of the work of Moshe Feldenkrais (1972, 1981) and similar to a test of hypnotic susceptibility. This technique entails slowly rolling one's eyes upward from the floor to the ceiling while steadily tapping the gamut spot (i.e., between the little finger and ring finger knuckles on the back of either hand, which is the third acupoint on the triple warmer meridian).

After a patient has been treated on a particular issue by utilizing an appropriate sequence of major treatments, this technique is employed to further lower the level of discomfort if any yet remains. On a 1 to 10 scale, if the patient is down to a 2 or 3 after being treated with a particular sequence, the eye roll can then be used to often lower the subjective units of distress to 1. Even if the subjective units of distress are down to 1 after the patient has completed the majors nine gamut majors, thought field therapy practitioners frequently find it beneficial to introduce the eye roll "for good measure."

The instructions for the eye roll are as follows:

> Now using your [dominant hand], continuously tap between your little finger and ring finder knuckles on the back of your other hand, keeping your head still, and slowly and steadily moving your eyes from the floor to the ceiling. Take about five to six seconds to do this.

This procedure can also be used alone or in combination with the nine gamut treatments for rapid relaxation purposes.* When used for stress reduction with the nine gamut treatments, the treatment is as follows:

$$er \rightarrow 9G \rightarrow er$$

I have also found this method helpful in facilitating hypnotic induction. The eye roll can be further enhanced by having the client lower his or her eyelids while the eyes remain raised to the ceiling level, taking a deep breath, stop tapping, and then

* See *Why Do I Eat When I'm Not Hungry* by R. J. Callahan and Perry (1991).

lowering the eyes down to the floor level while exhaling. At this point, the therapist might direct the client's attention to the floating sensation that tends to occur at such times, suggesting that this effect might be deepened.

PSYCHOLOGICAL REVERSALS

As noted in Chapter 6, psychological reversal is a negativistic condition whereby one's "motivation operates in a way that is directly opposed to the way it should work" (Callahan, 1991, p. 41). When psychological reversal is present, an effective treatment will be rendered ineffective. This is assumed to apply not only to energy psychology treatment but also to other psychological and even medical treatments. Further, this condition is relevant in a number of other areas including academic performance, technical skills, and sports. For example, Blaich (1988) reports that correction of psychological reversal accounted for "the greatest single change in reading" compared to other treatments provided in his study.

Specific Psychological Reversal

Psychological reversal (PR) occurs in various forms or degrees. Specific psychological reversal (or simply reversal) is the simplest and most common form and is generally present when no treatment effect is achieved at the onset of treatment. Its presence can be further corroborated by testing an indicator muscle while having the client state, "I want to get over this problem." If the indicator muscle tests "weak" on this statement, reversal is likely present. To check further, the muscle is tested again while the client says, "I want to continue to have this problem." In the latter instance, the presence of reversal is indicated if the muscle tests "strong." Instead of using the generic term *problem*, a more specific statement might be preferred (e.g., trauma, fear of flying, depression, etc.).

It must be emphasized that the test for reversal should not be interpreted too literally. That is, the presence of reversal does not really mean that the client wants to continue to have his or her problem. The purpose of the statement is to test for the presence of reversal only. While some may interpret reversal to mean that the client unconsciously wants to have the problem or is in conflict about achieving the expressed goal, Callahan's position is at variance with these views. Rather, reversal occurs primarily at an energy level and results in blockage to positive change. When reversal is present, it is assumed that the directionality of energy "flow" or "charge" is literally reversed.

If reversal is indicated, the treatment involves having the client stimulate or karate chop at SI-3, the little finger side of the hand, while stating the following three times: "I deeply accept myself even though I have this problem" (e.g., trauma, fear, etc.) (Figure 7.2). After providing the reversal treatment, the therapist should once again check by repeating the muscle test. When the correction has been made, treatment can proceed effectively.

In rare instances, the client will test strong or weak to both positive and negative statements (i.e., strong or weak to both "I want to get over this problem" and to "I want to continue to have this problem"). Assuming the client is not neurologically

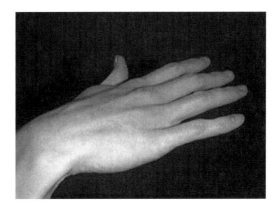

FIGURE 7.2 Psychological reversal treatment at small intestine-3 (SI-3), little finger side of hand.

disorganized at the time and the examiner has been able to calibrate the indicator muscle response to other conditions or statements (e.g., the subject's correct name as compared to wrong name) is also indicative of psychological reversal.

When the indicator is strong to "I want to keep this problem" and weak to "I want to get over this problem," an alternative treatment phrase might be "In spite of this reversal in attitude about my problem, I deeply and profoundly love, accept, and respect myself." When the indicator is strong or weak for both "I want to keep this problem" and "I want to get over this problem," an alternative treatment phrase might be "In spite of this conflict in attitude about my problem, I deeply and profoundly love, accept, and respect myself." These considerations about diagnosing and treating reversals are also applicable to the other forms of reversal discussed below.

Massive Psychological Reversal

While specific reversal relates to a specific issue or context, massive psychological reversal (MPR) is pervasive or across contexts, affecting many areas of a person's life. Its presence is corroborated in a couple ways, other than by the clinical observation that the client's problem tends to be chronic and multifaceted.

One muscle test involves having the client place the palm of his or her hand on the top of the head as compared to the back of the hand on top of the head while testing the indicator muscle. If the indicator muscle is relatively "weak" when the palm is on the head and relatively "strong" when the back of the hand is atop the head, massive reversal is likely present. The normally organized individual, on the other hand, evidences a "strong" indicator muscle with the palm down and a "weak" indicator muscle with the palm up. The reason for this phenomenon, and the reverse in the instance of massive reversal, is assumed to be a function of electromagnetic polarity, such that the back of the hand and the top of the head both have positive charges. Given normal organization, the electromagnetic flow is in the same direction when the palm is positioned above the head, whereas the poles repel when the back of the hand is positioned above the head. In the instance of massive reversal, the poles are reversed, thus accounting for the reversed response.

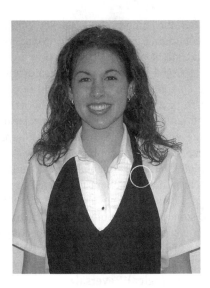

FIGURE 7.3 Neurolymphatic reflex (NLR) on the left side of the chest for treating psychological reversal. In thought field therapy, this reflex is also referred to as the "sore spot," because most people report a sore or tender sensation at the location. The neurolymphatic reflex is stimulated with rotating finger pressure.

Even if the above test suggests the presence of massive reversal, one should test further. After securing a strong indicator muscle, the therapist compares the relative strength of the indicator muscle while the client makes the following opposing statements: "I want to be happy (or have a happy life)." vs. "I want to be miserable (or have a miserable life)." "Weakness" on the former and "strength" on the latter is indicative of massive reversal. Again, if the client tests as having massive reversal, this is not to be interpreted as meaning that the client wants to have a miserable life.

The correction for massive reversal involves having the client continuously karate chop on the little finger side of either hand while saying three times, "I deeply and profoundly accept myself with all my problems and limitations." Alternatively, the client can make this statement three times while briskly rubbing the neurolymphatic reflex, otherwise referred to as the sore spot, in a circular motion on the left side of the chest (Figure 7.3). This reflex is associated with the lymphatic system and is often tender or sore. It is located between the second and third ribs away from the sternum on the left side of the chest.

After the massive reversal correction has been made, repeating the muscle tests will reflect the correction and treatment should be able to proceed effectively. However, it is possible that a specific reversal will become visible once the massive reversal has been corrected. In such an instance, the therapist then fixes the specific reversal before initiating treatment.

Mini Psychological Reversal

Mini psychological reversal (or mini reversal) (mPR) is evident when progress in treatment halts or stalls. That is, if a client reports subjective units of distress of 10, which descends to 5 after the appropriate sequence of meridian acupoints and remains at 5 even with continuing treatment, mini reversal is likely present. Therefore, this type of reversal might also be referred to as *intervening reversal*. This reversal can be further assessed by testing the indicator muscle while having the client say, "I want to be *completely* over this problem (e.g., trauma, phobia, etc.)" vs. "I want to continue to have (or keep) *some* of this problem." If the indicator muscle is "strong" on the latter and "weak" on the former, mini reversal is corroborated. Not to belabor the point, but again this is not interpreted to mean that the client really wants to keep some of the problem.

The treatment for mini reversal again entails the combination of an affirmation with tapping at a meridian point. The client is directed to continually karate chop on the little finger side of a hand while saying three times, "I deeply accept myself even though I still have some of this problem." After providing this treatment, the presence of mini reversal can again be assessed by repeating the muscle test. After mini reversal has been alleviated, progress in treatment will resume.

Deep-Level Reversal Psychological Reversal

Another level of psychological reversal is referred to as deep level psychological reversal (or simply deep level reversal) (PR2). While Callahan does not offer a cognitive or belief-oriented interpretation of this phenomenon, the diagnosis of this level entails testing the indicator muscle while having the client make the statement: "I *will* be over this problem (e.g., trauma, phobia, etc.)" vs. "I *will* continue to have this problem."

The treatment for deep-level reversal involves having the client continually tap directly under his nose (i.e., GV-27) while stating, "I deeply accept myself if I *never* get over this problem." Alternatively, an even stronger statement, such as the following, may prove more effective in some cases: "I deeply accept myself even though I'll *never* get over this problem."

Recurrent Reversal

Recurrent reversal is sometimes evident when treatment is proceeding effectively and suddenly there is resurgence or a spiking of the subjective units of distress. While resurgence can be due to another aspect of the problem coming to the fore, when recurrent reversal is present, the aspect has not changed.

In this instance, the treatment is more effectively conducted by stimulating the neurolymphatic reflex or sore spot on the left side of the chest while having the patient say one of the following: "I deeply accept myself even though this problem keeps coming back" or "I deeply accept myself even though I have this problem."

Criteria-Related Reversals

Several years ago I was treating a gentleman whose condition was not responding positively to the thought field therapy treatments being provided. He had committed a transgression for which he was experiencing severe guilt feelings, even though the event was over with and he appeared to have "learned his lesson." Regardless of the attempts to correct for specific and deep-level reversals, the subjective units of distress remained high and immovable. Perplexed by the state of affairs, the patient was asked what he thought might be going on. His report was quite revealing and heuristic: "I don't think I deserve to get over this."

"Thank you!"

As a result of the patient's report of the feeling under the feeling or the belief under the feeling, it was possible to discern a different type of reversal, one that entailed a criterion distinct from the other levels previously defined. The patient was thereupon asked to tap directly under his bottom lip (on the central vessel*) while stating three times aloud, "I deeply accept myself even though I don't deserve to get over this problem." Immediately, the subjective units of distress level decreased after resuming the algorithm that had not been working up until that point.

At the time, this was referred to as shame level reversal, since it seemed that the driving force was a sense of shame that the patient was reporting. The name has since been changed to deservedness or deserving reversal to more specifically highlight the issue or criterion involved.

Testing for and Correcting Criteria-Related Reversals

Since that initial discovery, a number of other criteria-related reversals have been explored that have proved beneficial to increasing the effectiveness of energy psychology treatment as well as other treatment approaches with a greater number of patients. Recently, the findings of James Durlacher, D.C., who independently made similar discoveries about what he refers to as "degrees" of psychological reversal, have been incorporated into this work (Durlacher, 1994). Durlacher, also an applied kinesiologist, learned Callahan's approach early on and has expanded on it in a variety of interesting ways.

Each of the following levels of reversal listed is defined in terms of a standard and mini version. It should be noted that this is merely a sampling of criteria-related reversals; other criteria can be involved depending on the individual client issues. The treatment statements are combined with manual muscle testing. For each of the types, the therapist should test opposite pairs of each of the test phrases. For example, "I deserve to get over this problem" vs. "I don't deserve to get over this problem." In most instances, combining the relevant treatment statement with tapping at small intestine-3 on the little finger side of either hand will make the correction. Alternatively, one may rub the neurolymphatic reflex, the sore spot, on the left side of the chest while stating the relevant affirmation.†

---

* According to Diamond (1985), the central vessel is associated with the emotional state of shame. With this in mind, I therefore directed the patient to tap at this point on that meridian order to restore balance and thus alleviate the sense of shame. Later, I found that the needed acupoint could be therapy localized.
† While these treatments for criteria-related reversals are generally effective, in many instances an alternative distinct treatment point is required. In such an instance, a diagnostic method is necessary to make this determination.

Deserving

Diagnosis: "I deserve to get over this problem."
Treatment: "I accept myself even if I deserve to have this problem."
Dx Mini: "I deserve to be completely over this problem."
Tx Mini: "I accept myself even if I deserve to have some of this problem."

Safety

Diagnosis: "It's safe for me to be over this problem."
Treatment: "I accept myself even if it isn't safe for me to be over this problem."
Dx Mini: "It's safe for me to be completely over this problem."
Tx Mini: "I accept myself even if it's unsafe for me to be completely over this problem."

Safety (Others)

Diagnosis: "It's safe for others (specify) for me to be over this problem."
Treatment: "I accept myself even if it isn't safe for others (specify) for me to be over this problem."
Dx Mini: "It's safe for others (specify) for me to be completely over this problem."
Tx Mini: "I accept myself even if it's unsafe for others (specify) for me to be completely over this problem."

Possibility

Diagnosis: "It's possible for me to be over this problem."
Treatment: "I accept myself even if it's impossible for me to get over this problem."
Dx Mini: "It's possible for me to get completely over this problem."
Tx Mini: "I accept myself even if it's impossible to get completely over this problem."

Permission

Diagnosis: "I will allow myself to get over this problem."
Treatment: "I accept myself even if I won't allow myself to get over this problem."
Dx Mini: "I will allow myself to get completely over this problem.
Tx Mini: "I accept myself even if I won't allow myself to get completely over this problem.

Motivation

Diagnosis: "I will do what's necessary to get over this problem."
Treatment: "I accept myself even if I will not do what's necessary to get over this problem."

Dx Mini: "I will do what's necessary to get completely over this problem."

Tx Mini: "I accept myself even if I will not do what's necessary to get completely over this problem."

Benefit

Diagnosis: "Getting over this problem will be good for me."

Treatment: "I accept myself even if getting over this problem is not good for me."

Dx Mini: "Getting completely over this problem will be good for me."

Tx Mini: "I accept myself even if completely getting over this problem is not good for me."

Benefit (Others)

Diagnosis: "My getting over this problem will be good for others (specify)."

Treatment: "I accept myself even if my getting over this problem is not good for others (specify)."

Dx Mini: "My getting completely over this problem will be good for others (specify)."

Tx Mini: "I accept myself even if my getting completely over this problem is not good for others (specify)."

Deprivation*

Diagnosis: "I will be (feel) deprived if I get over this problem."

Treatment: "I deeply accept myself even if getting over this problem is (feels) depriving to me."

Dx Mini: "I will be (feel) deprived if I get completely over this problem."

Tx Mini: "I deeply accept myself even if I am (feel) deprived if I get completely over this problem."

Identity†

Diagnosis: "I will lose my identity if I get over this problem."

Treatment: "I accept myself even if I lose my identity getting over this problem."

Dx Mini: "I will lose my identity if I get completely over this problem."

Tx Mini: "I accept myself even if I lose my identity if I get completely over this problem."

---

* Although this reversal is not mentioned in Dr. Durlacher's book (1995), *Freedom from Fear Forever*, he mentioned it to me in a conversation in 1997. When using muscle testing to diagnose this reversal, a strong muscle response indicates the presence of the reversal. This is distinct from the other reversals mentioned in this section.

† Similar to the deprivation reversal, a strong muscle response indicates the presence of psychological reversal associated with identity. I discovered identity reversal in my clinical work with clients.

NEUROLOGIC DISORGANIZATION AND
COLLARBONE BREATHING

The collarbone breathing exercise (CBB) is Callahan's answer to neurologic disorganization, a condition that applied kinesiologists refer to as polarity switching or simply switching.* In applied kinesiology, switching is assumed to entail left-brain/right-brain disorganization, among other features. Some of the signs that are frequently indicative of switching include reversals of letters and numbers, confusing left and right, saying the opposite of what one means, etc. Neurologic disorganization is also evident when an individual is significantly awkward or clumsy. When this condition exists, the client's psychological problem is generally slow to respond or recalcitrant to treatment sequences that should otherwise work to alleviate the problem.

The collarbone breathing exercises are designed to rectify this situation, at least long enough for the correct thought field therapy or other energy treatments to work.† Some clients are instructed to practice this procedure daily, sometimes several times a day, while other treatment procedures are being employed. In other instances, however, the need for collarbone breathing exercises is realized within a set of thought field therapy major treatments. This latter phenomenon appears to be at variance with traditional applied kinesiology lore in that certain conditions apparently have switching nested within them such that switching can be activated at various levels of the disturbance. This suggests that switching is more a function of energy disruption rather than a strictly neurologic event.

For example, a treatment sequence might proceed as follows:

$$CBB \rightarrow ue, ua, cb \rightarrow 9G \rightarrow CBB \rightarrow ue, ua, cb$$

The above notation indicates that switching was initially detected and then treated with the collarbone breathing exercises, after which the sequence ue, ua, cb and the nine gamut treatments were provided. At this point, switching was again detected and was again alleviated with the collarbone breathing exercises, after which the sequence of majors and the eye roll were provided.

This procedure entails simultaneous stimulation of the triple heater meridian at the gamut spot (tri-heater-3) and the kidney meridian at the collarbone points (kidney-27) while proceeding through an extensive breathing routine, which is described in detail below. While this procedure appears very odd and some may find it difficult to subscribe to, it is nonetheless highly effective. Oftentimes the value in correcting neurologic disorganization is found simply in that treatment proceeds more quickly

---

* A typical applied kinesiology approach to treating switching involves cranial-sacral work, a rather complex procedure employed by some osteopathic and chiropractic physicians, which addresses cranial faults. There are a number of other methods available for correct switching, with the collarbone breathing exercises among the most effective.

† The collarbone breathing exercises or other approaches for correcting polarity switching can be effectively used with other energy procedures, including emotional freedom techniques (EFT), negative affect erasing method (NAEM), energy diagnostic and treatment methods (ED×TM), etc. See the last section of this chapter for other approaches.

and efficiently afterward. In other instances, the collarbone breathing exercises are necessary in and of themselves to rectify conditions such as extreme awkwardness and clumsiness. At other times, treatment cannot proceed at all unless the switching is corrected. Frequently, this condition cannot be corrected at all, such as when an energy toxin or a structural imbalance is affecting the energy system. In such instances, correcting the primary cause of the energy disruption will simultaneously rectify the neurologic disorganization.

COLLARBONE BREATHING EXERCISES

The collarbone breathing exercises (CBB) are conducted by initially having the subject place the tips of the left index and middle fingers under the left collarbone next to the sternum while steadily tapping on the gamut spot of the left hand with the index and middle fingertips of the right hand. During the tapping procedure the subject engages in five distinct breathing positions, making sure to tap at least seven times during each of the following breathing positions:

1. Normal breathing in and out
2. Deeply filling the lungs with air
3. Exhaling half of the air out of the lungs
4. Exhaling nearly all the air out of the lungs
5. Half filling the lungs with air

After completing this phase of the treatment, the same tapping and breathing procedure is repeated while having the client place the tips of the left index and middle fingers under the right collarbone. Next, the procedure is continued with the tips of the right index and middle fingers under the left collarbone and then under the right collarbone.

While the procedure must certainly seem strange to this point, the next phase of the exercise is stranger yet. After the fingertips of each hand have stimulated each of the kidney-27 or collarbone points, the same process is conducted with the index and middle finger knuckles of each hand.

It is the position of applied kinesiology that the palm-side and backside of the hand have different electromagnetic polarities. Thus, the purpose of utilizing both the fingertips and the knuckles of each hand is to stimulate the collarbone points with every possible combination of polarities and to normalize polarities front to back and side to side. This is addressed in greater detail later.

To summarize, the fingertips and knuckles of each hand are sequentially placed under each collarbone point while the gamut spot is stimulated and the client goes through the five breathing positions (Figure 7.4). The fingertip and knuckle positions are listed on pages 141–142.

1. Left fingertips under left collarbone
2. Left fingertips under right collarbone
3. Right fingertips under left collarbone
4. Right fingertips under right collarbone

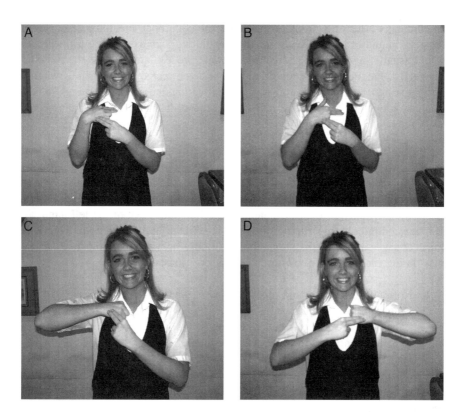

FIGURE 7.4 Four of the eight positions used for collarbone breathing exercises: tapping with the right hand on the left hand gamut spot with fingertips on the collarbone points (A, B) and knuckles on the collarbone points (C, D).

5. Left knuckles under left collarbone
6. Left knuckles under right collarbone
7. Right knuckles under left collarbone
8. Right knuckles under right collarbone

In all, the collarbone breathing exercises entail 40 separate treatments. That is, it involves 8 collarbone stimulation positions times 5 breathing positions for a total of 40 treatments. While it is perhaps easy enough to do all of the treatments as outlined, it should be noted that individual cases vary such that not all of the treatments are needed. A muscle testing diagnostic procedure makes it possible to discern which aspects of the collarbone breathing exercises are in need of treatment.

DIAGNOSING NEUROLOGIC DISORGANIZATION/POLARITY SWITCHING

The need for collarbone breathing exercises is evident from a number of signs. As noted, if treatment proceeds too slowly, such that the subjective units of distress lowers one point or less after each sequence, the need for collarbone breathing exercises is possibly indicated. Correcting switching with the collarbone breathing exercises will generally result in faster results as long as there is not something else blocking the treatment from working (e.g., see the section on energy toxins). The need for collarbone breathing exercises can be diagnosed by any of a number of interrelated methods.

Hand-over-Head Method

One way of diagnosing the presence of neurologic disorganization is by having the client place the palm of his or her right hand on his or her head while testing the strength in the extended left arm (middle deltoid muscle) or any other indicator muscle. The muscle should test strong. Now, having the client turn the right hand over so that the back of the hand is against the top of the head and the palm is pointing upward toward the ceiling should cause the indicator muscle to test weak. If the palm down is strong and the palm up is weak, the client is neurologically organized at the time. A useful mnemonic device offered by James Durlacher, D.C. (1994) is "palm is power, back is slack." If the indicator muscle is equally strong under both conditions, switching is probably present, and the collarbone breathing exercises can be employed to correct for this. After the collarbone breathing exercises are completed, the client should test normally organized if the correction has been successful.

The body appears to be variably polarized head to tail and front to back. If one is normally organized, the back of the hand is positively charged and the palm is negatively charged, while the head is positively charged and the charge becomes increasingly negative as it descends toward the feet. Thus, the electromagnetic flow is uninterrupted with the individual who is neurologically organized when the palm is placed atop the head with a "strong" muscle response evident.

If the polarity on the hand is reversed, but this is not the case at the apex of the head (or vice versa), a competing electromagnetic situation will exist, similar to when like magnetic poles are placed in contact with each other. This situation interferes with the normal electromagnetic flow, and thus we observe opposite effects. In order for the muscle to remain strong under both conditions, either or both the hand and head polarities must be neutralized.*

Index Finger Method

A second diagnostic test following the same basic principles as that of the previous method involves either the patient or tester placing the palm side of an index finger at the bridge of the patient's nose while the examiner tests the indicator muscle. The indicator muscle should be strong. Placing the ulnar (nail side) of the index finger on the bridge of the patient's nose should result in the indicator muscle testing weak. If the arm is strong under both conditions, switching is possibly present. Providing the collarbone breathing exercises should result in a change in the test and thus alleviation of the switched condition.

---

* If the palm-down position results in a weak indicator muscle response and the palm-down position results in a strong indicator muscle response, this may be consistent with massive psychological reversal.

K-27 Therapy Localization Method

A third test, based on opposite principles, involves either the therapist or patient therapy localizing to the kidney-27 (K-27), a method described by Walther (1988). This is done by placing the tips of the index and middle fingers underneath a collarbone point (the K-27 point under the clavicle next to the sternum) while testing the arm. If the arm is strong, switching is not present. If the arm is weak, switching is present, and a switching correction procedure, such as the collarbone breathing exercises, is needed. Note that one can test for switching at either collarbone point. If either collarbone point causes the indicator muscle to test weak, the subject is polarity switched. After providing the collarbone breathing exercises, repeating this test will reveal the muscle testing as strong when therapy localizing the collarbone points, and thus the neurologic disorganization will be at least temporarily alleviated.

True–False Method

Another indication of neurologic disorganization is evident when the client makes a true statement vs. a false statement, such as stating his or her correct name and then his or her incorrect name, while conducting a muscle test. The muscle should test strong on the true statement and relatively weak on the false statement. If the muscle is equally strong under both conditions, the possibility of switching exists. This is essentially equivalent to the first two methods in that there is no distinction in muscle strength. (This phenomenon is not specifically mentioned by Callahan as an indication of neurologic disorganization.) This test should then be verified further by conducting one or several of the aforementioned tests.

Other Corrections for Neurologic Disorganization/Polarity Switching

There are several simpler methods for correcting neural disorganization. The therapist may prefer to attempt a correction in one of these ways prior to advancing to the collarbone breathing exercises for especially recalcitrant cases. The advantage of these procedures, when they work for a client, is that clients tend to be more compliant with them.

Nasal Tap
Have the patient rapidly tap on both sides of the bridge of the nose for approximately 1 min and then reevaluate for neural disorganization. This will often alleviate the disorganization long enough for the other treatments to be effective. While it is not known why this technique works when it does, it has been proposed that the disorganization is the result of a cranial fault and that "the tapping affects the cranial primary respiratory mechanism" (Walther, 1988, p. 149).

Basic Unswitching Procedure
Switching/neural disorganization appears to involve body polarities. Think of this as a DC current that travels from a positive to negative pole. In this respect, there are three areas in which polarity can be switched: left-to-right polarity, front-to-back polarity, and top-to-bottom polarity. The collarbone breathing exercises specifically

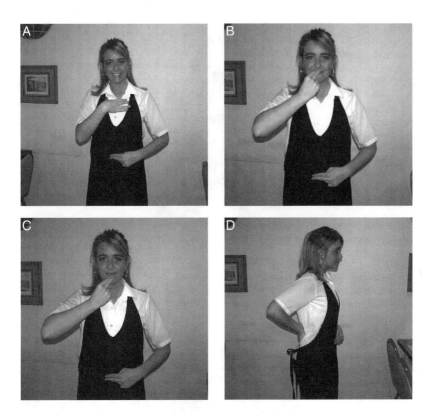

FIGURE 7.5 Basic unswitching procedure.

address left-to-right and front-to-back polarities, although it is conceivable that by rectifying these dimensions, the presence of top-to-bottom switching will also realign if present. However, the following procedure specifically addresses all three:

1. Have the patient stimulate the umbilicus by pressing on it with the first three fingers of either hand while briskly tapping or rubbing under both collarbones next to the sternum for about 10 seconds (Figure 7.5A).
2. Next, have the patient stimulate the navel while tapping under the nose for about 10 seconds (Figure 7.5B).
3. Next, have the patient stimulate the umbilicus while tapping under the bottom lip for about 10 seconds (Figure 7.5C).
4. Finally, have the patient stimulate the umbilicus while rubbing the coccyx for about 10 seconds (Figure 7.5D).
5. Reevaluate for switching.

Overenergy Correction

Neurologic disorganization can result from overenergy in the meridians. When the central vessel is overenergized, the individual may report feeling "confused," "spaced out," or unable to concentrate. The presence of overenergy can often be diagnosed

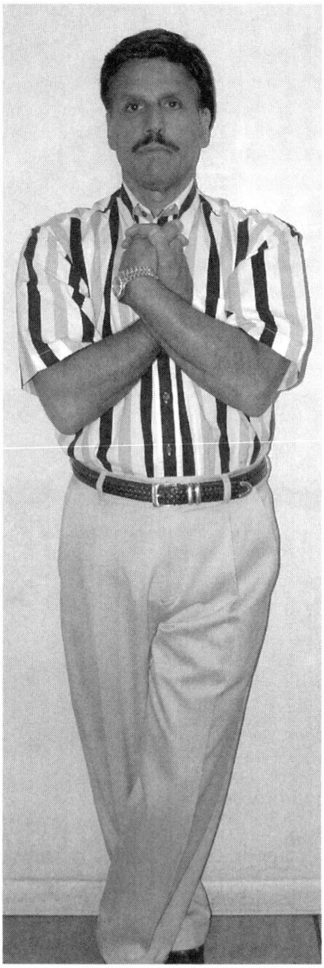

FIGURE 7.6 Overenergy correction position.

by finding a strong indicator muscle, tracing the meridian upward three times, and then rechecking the indicator muscle, which should test strong. Opposite results indicate overenergy. Next, tracing the meridian downward three times should result in the indicator muscle testing weak. Opposite results indicate overenergy.

One method of correcting overenergy and thus associated neural disorganization is as follows (Figure 7.6):

1. Place left ankle over right ankle.
2. Place hands out in front, arms extended, with backs of hands touching.
3. Bring right hand over left and on top of left.
4. Clasp/enfold fingers and fold hands and arms in and rest on chest.
5. Breathe deeply while resting tongue against palate behind top front teeth.
6. Reevaluate for switching after 1 to 2 min.

ESSENTIAL THERAPEUTIC METHOD*

The process of applying thought field therapy algorithms, as well as several of the other energy psychotherapy methods described in the following section, warrants a methodology in which the procedures can be nested. While there are instances in which simply guiding a client through an algorithm "in a vacuum" will prove effective, in reality therapy seldom takes place in such a vacuum. While the experienced practitioner will develop various effective protocols, the following method will afford the beginning practitioner the opportunity to effectively apply thought field therapy and related procedures and to develop a deeper sense of this approach to treatment.

After developing rapport, obtaining relevant history, and introducing the method as a possible treatment choice for the client's particular problem, one should obtain permission to provide the treatment and to conduct the basic muscle testing procedure to demonstrate the interaction of psyche and soma.† The muscle testing procedure is not absolutely necessary under all occasions, although it does often significantly facilitate the treatment process:

1. Initially determine the safety of pressing on the client's extended arm if one is using the deltoid muscles. This is referred to as qualifying the indicator muscle or the indicator muscle. That is, if the client has a physical problem that would prohibit pressing on the arm, such as an injured rotator cuff, that of course should not be done. In such instances, another muscle or muscle group should be isolated. (The triceps of the upper arm can be isolated by having the client bend the elbow with the arm partially flexed. Testing is conducted by exerting some pressure against the back of the wrist, attempting to push the hand in the direction of the shoulder while the client resists the pressure. The opponens pollicis longus can be isolated by having the client make a ring with the fingers by touching the tip of the thumb to the little finger. Testing is conducted by attempting to separate the thumb and little finger. Some separation is normal; however, a "strong" muscle is expected to lock.)
2. When testing with the middle deltoid muscle, have the client stand erect, looking down at the floor at a 45° angle (or to the side away from you), and extend the left or right arm directly out from the side and parallel to the floor. The elbow should not be bent, and the arm should not be rotated in either direction.
3. Face the client, avert your eyes, do not smile (because this appears to interfere with the test), and place one hand on the shoulder opposite the arm that is extended to steady the client. At the same time, place the fingers of your other hand on the client's wrist directly above the hand. Alterna-

---

* This therapeutic method is not equivalent to Callahan's thought field therapy diagnostic procedure. Rather, it is a procedural algorithm that I have found to be effective.

† This aspect of the methodology may not be applicable in some settings because some clients are averse to any level of physical contact. Additionally, there may be restrictions placed on some therapists in some jurisdictions.

tively, you may simply stand off to the client's side with your hand on the wrist and perhaps your other hand resting on the shoulder of the arm being tested. (This test may also be conducted while the client is sitting.)

4. Tell the client that you are going to press on the arm and ask the client to resist your force and attempt to hold the arm in the fixed position. However, the client should not attempt to raise the arm higher than the parallel position or twist the arm in order to rigidly brace it.

5. Test the indicator muscle *in the clear* by applying pressure slightly above the wrist away from the hand in an effort to push the client's arm down. This pressure should not be too great — moderate pressure at most. A good rule of thumb is to quickly apply approximately 2 lb of pressure for 2 seconds with two fingers. The goal is not to attempt to overpower the client's arm but rather to obtain a feel for the strength or the spring in the arm. When the arm is strong *in the clear,* there is a "locking" at the shoulder with an associated springing sensation. The reason this is referred to as testing *in the clear* is because the client is simply being asked to concentrate on resisting the pressure and not to touch any part of his or her body with the free hand or to simultaneously engage a thought field.*

6. Direct the client to think about something positive and then press on the arm in the same manner to evaluate the relative strength. The arm should test strong, perhaps even stronger than when the test was conducted *in the clear.*

7. Ask the client to think about something somewhat stressful. While the client is thinking about this "issue," ask the client to "hold" and again press on the arm. In most cases a "weakening" of the muscle will be evident. The shoulder may not lock, or some other aspect of weakness will be detectable. It is important to not press any harder than you did when testing *in the clear.* In this respect, the test is not only a test of the effects of the disturbing issue (i.e., the perturbed thought field) on the client's body; it is also a test of your own precision or integrity in conducting the test.

8. Alternatively, ask the client to say his or her right name and wrong name, correct age and incorrect age, etc., each time noting the distinction in muscle strength. On each occasion the muscle should test "strong" when the person makes a true statement and "weak" in response to a false statement. If there is no distinction in that the muscle tests equally "strong" under both conditions, the client is likely neurologically disorganized (ND).

9. To test further for neurologic disorganization, take the client through the hand-over-head test. When the palm is over the head, the indicator muscle should test "strong," whereas the indicator muscle should test weak when the back of the hand is positioned on top of the head. If both positions are equally strong, neurologic disorganization is probably present. If the

---

* *In the clear* has a wider implication for applied kinesiology in that it relates to therapy localization in a variety of ways.

reverse condition exists (i.e., the muscle is strong with the back of the hand and weak with the palm), this suggests massive reversal.

10. If neurologic disorganization is suggested, test further by therapy localizing to the kidney-27 points and testing the indicator muscle. That is, have the client place the tips of the index and middle fingers of the right hand under the right collarbone point while testing the indicator muscle and then under the left collarbone point while testing the indicator muscle. If the indicator muscle tests weak in either instance, neurologic disorganization is present. Correct by using the collarbone breathing exercises. (See collarbone breathing exercises section earlier in chapter.)

11. Note that sometimes the client's indicator muscle is strong under all conditions for other reasons. Among the possibilities are that the therapist is psychologically reversed for being able to test the client, both the client and the therapist may be psychologically reversed, or the patient simply cannot be tested.

12. If massive reversal is suggested, test further by evaluating muscle strength while the client says, "I want to be happy" vs. "I want to be miserable." If the latter tests relatively stronger, have the client correct for massive reversal by either stimulating the neurolymphatic reflex (NLR) on the left side of the chest (i.e., the tender spot at the intercostal space between the second and third ribs proximal to the sternum) or karate chopping the little finger side of either hand (small intestine-3) while saying three times, "I deeply and profoundly accept myself with all my problems and limitations." Then test again to be certain that the massive reversal has been corrected before proceeding.

13. Have the client attune the relevant issue to be treated (e.g., phobia, trauma, depression, addictive urge, etc.) and test the indicator muscle, which should be relatively weak compared to the test *in the clear.* Remember the relative weakness in the problem state because once the condition has been resolved, the muscle should no longer test weak. Also, have the client give a subjective units of distress rating of 1 to 10, with 1 representing an absence of distress and 10 indicating maximum distress.*

14. Test for specific reversal by evaluating the indicator muscle after the client says, "I want to get over this problem (e.g., phobia, trauma, etc.)" vs. "I want to continue to have this problem (e.g., phobia, trauma, etc.)." If the muscle is strong on the latter, specific reversal is present and must be corrected. If the muscle is strong on the former, specific reversal is not present. If there is no distinction, test again for neurologic disorganization and correct before proceeding. Alternatively, when the client tests "strong" under both conditions, both the therapist and the client may be psychologically reversed, in which case both should be treated for reversal.

---

* It is important to note that not all problems result in a weakening of the indicator muscle. If a positive emotion is associated with the problem (e.g., excitement, pleasure, etc.), it is likely that the indicator muscle will test "strong" instead. When this is the case, a different approach to therapy localization is needed. See *Energy Diagnostic and Treatment Methods* (Gallo, 2000) for further details.

15. If specific reversal is present, have the client stimulate the neurolymphatic reflex (i.e., "sore spot") or tap the little finger side of the hand while saying three times, "I deeply accept myself even though I have this problem (phobia, trauma, etc.)." Then test again to be certain that the reversal has been corrected before proceeding.

16. Assuming that all is well at this point, proceed with the following basic formula when using a thought field therapy algorithm:

$$SUD \rightarrow Majors \rightarrow SUD \rightarrow 9G \rightarrow SUD \rightarrow Majors \rightarrow SUD \rightarrow er$$

Translated, this means that subjective units of distress 1 to 10 are initially determined. Next, the sequence of majors is provided (e.g., ue, ua, cb) and the distress is again evaluated. There should be a lowering of the distress level. (If there is no change in the distress, a reversal is present, the sequence of majors is ineffective, or perhaps the target is too broad. These matters must be addressed before proceeding.) Then, the nine gamut treatments are conducted, after which the distress is again evaluated. (After the nine gamut treatments, the distress is usually lower, albeit not necessarily lower, because the nine gamut treatments often merely tune in relevant aspects of the material or thought field being treated.) Next, provide the majors again and reevaluate the distress. If the subjective units of distress are within the 1 to 3 range, the client is taken through the "er" one to three times. If the subjective distress is not within this range, repeat the nine gamut treatments and majors to lower the distress within this range. Treatment is complete when the subjective distress remains stable at 1.

17. If at any point treatment stalls, meaning that the distress does not lower after a sequence of majors or the eye roll, a mini reversal is likely present. Evaluate the indicator muscle after the client says, "I want to be completely over this problem (phobia, trauma, etc.)" vs. "I want to continue to have some of this problem." If the latter is stronger, mini reversal is present. Correct by having the client tap on the little finger side of the hand (SH) while saying three times, "I deeply accept myself even though I still have some of this problem." Test again to be certain that the mini reversal has been corrected before proceeding.

18. Treatment can also stall or not even start because of deep-level reversal. To determine if a deep-level reversal is present, test the indicator muscle while having the patient say, "I *will* be over this problem" vs. "I *will* continue to have this problem." If the indicator muscle is strong on the latter and weak on the former, have the patient tap directly under his nose (un) on the governing vessel while saying three times, "I deeply accept myself even if I never get over this problem."

19. To test for mini deep-level reversal, evaluate the indicator muscle after the patient says, "I will be completely over this problem" vs. "I will continue to have some of this problem." Obviously, mini deep-level reversal is present if the indicator muscle is strong on the latter and weak on the former. The correction again entails having the patient tap under his

or her nose while saying three times, "I deeply accept myself even if I never get completely over this problem."

20. During treatment, recurrent reversal may also occur. This condition is evident when the subjective units of distress have been decreasing and then "shoot" back up. The recurrence can be further confirmed by testing the indicator muscle while having the client say, "I want to get over this problem" vs. "I want to continue to have this problem." If psychological reversal is revealed, direct the client to briskly stimulate with a circular motion the neurolymphatic reflex on the left side of the chest while saying three times, "I deeply accept myself even though this problem keeps coming back." (See section on psychological reversals.)

21. Other than recurrent reversal, a resurgence of subjective units of distress can also occur as a result of a shift in focus to other distressing material. The client may spontaneously or upon inquiry report that another aspect of the trauma, phobia, etc. came to mind. In this instance, one should direct the client to return focus to the initial issue if possible before moving on to other material. If the secondary matter continues to intrude, alternatively treat it before returning to the original target.

22. In many instances it is appropriate to challenge the results at this point. In essence, this involves either overtly or covertly directing the client to attempt to feel bothered about the issue. If the client can resurrect negative emotions, treatment is not yet complete. However, with especially stressed or fragile clients, it may not be advisable to challenge in this way, since such clients may require some time for the treatment effects to settle in or stabilize. (See section on challenging.)

23. When treatment is complete, it is generally important to debrief the client. This includes information about the possibility of recurrence, energy toxins, etc. At this point it is also useful to provide the client with a "prescription" of the algorithm that succeeded in alleviating the distress. In this way, the client is empowered for self-treatment if necessary.

24. Some problems require *in vivo* treatment in addition to that which has been provided in the office while the patient merely "thinks about" the problem. It is recommended that *in vivo* treatment only be offered after office treatment has been successfully completed and that the *in vivo* treatment not be conducted in such a fashion that promotes painful exposure. Rather, especially with highly distressing issues, the treatment is conducted in a gradual, piecemeal manner, only allowing the patient to approach the stressful situation as discomfort is alleviated (e.g., similar in protocol to *in vivo* systematic desensitization).

25. Sometimes progress can be blocked by other levels of reversal or criteria-related reversals. It appears that issues related to shame or deserving, deprivation, safety, etc. can interfere with the treatment working. These reversals have not been an aspect of Callahan's approach to thought field therapy, although they have been an aspect of the therapeutic work of other practitioners (Durlacher, 1995; Gallo, 1994b, 1997b). (See earlier section on criteria-related reversals for details.)

ENERGY PSYCHOTHERAPY PROCEDURES

TREATMENT POINTS*

The following chart of treatment points is provided to facilitate understanding of the subsequent algorithms or therapeutic recipes:

Treatment Points and Meridians

T   Lung: Radial nail point of thumb (LU-11)
IF   Large Intestine: Radial nail point of index finger (LI-1)
UE   Stomach: On the intraorbital ridge directly below the center of the pupil, under the eye, with the eye looking straight ahead (St-1)
UA   Spleen/Pancreas: On lateral thorax at level of sixth intercostal space on the mid-axillary line; 6 in. below armpit on side (Sp-21)
LF   Heart: Radial nail point of the little finger (Ht-9)
SH   Small Intestine: Ulnar side of hand at crease from palm when fist is made (SI-3)
EB   Bladder: Eyebrow point; beginning of eyebrow at bridge of nose (Bl-2)
CB   Kidney: Juncture of first rib, clavicle, and sternum; collarbone point (K-27)
MF   Circulation-Sex/Pericardium: Radial nail point of middle finger (CX-9)
BH[a]   Tri-Warmer: Back of hand proximal to and on ulnar side of the fourth metacarpal head; gamut spot (TH-3)
SE   Gallbladder: $^{1}/_{2}$ in. lateral to the lateral eye canthus; outside of eye or side of the eye (GB-1)
R   Liver: Upper edge of the eighth rib inferior to nipple; lower rib (LV-14)
BL   Central Vessel: Depression between lower lip and chin; under bottom lip (CV-24)
UN   Governing Vessel: Juncture of the philtrum and upper lip; under nose (GV-27)

[a] The BH point is also referred to as the gamut spot or G in Callahan's thought field therapy.

TREATMENT RECIPES OR ALGORITHMS

The original position of thought field therapy is that a specific order or *sequence* of acupoints must be stimulated (tapped) to achieve a therapeutic result. Callahan offers the metaphor of a combination lock, noting that the precise order is essential if the lock is to be opened. This sequence tradition is followed in the subsequent sections, especially when two or more algorithms are presented that contain the same acupoints but with a different sequence or syntax (e.g., ue, ea, cb *and* ue, ua, cb). However, it should be noted that this position is not maintained by all energy psychology approaches. In other systems, for example, there would not be a fundamental difference between ue, ea, cb *and* ue, ua, cb.†

SPECIFIC PHOBIAS

The *Diagnostic and Statistical Manual-IV* defines specific phobias as characterized by "marked and persistent fear of clearly discernible, circumscribed objects or

* Several of the abbreviations presented here are not identical to those employed by Callahan.
† See *Energy Diagnostic and Treatment Methods* (Gallo, 2000) and *Energy Psychology in Psychotherapy: A Comprehensive Source Book* (Gallo, 2002) for further details.

situations" and indicates that exposure to such "stimulus almost invariably provokes an immediate anxiety response" (American Psychiatric Association, 1994, p. 405). To receive a diagnosis of specific phobia, the condition must be sufficiently severe that it results in avoidance of the object or situation or in endurance with intense discomfort. Additionally, the person is cognizant of the irrationality of the fear, but rational words appear to do little to eliminate or reduce the intensity of the condition. It is reported that only about 20% of "phobias that persist into adulthood remit" (p. 408).

While many etiologies for the development of specific phobias have been recognized in the field (e.g., trauma, informational transmission, panic attacks while in specific situations, and observation of others experiencing trauma), it has been Callahan's position that the vast majority of phobias are inherited (Callahan, 1994). The rationale offered is that phobias do not appear to be randomized; they appear to be quite delimited for the most part. Specifically, we find phobias for various animals such as snakes, cats, dogs, spiders, moths, etc.; natural environmental phenomena including storms, water, heights, etc.; situations such as elevators, enclosed places, driving, etc.; as well as blood-injection-injury type phobias. We do not encounter phobias of books, street lights, roadmaps, etc., even though it is conceivable that people could develop phobias for these items since there are bound to be instances where people have had negative experiences associated with them.

A recent review of the literature is not supportive of an associate model for the etiology of specific phobias in general (Menzies and Clarke, 1995a). Additionally, research has not been supportive of an associative model for the etiology of water phobia or acrophobia (Menzies and Clarke, 1993, 1995b).

Assuming that phobias are inherited, a seemingly interesting paradox exists. How is it, then, that various psychological treatments, such as thought field therapy, can cure the phobia? Could a psychological treatment actually alter the DNA? That is, is not heredity a function of genes, which are basically protein structures?

The answer offered by Callahan is that although phobias are inherited, the inheritance route is by way of energy, not protein. In this respect, past traumas are stored in a resonance for the species to access for survival purposes. This is in line with Sheldrake's speculations about formative causation (Sheldrake, 1981, 1988) as well as McDougall's earlier research discussed in Chapters 1 and 3 (McDougall, 1927, 1930, 1938).

The essential algorithm for treating most specific phobias includes variable stimulation of points on the stomach, spleen/pancreas, and kidney meridians. Callahan's algorithm for most specific phobias is the following:

eye, arm, collarbone → 9 Gamut → eye, arm, collarbone → eye roll

or

ue, ua, cb → 9G → ue, ua, cb → er

or

ue, ua, cb → 9G Sq* → er

These formulas indicate that the stomach meridian is stimulated or activated by tapping directly on the bony orbit directly under the eye (ue), followed by tapping 6 in. under the armpit (ua) on the spleen/pancreas meridian, and then tapping under the collarbone next to the sternum (cb) on the kidney meridian. After this sequence has resulted in a decrease in subjective units of distress by at least two points, the nine gamut treatments are done (refer to relevant section). After the nine gamut treatments, the sequence (Sq) ue, ua, cb is repeated. Finally, the eye roll (er) is done if the subjective units of distress are within the 1 to 3 range.

According to Callahan, some specific phobias require a different sequence of meridian points, especially claustrophobia, fear of spiders, and anxiety related to flight turbulence. In these instances, the following alternative sequence may be necessitated:

arm, eye, collarbone → 9G → arm, eye, collarbone → eye roll

or

ua, ue, cb → 9G → Sq → er

In this instance the patient is directed to initially tap under the arm (ua) on the spleen meridian, then under the eye (ue) on the stomach meridian, and then under the collarbone (cb) on the kidney meridian. Again, after a decrease of at least two subjective units of distress points, the nine gamut treatments are provided, after which the sequence of majors is repeated (i.e., ua, ue, cb), followed by the eye roll (er) when the subjective units of distress are within the 1 to 3 range.

Frequently, individuals suffering from specific phobias will evidence reversals, especially recurrent and mini reversals during the course of treatment. Typical criteria-related reversals include those for safety, identity, and possibility. Additionally, some specific phobias are more complex than others, requiring treatment of many aspects or holons prior to realizing a cure. For example, fear of flying may require directing treatment to a number of features including claustrophobia, take-off, landing, flight turbulence, being at a high elevation, fear of crashing, etc. Frequently, these various aspects emerge in order of importance one by one as each previous aspect has been successfully treated. At other times, it is necessary for the client–therapist partnership to uncover and treat the specific aspects.

The algorithms for specific phobias have been presented initially, since historically Callahan developed treatments for these conditions first. However, the remainder of this section is presented in alphabetical order for ease of location.

ADDICTION AND ADDICTIVE URGE

Addictive urges may be classified as anxiety. The anxiety is a manifestation of perturbations in the thought field. The perturbations trigger specific "vibrations" in

---

* Sq stands for *sequence*, indicating the sequence of treatment points or majors conducted prior to and after the 9G. Henceforth, the Sq abbreviation is used rather that repeating the sequence of majors.

the energy system, which in turn affect the other relevant systems (i.e., neurologic, hormonal, endocrine, cognitive) and culminate in the gestalt that is referred to as anxiety.

There is an obvious distinction between addiction and addictive urge. The urge is simply the craving anxiety. It is an aspect of addiction, but it is hardly the whole of the problem. Alleviating an addictive urge, while beneficial to the overall therapy of addiction, cannot be expected to be sufficient in alleviating the addiction. The latter includes a number of other factors, such as a history of trauma, social anxiety, camaraderie, compulsion to self-sabotage, clinical depression, obsessive-compulsive features, and so on.

To alleviate an addictive urge, first have the patient attune the urge by thinking about or being in the presence of the substance to which he or she is addicted (i.e., alcohol, drugs, chocolate, gambling, etc.). Following the essential therapeutic process, check for and correct reversals and then employ the following algorithm:

$$ue, ua, cb \rightarrow 9G \rightarrow Sq \rightarrow er$$

As with all thought field therapy treatments, it is important to recognize the reactivation of reversal: recurrent, mini, or otherwise. Generally, the addicted person is not psychologically reversed for getting over the addictive craving, although the addiction as a whole is an entirely different matter, which often gives rise to reversals. Obviously, the addict wants to alleviate the addictive urge or craving, and thus he or she turns to the favorite substance (rather than tapping) to accomplish this end.

Given extensive treatment of patients with addictive disorders, I have found a number of effective alternative sequences that should prove helpful when the basic urge reduction sequence does not alleviate the urge:

$$ue, ua, cb, lf, cb \rightarrow 9G \rightarrow Sq \rightarrow er$$

This sequence adds the heart meridian point, lf, possibly in those instances where anger is an aspect of the urge. While anger is not considered to be an aspect of the heart meridian in traditional acupuncture lore, the liver and gallbladder meridians are the more likely candidates for this affect. Consistent with Diamond's findings (1985) that the heart meridian is active with anger, stimulation of this point nonetheless seems to do the job when anger is an aspect of the condition being treated.

$$ue, cb, ue \rightarrow 9G \rightarrow Sq \rightarrow er$$

This sequence is useful with patients who consistently experience an increase in urge after the "under the arm" point (ua) is tapped. In such instances, it may be advisable to delete this treatment point when treating addictive urges.

$$ue, cb, ua, cb, ue \rightarrow 9G \rightarrow Sq \rightarrow er$$

This sequence includes a repetition of treatment points such that various sequences are nested within it, thus taking a number of possibilities into account. The relevance of this design is to reduce the need for diagnosis when the basic sequence proves inadequate to eliminate the urge.

$$ue, cb, ua, lf, ua, cb, ue \rightarrow 9G \rightarrow Sq \rightarrow er$$

This sequence is similar to the previous algorithm, although it adds the heart meridian point (lf) before reversing the order.

$$ue, ua, cb, ua, ue, cb \rightarrow 9G \rightarrow Sq \rightarrow er$$

Similar to the previous two algorithms, this sequence repeats treatment points in various orders to eliminate the need for diagnosis when the basic sequence proves incapable of reducing the urge.

Concerning addiction, it is important to assess the patient with regard to massive reversal, as well as specific and deep-level reversals. Various levels of reversal are invariably present with addiction and serve to promote the self-sabotaging aspects of the condition and to interfere with any inclination to treat oneself when addictive urges arise.

To increase the patient's chances of success in treatment, it is recommended that regular treatment for massive reversal and specific reversal be prescribed. In this respect, we advise our patients who have addictive disorders to treat themselves perhaps five or more times daily at regular intervals. For example, the patient may benefit from rubbing the neurolymphatic reflex (i.e., "sore spot") spot while saying three times, "I deeply accept myself with all my problems and limitations and even though I'm addicted to alcohol." This affirmation efficiently combines massive reversal and specific reversal.

Additionally, many addicted patients simply do not believe that they will ever get over their addiction. In such instances, it is recommended that the patient treat himself or herself regularly for deep-level reversal by tapping under the nose (un) while saying three times, "I deeply accept myself even if I never get over this problem."

Another level of reversal, pertaining to deserving, is referred to as deservedness reversal (Gallo, 1994b). Here, the patient seems to deeply believe that he or she is not worthwhile and that he or she does not deserve to get over the addiction. In other words, the addict may believe that he or she deserves to be addicted. This level of reversal can be effectively treated by having the patient tap under the bottom lip (central vessel) while saying three times, "I deeply accept myself even if (or though) I don't deserve to get over this problem (e.g., my addiction to cocaine, alcohol problem, etc.)."

Another level of reversal that seems to be relevant in the treatment of addiction relates to the issue of deprivation (Durlacher, 1997). In this regard, the addicted person experiences a sense of being deprived if he or she cannot use the substance and will therefore wane in resolution to remain abstinent of the alcohol, drugs, chocolate, etc. This reversal can be diagnosed via muscle testing. The treatment involves tapping at small intestine-3 (the SH point) while saying three times, "I deeply accept myself even though I'll feel deprived if I get over this problem."

Addiction should not be taken lightly. One would be professionally and morally remiss to convey to the addict that all he or she has to do is tap at various points on the body and say a few affirmations. Rather, addiction, like many conditions, needs to be treated in a comprehensive manner. The patient should be involved in therapy and support groups directed at teaching various coping mechanisms, addressing relevant life experiences and issues and clinical depression, etc. To recommend otherwise would be to foolishly play into the denial and empty promises that are the hallmarks of addiction.

ALLERGY (INHALANT TYPE)

Frequently, I have found this treatment approach helpful in temporarily reducing and even eliminating inhalant allergy symptoms, such as to pollen, dust, mold, etc. Here is an algorithm that is frequently effective:

$$mf, ua, cb \rightarrow 9G \rightarrow Sq \rightarrow er$$

ANGER

While there may be some value in the momentary experience of anger, to harbor anger surely does more damage to oneself than to the person or circumstance for which one holds the anger. Buddy Hackett, the famed comedian, said many times that he could not see being angry at someone because "While you're angry at them, they're out dancing." Besides this practical truth, anger interferes with one's mental functioning at the time and often leads to disturbing actions if one becomes sufficiently hoodwinked by the thoughts of anger. There is also evidence that sustained hostility is a factor in one's physical health, especially in the development of coronary disease.

Certainly one can come to even deeper philosophic and spiritual understandings of anger. Harboring anger often prevents one from healing and getting on with life in a more serene manner. Following the precepts of *A Course in Miracles* (Foundation for Inner Peace, 1975), our primary objective in life is peace of mind, which we arrive at through the process of forgiveness.

Even though the angry person may come to realize the validity of these philosophical and practical issues concerning anger, often this knowledge is insufficient to eliminate or transcend the state of anger. Every time the person thinks about the object of the anger, anger is experienced. While it may be important to come to the realization that the anger is a function of one's own thought process, that the anger is essentially an internally created experience, and that it is possible to attain a level of realization that makes it possible to transcend anger, it is often helpful, if not essential, to assist the patient in dissolving the anger via elimination of the anger-laden perturbations.

While acupuncture literature cites the liver and gallbladder meridians as relevant to anger, both Diamond and Callahan have indicated the importance of the heart meridian with respect to anger. This meridian may also be important in terms of alleviating anger because it also appears to be relevant with regard to forgiveness. Many healers have cited forgiveness as essential before healing can begin.

Similar to Diamond, the thought field therapy approach often includes an affirmation in addition to tapping directed at the heart meridian. The thought field therapy treatment point is the last or ninth acupoint on the heart meridian (Ht-9, abbreviated lf), located at the radial nail point of the fifth or little (pinkie) finger. This point is located by looking at the back of either hand and noting the inside aspect of the little fingernail where the nail meets the cuticle on the side facing the fourth or ring finger.

Additionally, the procedure involves stimulating the remaining meridians via the K-27 (collarbone point) after treating the heart meridian. While tapping at the lf point, the standard affirmation employed by Callahan is as follows: "I forgive (person's name), I know you can't help it." This affirmation is stated three times while repeatedly tapping at the lf point.

Many patients object to the affirmation attached to this treatment. Some will emphasize that the person "could" or "should" have been able to help it. One response might be to observe that if the person could have helped it and if the person had been sufficiently enlightened at the time, then the transgression would never have occurred in the first place. Of course, here we would be attempting a cognitive strategy that does not always make emotional sense to the patient who is experiencing chronic or even acute anger. We could pursue various lines of logic, but the emotional aspect wards off the reasoning, as reasonable as it might be.

Alternatively, the anger can be treated without even utilizing an affirmation. In this regard, the sequence of tapping is often independently effective. However, because an appropriate affirmation can enhance the effectiveness of the treatment, the following are offered as they have proved just as effective:

"I forgive you (insert name), I know you're doing the best you can."
"There is forgiveness in my heart" (adapted from Diamond, 1985).
"I release myself of this anger."

In addition to anger at another person or situation, obviously one can experience anger toward oneself. This treatment for anger is effective in these respects as well. Further, it should be noted that often a person will be psychologically reversed for getting over the anger toward self or others, and in such cases treatment for psychological reversal will be needed.

The anger (forgiveness) algorithm is as follows:

$$\text{lf (I forgive ...), cb} \rightarrow \text{9G} \rightarrow \text{Sq} \rightarrow \text{er}$$

ANTICIPATORY AND PERFORMANCE ANXIETY

While anticipation of an anxiety-producing situation (e.g., public speaking, sexual performance, etc.) may be different from actually being in the situation, from the standpoint of thought fields and the body's energy system, there is often little distinction. In most cases the structure of the field is similar, entailing disruptions associated with same meridians. In these instances perturbations associated with the stomach, spleen, and kidney meridians are quite common. Generally, I have found that the typical sequences for treating these conditions will be the following:

$$\text{ue, ua, cb} \rightarrow 9G \rightarrow Sq \rightarrow er$$

The standard therapeutic procedure involves asking the client to "think about" the situation or circumstance that produces discomfort and to rate the subjective units of distress 1 to 10, after which the treatment sequence is provided (after assessing for preliminaries such as psychological reversal).

ATTENTION-DEFICIT/HYPERACTIVITY DISORDER

The patient with attention-deficit/hyperactivity disorder (ADHD) can be classified as primarily inattentive, primarily hyperactive-impulsive, or combined. While these diagnoses are estimated to occur in 3 to 5% of younger school-age children, and there are limited data concerning the prevalence among adolescents and adults (American Psychiatric Association, 1994), it seems likely that the frequency of diagnosing these conditions has been on the upswing since the publication of the fourth edition of the *Diagnostic and Statistical Manual of Mental Disorders.*

While there are no specific thought field therapy algorithms for treating these conditions, a number of procedures and considerations have been helpful in many instances. Many children with attention-deficit/hyperactivity disorder have been helped by tracking down energy toxins and allergies that produce the symptoms. Some of the typical "allergens" include mold, dust, corn, wheat, herbs, pepper, refined sugar, milk products, caffeine, noxious chemicals, perfume, and detergents. Essentially any food that a child craves excessively may be an energy toxin or allergen (see Rapp, 1991).

Interestingly, in many cases of hyperactivity, psychostimulant medications such as methylphenidate paradoxically alleviate the symptoms. Callahan has indicated that this paradoxical phenomenon calls to mind psychological reversal.* Also a primary thought field therapy position about energy toxins is that they result in reversal, accounting for their tendency to block treatment effectiveness or to cause a regression after positive treatment effects.

In addition to removing toxins, treatments for reversal and criteria-related reversals will be beneficial in some instances. However, as long as the toxin is significantly present, few permanent effects in this way would be expected. When the level of the toxin is minimal, the chances of reversal corrections holding will be more likely.

Corrections for neurologic disorganization/switching will also be helpful in many instances of attention-deficit/hyperactivity disorder. Again, this follows similar lines to reversal. One way to diagnose the presence of toxins is by observing that after neurologic disorganization has been diagnosed, correction for this condition fails to take effect or hold for very long. Again, it is the energy toxin that is causing the switching problem.

Assuming that the toxins have been alleviated, residual attention-deficit/hyperactivity disorder symptoms, which may be more purely in the learned behavior category, will perhaps respond to standard energy psychotherapy methods. Consider

---

* However, it should be noted that psychostimulant medications such as Ritalin, Adderall, and Concerta frequently improve focusing and this accounts for their effective utilization with these conditions.

a relatively complex algorithm or a more global treatment such as the negative affect erasing method (NAEM) or emotional freedom techniques (EFT) discussed later in this chapter. Perhaps the Tapas acupressure technique (TAT), also discussed later, would prove beneficial toward alleviating the negative effects of some substances. Alternatively, an energy diagnostic procedure will be needed for effective treatment.

AWKWARDNESS AND CLUMSINESS

Momentary or chronic awkwardness and clumsiness may be indicative of neurologic disorganization or switching. In such instances, the collarbone breathing exercises or other corrections for switching may prove beneficial. Alternative correction methods such as the basic unswitching procedure or the overenergy correction may be used. Some people may need to do these treatments on a regular basis.

CLINICAL DEPRESSION

Clinical depression often responds quite well to an amazingly simple algorithm. After addressing psychological reversals, especially massive reversal ("I deeply accept myself with all my problems and limitations") and specific reversal ("I deeply accept myself even though I'm depressed"), the patient is directed to tap at tri-heater-3 (the gamut spot) for an extensive period of time, perhaps a minute or so, until a decrease in depression is experienced. The target may be a feeling of depression, a feeling of emptiness, a sense of despair, etc. After a decrease is evident, the patient then taps at the collarbone point for approximately five taps and then returns to the gamut spot. This alternating sequence is repeated until the depression is significantly decreased or alleviated, at which point the nine gamut treatments are provided. At this point the original sequence is repeated followed by the eye roll when the subjective units of distress are within the 1 to 3 range.

Callahan's depression algorithm is as follows:

$$bh \text{ (extended*)}, cb \rightarrow 9G \rightarrow Sq \rightarrow er$$

While this basic depression algorithm is frequently effective in alleviating symptoms of depression, at other times it is insufficient. When it proves insufficient, it should be "front loaded" with an extensive "trauma" algorithm such as the following:

$$eb, ue, ua, cb, lf, cb, if, cb, bh(\text{extended}), cb \rightarrow 9G \rightarrow Sq \rightarrow er$$

Frequently, there will be no remaining traces of depression after either of these treatments has been provided. While this hardly guarantees that there will not be a recurrence of symptoms, the fact that the depression can be even temporarily eliminated in this manner is no small thing. However, frequently a single treatment in this manner will result in elimination of the depression without return.

Generally, the patient needs to be treated many times before sustained improvement is realized. It is advisable to repeat the treatment in the office and to be available

---

* "Extended" indicates extensive stimulation of 50 or more taps.

to even repeat the treatment over the phone if necessary. Certainly, it is appropriate to teach the patient how to self-treat, but often patients need to experience the success of the treatment via therapist administration before feeling comfortable and confident with self-treatment.

As far as antidepressant medication is concerned, utilization of the thought field therapy treatment is a fairly simple matter when the medication is not alleviating the depression. At such times, the efficiency of the thought field therapy treatment will be readily apparent. Nonetheless, as the medication is titrated, regular utilization of the algorithm is indicated.

The issue of medication becomes more relevant in cases where the antidepressant is effective. At such times it will be difficult to know if the thought field therapy algorithm is accomplishing anything. Therefore, the protocol will involve extensive treatment with the algorithm while having the patient think about what it was like to feel depressed. After a period of treatment in this manner, resulting in various positive changes in the patient's behavior, titration of the medication can begin. Again, regular use of the algorithm will be necessitated during and after discontinuation of the antidepressant.

EMBARRASSMENT

This emotional state is discussed by Diamond (1985) as associated with the governing vessel, the meridian that begins at the tip of the coccyx, ascends the spine, enters the brain, traverses the back of the head, and terminates at the upper gingiva. I have found that embarrassment can often be relieved by having the patient tap directly under the nose (un) at the juncture of the philtrum and upper lip, which is at GV-26. Results can often be enhanced by employing the following algorithm:

$$un, cb \rightarrow 9G \rightarrow Sq \rightarrow er$$

FATIGUE

Fatigue associated with insufficient sleep, jet lag, or perhaps even chronic fatigue syndrome can benefit from these kinds of procedures. The following algorithm, which I developed, frequently has been found to be beneficial in reducing fatigue and promoting a state of alertness and energy:

$$ue, cb, eb, cb \rightarrow 9G \rightarrow Sq \rightarrow er$$

FRUSTRATION, IMPATIENCE, AND RESTLESSNESS

Diamond (1985) reports that frustration, impatience, and restlessness are consistent with bladder meridian imbalances. With this in mind, supported by clinical tests, I developed the following algorithm, which has generally proved of value in treating these states:

$$eb, cb \rightarrow 9G \rightarrow Sq \rightarrow er$$

GENERALIZED ANXIETY DISORDER

Generalized anxiety disorder (GAD) also responds to thought field therapy treatments, frequently the same ones used in the treatment of addictive urges (for example):

$$\text{ue, ua, cb} \rightarrow 9G \rightarrow Sq \rightarrow er$$

or

$$\text{ue, cb, ua, cb, ue} \rightarrow 9G \rightarrow Sq \rightarrow er$$

The treatment must be consistently repeated over time if the client is to realize stable improvement. In this regard, the client is taught effective algorithms for self-treatment whenever significant anxiety arises. This same strategy should be employed with addictive urges.

Additionally, generalized anxiety disorder frequently seems to entail ingestion of energy toxins and other substances that stimulate the nervous system, such as caffeine, nicotine, psychostimulants, etc. When such substances are identified as relevant in a particular case, abstinence is generally necessary if treatment is to be effective. Treatment directed specifically at addictive craving and the addiction is often necessitated in instances when the toxic substance is also one to which the patient is addicted.

GUILT FEELINGS

The word guilt is from the old English *gylt*, meaning crime. While guilt is defined as "remorseful awareness of having done something wrong," a distinction between the guilt affect and ontological guilt should be kept in mind. While one may feel guilty for having violated one's morals, obviously it is possible to feel guilty without having done anything wrong at all. Also, it is possible not to feel guilty and yet be "guilty as hell." Furthermore, there are instances where the affect of guilt has worn out its welcome or usefulness, leading to more harm than good.

When a patient suffers from chronic feelings of guilt for real or imagined sins, it is beneficial to alleviate the torment. Chronic guilt can seriously interfere with one's peace of mind and can also lead to self-destructive behaviors. While the therapist may wish to address the cognitive, philosophic, and moral aspects, this is often insufficient to neutralize the negative affect.

Guilt feelings appear to be associated with the large intestine meridian. The thought field therapy treatment point for this meridian is at the tip of the index finger (abbreviated if). It is the first point on the large intestine meridian (LI-1), located at the radial nail point of either index finger. Facing the palm of the hand, the side of the index fingernail closest to the thumb is where the point is located, the corner of the nail where it meets the cuticle.

Similar to Diamond's approach, treatment of guilt feelings often includes an affirmation while tapping at the "if" point. The standard affirmation employed by Callahan is as follows: "I forgive myself because I can't help it." Alternatively, affirmations such as the following might be substituted: "I forgive myself; I'm doing the best that I can" or "I release myself of this guilt."

Additionally, the procedure involves stimulating the remaining meridians via the kidney-27 (i.e., collarbone point) after tapping on the "if" point and saying or thinking the affirmation three times.

The thought field therapy algorithm for guilt feelings is as follows:

$$\text{if (I forgive myself ...), cb} \rightarrow 9G \rightarrow Sq \rightarrow er$$

INSOMNIA

There are a variety of causes of insomnia, and again there is no one energy psychotherapy procedure that is suited to the task. Insomnia can be related to sleep apnea, restless leg syndrome, biochemical disturbances, toxins, etc. In some instances, a thorough medical workup will be needed. However, insomnia can also be a symptom of depression, stress, worry, and anxiety. In such instances, employing an appropriate algorithm or other energy treatment will frequently alleviate the problem.

JEALOUSY

As Diamond elucidates, "Jealousy is derived from the Latin *zelus*, meaning zeal or fervor. The idea behind jealousy is that we act and even fight with zeal to protect and regain what we feel is rightfully ours" (1985, p. 146). Although some may see jealousy as a sign of love, or may reframe it as love, this likely blurs the issue. Chronic feelings of jealousy are nonetheless painfully pathologic and worth alleviating.

Frequently, jealousy is associated with a trauma of sorts. A patient complains of love pain due to a romantic breakup, separation, divorce, etc. Additionally, the pain includes having observed or knowing that the lover is involved with another person. How do we treat this situation? How do we afford the patient with a sense of relief?

I have found that jealousy is frequently consistent with an imbalance within the circulation-sex meridian. While any of the trauma algorithms may prove beneficial for treating traumas that include feelings of jealousy, the following algorithm I developed, which includes treatment of the circulation-sex meridian, has been helpful to many patients:

$$\text{mf, ua, cb} \rightarrow 9G \rightarrow Sq \rightarrow er*$$

This algorithm begins with tapping at the index finger side of the middle fingernail (mf), followed by tapping under the arm at spleen-21 (ua), and then under the collarbone (cb) at kidney-27. As usual, the eye roll procedure (er) is added when the subjective units of distress are within the 1 to 3 range.

Additionally, it should be obvious that feelings of jealousy frequently entail psychological reversals and these will need to be corrected if the algorithm is to

---

* I developed the jealousy algorithm as a result of personal work as well as my work with clients.

prove of any benefit. Furthermore, it is generally necessary to treat jealousy in a comprehensive manner, attending to various painful memories at the root of this affect. This may include memories from childhood as well as those specific to the current traumatic circumstances.

JET LAG

I have frequently found this approach helpful in eliminating symptoms of jet lag. The following algorithms can be used once jet lag has set in or they can be used to prevent jet lag from occurring by using them regularly while flying to your destination.

Flying east:

$$ue, cb \rightarrow 9G \rightarrow Sq \rightarrow er$$

Flying west:

$$eb, cb \rightarrow 9G \rightarrow Sq \rightarrow er$$

NASAL STUFFINESS/CONGESTION

Here's an algorithm that has frequently been helpful in temporarily reducing or eliminating nasal stuffiness and congestion. For greater effectiveness, I have often found that this treatment should be combined with the one for inhalant allergy symptoms.

$$un, cb \rightarrow 9G \rightarrow Sq \rightarrow er$$

OBSESSION AND OBSESSIVE-COMPULSIVE DISORDER

Obsession and obsessive-compulsive disorder (OCD) do not respond easily to any psychotherapeutic approach. However, the treatment of these conditions can often be accelerated with thought field therapy, given appropriate protocols.

At a minimum, frequently there are some minor traumas at the source of the obsession, and it is hardly news that, as such, the patient suffers from a sense of guilt. Tracking down the relevant traumas for treatment with the appropriate trauma algorithms is often the first step in successful treatment.

The obsessive process itself can often be treated with the following algorithm developed by Callahan:

$$cb, ue, cb \rightarrow 9G \rightarrow Sq \rightarrow er$$

Alternatively, the therapist may find one or a combination of the following sequences to be effective in those instances where the basic algorithm proves insufficient:

$$ue, cb, ue, cb \rightarrow 9G \rightarrow Sq \rightarrow er$$

Additionally, the compulsive behaviors can be effectively treated with the same algorithms. They can also be treated similarly to addictive urges with algorithms such as the following:

$$ue, ua, cb \rightarrow 9G \rightarrow Sq \rightarrow er$$

$$ue, ua, cb, lf, cb \rightarrow 9G \rightarrow Sq \rightarrow er$$

and so forth.

PANIC DISORDER AND AGORAPHOBIA

Panic, agoraphobia, and other complex anxiety conditions frequently do not respond to the algorithms listed for specific phobias or generalized anxiety disorder. Often, the sequence must be varied and the bladder (eb point) and heart (lf point) meridians are frequently involved. Additionally, traumas frequently need to be neutralized in cases of complex anxiety (see section on trauma and post-traumatic stress disorder later in the chapter). For example, an initial panic attack is often traumatic, and the patient may become preoccupied with the thought of having another one. This can lead to a recurrent panic condition, agoraphobia, social phobia, etc.

The following algorithms for the treatment of complex anxiety are listed in a related format by Callahan (1990). If the initial sequence does not alleviate the anxiety, the therapist should attempt the subsequent ones in the order of presentation.

1. ue, ua, eb, cb, lf → 9G → Sq → er
2. ua, ue, eb, cb, lf → 9G → Sq → er
3. eb, ua, ue → 9G → Sq → er
4. ue, eb, ua, lf → 9G → Sq → er
5. cb, ue, ua → 9G → Sq → er

PHYSICAL PAIN

Physical pain also often responds quite well to the same algorithm(s) used for clinical depression. Headaches seem to respond quite well to this treatment, whereas other types of pain at other areas of the body are less thoroughly responsive to this approach.

It should be noted that Goodheart developed a meridian-based pain alleviation treatment, which he refers to as the Melzak–Wall pain treatment (Walther, 1988). In this regard, he utilizes tonification points, which, according to acupuncture literature, increase the level of energy, or chi, within the meridian. After therapy localization directed at the wrist pulses to determine which meridian or meridians are deficient in chi, the procedure involves tapping on the respective tonification points. Goodheart found that after the pain was alleviated in this fashion, the pain could be resurrected by tapping on the meridian's respective sedation point (i.e., the point along the meridian that, when stimulated, decreases the amount of energy available within the meridian).

Callahan's method merely utilizes the same tonification point, triple-warmer-3 or the gamut spot, regardless of the location of the pain. Additionally, this is combined with stimulation of the kidney meridian at kidney-27 or the collarbone point.

The essential protocol initially involves correcting for neurologic disorganization and psychological reversals when present. The patient is then directed to focus his or her attention on the physical location of the pain. In this respect, it is often helpful to have the patient close his or her eyes and verbally describe the pain in terms of precise location, shape, type of pain (e.g., burning, stabbing, sharp, etc.), and so forth. Also, as is the case with all algorithms, the subjective units of distress must be designated to determine treatment progress. For convenience sake, the algorithm is as follows:

$$\text{bh (extended), cb} \rightarrow 9G \rightarrow Sq \rightarrow er$$

While this basic algorithm is frequently effective in alleviating physical pain symptoms, similar to its use with clinical depression, at other times it is insufficient. In such instances, "front loading" with an extensive algorithm such as the following is often helpful:

$$\text{eb, ue, ua, cb, lf, cb, if, cb, bh (extended), cb} \rightarrow 9G \rightarrow Sq \rightarrow er$$

Often, there will be no trace of pain after either of the above treatments has been provided. While this does not guarantee that there will not be a recurrence of pain, the fact that the pain can be alleviated in this manner is noteworthy. However, sometimes a single pain treatment in this manner will eliminate the pain altogether without the need for additional treatment.

In most instances, the patient requires repetition of treatment over time to obtain sustained improvement. It is advisable to repeat the treatment in the office and to be available to repeat the treatment over the phone if necessary. It is also appropriate to teach the patient how to self-treat, but frequently the patient must undergo several treatments administered by the therapist before achieving the comfort and confidence for self-treatment.

As far as pain medication is concerned, utilization of the thought field therapy treatment is a fairly simple matter when the medication is not alleviating the pain altogether. At such times, the efficiency of the thought field therapy treatment will be readily apparent. Nonetheless, as the medication is gradually discontinued, regular utilization of the algorithm is needed.

The issue of medication becomes more relevant in cases where the pain medication is effective and the patient has become dependent on it. At such times it will be difficult to know if the thought field therapy algorithm is accomplishing anything, as the patient will often attribute the results to the medication and may be reluctant to reduce the medication. Thus, the protocol necessitates significant modifications, including extensive treatment with the algorithm at the least signs of pain, treatment for urges or desires for the effects of the pain medication, regular treatment for psychological reversals, etc. After a period of treatment in this manner and various positive changes in the patient's behavior, discontinuation of the medication can begin. Again, regular use of the algorithm will be necessitated during and after the pain medication has been eliminated.

Another consideration worth noting is the events that led to the development of the pain problem, specifically with regard to chronic pain conditions.

RAGE

While rage may be rooted in anger, it is far more extreme and entails obvious behavioral aspects. It is a violent, explosive, often destructive form of anger. Rage is from the Latin root *rabere*, meaning "to be mad." This is the same root from which we derive "rabies."

From a meridian standpoint, rage is a manifestation of the gallbladder meridian. The thought field therapy treatment point is the first acupoint on the gallbladder meridian (GB-1, abbreviated se). It is located $1/2$ in. lateral to the lateral eye canthus. This point is located by placing a finger at the temple side of the bony orbit of the eye socket and sliding the finger $1/2$ in. in the direction of the temple.

After tapping five times at the se point, the patient taps five times at the collarbone point. This is similar to the treatment for anger as well as several other algorithms. While an affirmation is not employed by Callahan for the treatment of rage, I have found the application of Diamond's (1985, p. 117) affirmations (individual or combined) for balancing the gallbladder meridian effective: "I reach out with forgiveness." "I reach out with love." "I reach out with forgiveness and love."

The thought field therapy rage algorithm is as follows:

$$\text{se (I reach out ...), cb} \rightarrow 9G \rightarrow Sq \rightarrow er$$

SHAME

According to Diamond, shame is the emotion associated with what is referred to as the central or conception vessel. This meridian begins at the perineum and ends at the depression between the chin and lower lip (bl). I have found that this emotional state can often be relieved by having the patient tap directly under the bottom lip at central vessel (CV)-24:

$$\text{bl, cb} \rightarrow 9G \rightarrow Sq \rightarrow er$$

STRESS REDUCTION

Essentially, all of the algorithms reduce stress. However, for rapid, uncomplicated stress (if there can be such a thing), the eye roll (er) can often do the job.

As always, the individual begins by rating the subjective units of distress in the range of 1 to 10. Next, the eyes are pointed downward, while the head is held erect. While the eyes are in this position, one steadily taps on back of hand (bh) point between the little and ring finger knuckles on the back of either hand (i.e., triple-warmer-3). Then slowly and steadily the eyes are raised toward the ceiling and held there for a moment while continuing to tap at the gamut spot. After taking a stress reading again (1 to 10), assuming that the subjective units of distress have decreased, it may prove beneficial to do the nine gamut treatments and then repeat the eye roll procedure. As this section of the chapter on thought field therapy algorithms comes to a close, interested readers are invited to enjoy a bit of stress reduction by practicing the following algorithm;

$$er \rightarrow 9G \rightarrow er$$

Trauma and Post-Traumatic Stress Disorder

The thought field therapy treatments for trauma and the various trauma-based conditions, such as post-traumatic stress disorder (PTSD), are among the most powerful thought field therapy algorithms available. While trauma may be effectively treated via a combination of flooding and cognitive restructuring, such an approach is wrought with undesirable side effects and is seldom efficient. Additionally, while eye movement desensitization and reprocessing effectively treats trauma, it has been the experience of many that this method also frequently results in painful abreaction, which is seldom experienced with thought field therapy if the therapist is sufficiently expert in the technique.

The thought field therapy algorithms for trauma invariably involve treatment of the bladder meridian or the eyebrow point (eb). The most basic algorithm for trauma and painful memories is the following:

$$eb, cb \rightarrow 9G \rightarrow Sq \rightarrow er$$

While this sequence is often effective as the trauma becomes increasingly complex, the algorithm is also more complex because several meridians are often disrupted by their respective thought field perturbations. Therefore, the basic complex sequence additionally addresses the stomach and spleen meridians as follows:

$$eb, ue, ua, cb \rightarrow 9G \rightarrow Sq \rightarrow er$$

Frequently, the traumatized person understandably harbors considerable anger about the traumatic event, including anger about the circumstance, anger about and at other people involved, and anger about one's own real or imagined responsibility in the matter. In such instances this is better treated with the following algorithm:

$$eb, ue, ua, cb, lf, cb \rightarrow 9G \rightarrow Sq \rightarrow er$$

Additionally, the traumatized patient may suffer guilt feelings about the traumatic event. If the event was a date rape, for example, the victim might become obsessed with the erroneous thoughts of having somehow caused the event. These thoughts and guilt feelings are likely cybernetically related such that the thoughts elicit the affect and the affect in turn stimulates the production of additional guilt-ridden thoughts, and so on. These features can be addressed with the following algorithm, which additionally treats the large intestine imbalance that is frequently found with guilt feelings (treated by stimulating the index finger point or "if"). As with the case of anger not being considered associated with the heart meridian in traditional acupuncture, so, too, the large intestine meridian in traditional acupuncture is not connected with guilt feelings but rather with grief and sadness. Not withstanding the possibility that there are other acupoints that can achieve the desired results as well, activating this point on the index fingernail appears to promote the alleviation of guilt feelings.

$$eb, ue, ua, cb, if, cb \rightarrow 9G \rightarrow Sq \rightarrow er$$

Alternatively, aspects of both algorithms 3 and 4 (listed previously in the panic disorders and agoraphobia section) can be combined to alleviate the anger (lf) as well as the guilt (if) associated with the traumatic event:

$$eb, ue, ua, cb, lf, cb, if, cb \rightarrow 9G \rightarrow Sq \rightarrow er$$

Trauma and post-traumatic stress disorder require variable protocols. Sometimes it is sufficient simply to ask the patient to think about the trauma as a whole or globally and then to provide the appropriate algorithm. In such instances we find that the patient's trauma is immediately alleviated or that different aspects of the trauma emerge, one after another, until the entire trauma is neutralized.

At other times it is necessary to assist the patient in tuning into various aspects of the trauma, each in turn for treatment. The trauma might be treated linearly as it actually occurred in time. Alternatively, it often proves effective in many cases to ask the patient to bring up various aspects as he or she so chooses. Thus, the patient may begin with the most devastating aspect or perhaps a much less anxiety-provoking element. In this regard, we believe that the person's interest is of great relevance to the effectiveness of the treatment.

VISUALIZATION ENHANCEMENT

Visualization has been employed extensively throughout the therapy and performance fields. It is based on the assumption that if one is able to visualize vividly an outcome, then the outcome, within reason, will be more readily achievable in reality. This is consistent with Maxwell Maltz's (1960) psychocybernetics, which holds that the nervous system cannot distinguish between a reality and an event imagined vividly, and it is also a major feature of many types of hypnotic suggestion. Also, there have been reports of the benefits of visualization in a variety of areas, including immune system augmentation in the treatment of cancer (Simonton and Creighton, 1982).

Assuming that one is able to visualize, frequently there is impairment of this facility in the area for which one is seeking improvement. That is, if the patient desires to overcome a particular psychological problem, such as the fear of flying, he or she will be unable to adequately visualize being over the problem. He or she will not be able to see himself or herself seated comfortably in the airplane as it speedily takes off, flies some distance, turbulence and all, and finally lands at the desired destination. Either the internal images will not be available or they will be "fuzzy" or of otherwise poor quality, thus precluding the feasibility of using this procedure as an aspect of treatment. Perhaps it is the stress of so strongly desiring the outcome or disbelief in one's ability to achieve it that interferes with the ease of visualization in the specific area.

Nonetheless, Callahan (1990) has found that visualization often can be enhanced by "balancing" the energy system. What follows is a protocol that combines aspects of his work with other useful features. This protocol also can be used to enhance therapeutic effects of other conditions described in this chapter.

1. Establish visualization ability by having the client visualize an innocuous event, such as imagining an orange flying through the air. Have the client also rate how well he or she is able to visualize, using a range of 0 to 10, with 0 representing not being able to visualize the orange at all and 10 representing impeccable visualization.
2. If the client is unable to visualize well, having the client proceed through the following treatment will often result in improvement in this area: PR → ua, eb → 9G → Sq → er. At the psychological reversal point have the client say, "I deeply accept myself even though I am not able to clearly visualize an orange." (Alternatively, correction for deep-level or a criteria-related reversal could be needed. See previous relevant sections.) Next, the client taps about five times 6 in. under either armpit (ua), followed by tapping five times at the beginning of either eyebrow at the bridge of the nose (eb). At this point, the rating is reviewed before proceeding with the nine gamut treatments, repeating the ua, eb sequence, and then doing the eye roll (er). Sometimes this treatment sequence must be repeated a few times to assist the client in visualizing within the 8 to 10 range.
3. Assuming that the client is now able to visualize well, proceed by having the client imagine being over the psychological problem, and again rate the visualization adeptness 0 to 10. This might involve seeing oneself seated comfortably in the seat of a passenger jet as it takes off, shooting a basketball into the net with ease, being able to talk with confidence before a large audience, etc.
4. Assuming that the client is unable to adequately visualize the desired outcome, have the client perform the same visualization enhancement procedure described in item 2: PR → ua, eb → 9G → ua, eb → er. Of course, the psychological reversal treatment will be specific to the issue being treated (e.g., "I deeply accept myself even though I have this problem making a basket" or "I deeply accept myself if I never get over this problem of making a basket" or "I deeply accept myself even if I don't deserve to make a basket").
5. When the client is able to visualize the outcome clearly, assist the client in visualizing the outcome from an associated position. For example, rather than visualizing oneself over there seated in the plane, the client now develops visualization consistent with being seated in the plane. In this respect, the client would imagine the backs of the seats in front, the sensation of the seat against the back, the passenger seated at the left or

right, the scenery rapidly moving past the window as the jet speeds down
the runway, the sound of the jet's engines, etc. This phase of the protocol
may also require the visualization enhancement procedure.

6. Depending on the client's speed of integration, several aspects of the
   outcome may need to be targeted in this fashion.

RELATED TREATMENT METHODS

Although the thought field therapy algorithms represent an attempt to define treatment
needs by providing precisely defined sequences of meridian points, other treatment
procedures exist that generally take a more global approach to treatment. These
methods do not proceed on the assumption that sequence or even specific meridian
acupoints necessarily matter. Rather, they simply focus on activating the energy
system as a whole, thus removing or overriding energy blocks or perturbations.

EMOTIONAL STRESS RELEASE

In the 1930s, Terrence Bennett, D.C., discovered a number of neurovascular reflexes
about the cranium that he believed affect vascular flow throughout the body (Walther,
1988). In the 1960s, Goodheart investigated these reflexes and concluded that they
also related to specific muscles (Goodheart, 1987). He found that muscle functioning
could be improved by stimulating the respective Bennett reflexes. Additionally, he
observed that the Bennett reflexes located at the frontal eminence were associated
with a large number of muscles and that by stimulating these reflexes, emotional
conditions could also be effectively treated.* In that these emotional neurovascular
reflexes improve muscle functioning, it follows that they also affect meridian functioning. Therefore, this method may also be considered within the realm of energy
psychology and psychotherapy.

The emotional neurovascular reflexes are located on the small protrusions on
the forehead, the frontal eminence, halfway between the middle of each eyebrow
and the normal hairline (Figure 7.7). A modified protocol that I have been effectively
using with a variety of patients over the past few years follows:

1. The subject closes the eyes and lightly places the fingertips on the emotional stress release points. The skin over the emotional stress release points
   should be pulled lightly in the direction of the sides of the head. Alternatively, the therapist can hold the reflex points. In either case, the thumbs
   should not be touching the emotional stress release points, as the thumbs'
   pulses will confound perception of the emotional neurovascular pulses.
2. The subject directs attention on these points and attempts to locate a pulse,
   which is approximately 72 beats per minute. This pulse is independent of
   the heart rate (see Chapter 4). The subject continues to focus on the pulse

---

* The neurovascular reflexes on the frontal eminences, also referred to as the emotional neurovascular
reflexes, are related to the following muscles: supinator, pectoralis clavicular, sacrospinalis, peroneus
tertius, peroneus longus, peroneus brevis, tibialis anterior, rhomboids, biceps brachii, flexor hallucis
longus, and flexor hallucis brevis.

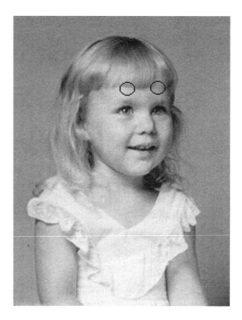

FIGURE 7.7 Emotional stress release neurovascular reflexes. The reflex points are touched lightly with the fingertips of both hands while the subject holds the distressing issue in mind. One or several sets of the emotional stress release often alleviate the associated distress.

of each reflex point until they are synchronized, pulsating in unison. (If the subject cannot feel the pulses after a few attempts, proceed without taking pulse perception into account.)

3. The subject thinks about the specific emotionally charged issue (e.g., phobia, trauma, etc.) and rates the subjective units of distress in the range of 1 to 10. Frequently, the pulse at the frontal eminence will not be synchronized when the stress is initially accessed.
4. The subject remains focused on the issue and the pulses until the pulses synchronize again and the issue becomes difficult to keep in mind. Generally, there will be a shift in a more relaxed, more accepting or otherwise more positive direction. This will generally occur within a few seconds to a few minutes.
5. Discontinue stimulation of the points and reevaluate the subjective units of distress.
6. If the distress is not down to a "1," repeat the process until the emotional stress is entirely released.
7. If the process stalls at any time, consider the various psychological and criteria-related reversals outlined earlier.

FRONTAL/OCCIPITAL HOLDING

Frontal/occipital (F/O) holding is one of the stress-defusing methods used in three-in-one concepts (also referred to as *one brain*) to alleviate trauma. It may also be employed to alleviate a variety of other stress-related conditions. It is similar to emotional stress release in that the neurovascular reflexes on the forehead are activated while the patient visualizes or otherwise thinks about the trauma or stressful situation. However, with frontal/occipital holding, the therapist or client places the palm of one hand on the forehead, while the other palm rests on the occipital bone at the back of the head (Figure 7.8). This method elaborates the details of the trauma while the patient is assisted in reexperiencing it in a detached manner. (It is assumed that the hand on the occipital region activates visual memories in visual centers of the brain and sends them forward into the frontal lobes of consciousness.) The therapist can also assist the client at this point in visualizing or thinking about the historical information in an altered form, rewriting history so to speak, or revising one's decisions in relationship to the event.

EMOTIONAL FREEDOM TECHNIQUES*

Gary Craig, a Stanford-trained engineer, began studying Callahan's methods in the early 1990s, learning muscle testing diagnosis as well as voice technology. In time, he came to develop a pragmatic comprehensive algorithm, referred to as the "basic recipe," after tallying the treatment points that came up most frequently through diagnosis. He reported that he found the basic recipe to be effective approximately 80% of the time for the people with whom he tried the approach. Initially, he also employed a sequence within a sequence that involves going back and forth along a defined group of points so as to take into account a wide array of sequences of meridian points nested within the whole. The initial basic recipe included the following treatment points, as designated by Craig (1993):

EB = Beginning of the Eye Brow
UE = Under the Eye
CB = Beneath the Collarbone
UA = Under the Arm
 IF = Index Finger
LF = Little Finger
9G = 9 Gamut Procedure†
PR = Psychological Reversal Treatment

With these treatment points, the basic recipe proceeds as follows. It should be observed that the treatment for specific reversal is conducted at the beginning of the sequence without diagnosing its presence. This does not pose a problem, since the procedure will alleviate reversal if it is present and will not install a reversal if one is not present:

---

* Gary Craig has developed a training package that includes a manual, 4 audio tapes, and 11 video tapes (or CDs), detailing the application of emotional freedom techniques to a wide array of areas. This program, as well as information about seminars and other products, can be obtained directly from Gary H. Craig, Emotional Freedom Techniques, 38802 Breaker Reach, The Sea Ranch, CA 95497, 707-785-2848, Fax: (707) 785-2600, e-mail: ghcraig@mcn.org, www.emofree.com.
† This is identical to Callahan's nine gamut treatments.

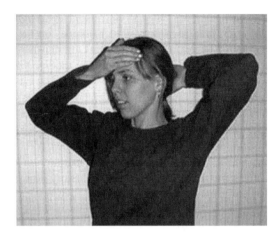

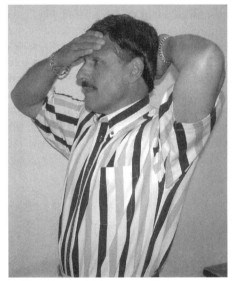

FIGURE 7.8 With frontal/occipital holding, the palm of one hand is placed on the forehead while the other palm rests on the occipital bone at the back of the head. This position is maintained while stressful material is held in mind.

PR → CB, EB, UE, CB, UA, IF, LF, CB

(reverse) LF, IF, UA, CB, UE, EB, CB

(reverse) EB, UE, CB, UA, IF, LF, CB → 9G

(reverse) CB, EB, UE, CB, UA, IF, LF, CB

(reverse) LF, IF, UA, CB, UE, EB, CB

(reverse) EB, UE, CB, UA, IF, LF, CB

Craig found that with persistence, the basic recipe made it possible to effectively treat a wide array of problems. He also incorporated having the client repeatedly state the issue being treated while tapping at each of the treatment points (e.g., "My fear of heights." "This depression." "This craving.").

In time, Craig came to find that the basic recipe could be streamlined by simply proceeding down the body on the Callahan treatment points, excluding the liver meridian point under the breast, and generally excluding the treatment points on the fingers as well (Craig and Fowlie, 1995). The revised basic recipe includes the following treatment points as abbreviated by Craig and Fowlie:

EB = Eye Brow
SE = Side of the Eye
UE = Under the Eye
UN = Under the Nose
Ch = Chin*
CB = Under the Collarbone
UA = Under the Arm
Th = Thumb
IF = Index Finger
MF = Middle Finger
BF = Baby Finger†
KC = Karate Chop

The revised basic recipe is as follows:

Setup‡ EB, SE, UE, UN, Ch, CB, UA, (Th, IF, MF, BF, KC) → 9G → EB, SE, UE, UN, Ch, CB, UA, (Th, IF, MF, BF, KC)

This already incredibly brief treatment can be shortened even further by not including the treatment points within parentheses, which are often unnecessary. Additionally, Craig advises that the setup is indicated only about 40% of the time and the nine gamut treatments are necessary only about 30% of the time.

When providing emotional freedom techniques (EFT), the treatment protocol proceeds as follows:

1. Take a subjective units of distress rating (1 to 10) after having attuned the issue and associated distress.
2. Next, provide the setup. This is treatment for specific reversal. Here, the client karate chops the little finger side of either hand while stating three

---

* The Ch point is equivalent to the UL point in thought field therapy. It is on the central or conception vessel at CV-24.
† The BF point is equivalent to the LF point in thought field therapy.
‡ Setup is Craig's term for correcting psychological reversal at the onset of treatment.

times an affirmation such as "Even though I have this (problem), I deeply and completely accept myself."*

3. At this point proceed with the sequence, tapping five to seven times at each of the treatment points in order while stating the problem aloud. This is referred to as the "reminder phrase," e.g., EB ("fear of heights"), SE ("fear of heights"), UE ("fear of heights"), etc.

4. After tapping at the UA point, reevaluate the subjective units of distress. If the subjective units of distress are down significantly (2 or more points), perform the nine gamut treatments. Otherwise, continue with tapping the treatment points on the hand before evaluating again and initiating the nine gamut treatments (given a significant decrease in the subjective units of distress).†

5. If there is no significant decrease in the subjective units of distress after tapping on the various treatment points, consider that there may be a reversal. At this point, repeat the setup before resuming treatment.

6. Note that a psychological problem may be relatively simple, requiring merely a single run or two of the basic recipe to reduce the subjective units of distress to "1." Other problems are more complex, entailing a variety of aspects. Persistence with the basic recipe often pays off.

7. Similar to standard practice in thought field therapy, when the subjective units of distress level is within the 1 to 3 range, consider using the eye roll procedure as a kind of shortcut to lower the subjective units of distress further without having to repeat the basic recipe.‡

8. Note that Craig also recommends Callahan's collarbone breathing exercises in those instances where the basic recipe has to be repeated frequently and progress is slow, approximately 5% of cases.**

9. Keep in mind that while energy toxins may block treatment effectiveness, Craig indicates that this is rare and that persistence on the part of the client with the basic recipe will frequently result in significant improvement in time. He notes that there are "windows of opportunity" in which the toxin is not exerting its deleterious effects and the basic recipe will work.

Tapas Acupressure Technique

The Tapas acupressure technique (TAT) was developed by Southern California acupuncturist Elizabeth (Tapas) Fleming, L.Ac., who maintains a practice in traditional Chinese medicine. She studied acupuncture in the United States and China, as well as the work of Devi Nambudripad, D.C., L.Ac., R.N., Ph.D., developer of

---

* As an alternative, Craig recommends rubbing the neurolymphatic reflex ("sore spot") on either the left side of the chest or right side of the chest, beneath the collarbones and above the breasts, while stating the appropriate affirmation.

† It should be noted that Gary Craig discontinued using the nine gamut treatments since the publication of the first edition of *Energy Psychology*. The procedure is included in this second edition for therapists who wish to evaluate for themselves if the nine gamut treatments are needed.

‡ Craig has also discontinued using the eye roll procedure, since he believes that it is unnecessary.

** Again, the collarbone breathing exercises have been pruned from emotional freedom techniques since the first edition of this book.

the Nambudripad allergy elimination technique (NAET) (Nambudripad, 1993). She developed the procedure in 1993, originally referring to the method as making peace with your trauma (MPT) (Fleming, 1996a). By 1996, she renamed it the Tapas acupressure technique, apparently to better reflect the scope of its applicability, which is not limited to the treatment of trauma (Fleming, 1996b). The Tapas acupressure technique also entails a treatment philosophy/theory that is consistent with traditional Chinese medicine. The Tapas acupressure technique is described as alleviating duality, which is seen at the heart of traumatic stress and other psychological problems. With respect to trauma, Tapas states the following:

> A trauma occurs when life becomes unbearable and you tell it "No." Or variations on the theme which could include: "Hold it right there." "This is too much for me." "If this happens, I won't survive." This is not necessarily a conscious choice. It is a natural response to your life in that moment. This response sets up patterns of mental, emotional, and physical behavior and health. A blockage, or energy stagnation has just been put in place and your life has been impacted. It seems like a good idea at the time, but you lose the ability of distinguishing the difference between a truly life-threatening event and an event that merely has certain aspects that resemble the original traumatic event. It is as if life were a flowing stream, and at one point, out of fear, you roll a boulder into it to try to dam the flow in order to keep a traumatic event from happening to you. The water, of course, simply flows around the boulder, but in your life — in your body, mind and emotions — there is a blockage that wasn't there before.

> TAT is a way of saying to your whole body-mind: "Have another look at this." It is an opportunity to change, based on taking a new look, rather than continuing to look away. By taking another look, within the context of TAT's direction of the body's energy flow, the charge that is still being held is removed from the past event and the event can now be integrated into your whole system. (Fleming, 1996b, p. 5)

Although it is strongly recommended that the reader study Tapas's method in greater detail by referring to her manual and attending her seminars, the following provides a basic overview of the treatment process.*

1. The client chooses a trauma, phobia, or other issue to treat. Tapas recommends that the person determine if it is permissible to work on this issue at the time, an ecological check so to speak. This may be assessed by checking one's visceral sensations, by an internal image, or perhaps by a therapist-administered or self-administered manual muscle test.
2. The client rates the subjective units of distress in the range of 1 to 10, with 10 the highest level of distress.
3. The client pays attention to the trauma, phobia, or whatever the issue may be. At this point, the Tapas acupressure technique pose is assumed.

---

* Information on Tapas Fleming's seminars and *The Tapas Acupressure Technique (TAT) Workbook* may be obtained directly from Tapas Fleming, L.Ac, 5031 Pacific Coast Hwy. #76, Torrance, CA 90505, 301-378-2318, e-mail: <TAPASVINI@aol.com>.

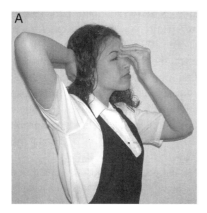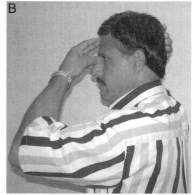

FIGURE 7.9 Demonstration of the TAT pose.

4. The client assumes the pose as follows (Figure 7.9): With either hand, place the tip of the thumb under the same side eyebrow next to the nose. Place the ring finger of the same hand under the other eyebrow next to the nose. This is a light pressure, as the person touches both sides of the upper section of the nose beneath the eyebrows. Also place the middle finger of the same hand 1/2 inch above and between the eyebrows (i.e., the third eye point). The index finger may rest on the middle finger. Additionally, gently rest the other hand on the back of the head on the occipital ridge, the base of the skull (e.g., as is done with frontal/occipital holding).

5. If the person is unable to hold this pose, another person may hold the pose for the person.

6. The client holds the pose until a positive change is noticed or for 1 min, whichever comes first. "Some people notice no change while doing TAT. Common changes include a sigh, a sense of relaxation, not being able to easily focus on the trauma [or other issue] anymore, hands automatically wanting to come out of the TAT position, subtle energy movements in the body, or a sense of peace" (Fleming, 1996b, p. 8).

7. The subjective units of distress using 1 to 10 are reevaluated. If the rating is not yet a "1," any aspect that may be "stuck" is attended to. This may involve a feeling, sensation, thought, sound, etc. The client repeats the pose with this aspect and continues this process until the subjective units of distress rating is "1."

8. Next, a positive, opposite statement about the issue is devised. For example, if the issue was a fear of mice, after the subjective units of distress are at "1," a feasible positive statement might be "I'm comfortable with mice." If the issue was having been in a severe automobile accident, an appropriate statement might be "I survived." After alleviating feelings of depression, it might be appropriate to attend to the statement, "I'm happy with life." The pose is repeated while thinking of this statement.

9. Next, the client pays attention to the "storage place." Metaphor or otherwise, this represents the "place" where the trauma, phobia, etc. was "stored." Tapas advises: "Your 'storage place' is unique to you. It could be your nervous system, your stomach, your shoulders, another person or group of people, or even a city or country: wherever was 'home' for your trauma [phobia, depression, etc.]... You don't need to know where it was stored; you just need to have the intention that wherever it was, that's where you are open to having healing occur" (Fleming, 1996b, p. 8).

10. Finally, Tapas advises the client to drink a lot of water over the course of the following 24 hours. In her view, the Tapas acupressure technique releases not only the mental aspects of the trauma, phobia, etc. but also something physical (toxins) and the water helps to wash it out of the system.

ENERGY DIAGNOSTIC AND TREATMENT METHODS

Energy diagnostic and treatment methods (EDxTM)* is the therapeutic approach that I developed in the early 1990s. It involves various meridian-based protocols in addition to other treatments such as the healing energy light process (HELP) (see below) and modalities that focus on other aspects of the energy system and methods to elevate the client's consciousness of thought. The approach stems from my study and practice of phenomenology, cognitive-behavioral therapy, neurolinguistic programming, thought field therapy, behavioral kinesiology, other approaches to psychotherapy, and various clinical findings.

In addition to discovering various permutations of psychological reversal, discussed earlier in this book, energy diagnostic and treatment methods stemmed from several serendipitous events. For example, one patient complained of unhappiness, which he rated an 8 on a 0 to 10 scale measuring subjective units of distress. Using manual muscle testing, we therapy-localized the liver meridian alarm point, which suggested that the liver meridian was involved in his disturbance. Using the standard treatment point, which is also the liver alarm point in thought field therapy (i.e., the 14th liver point directly under either breast), we did not obtain a decrease in subjective units of distress and he did not evidence psychological reversal. Rather than assuming that we needed to find a sequence before his distress would decrease appreciably, I explored the possibility that simply treating the liver meridian at some other location would achieve a result. We then identified the eighth liver acupoint on the inside of the knee, and after the patient tapped the acupoint several times his distress dropped to 4. Alleviation of distress altogether was obtained after he additionally tapped on the third liver acupoint on the dorsal side of the foot between the great and second toes. Obviously, these results were consistent with a sequence of sorts, albeit within the same meridian and with the points stimulated for an extended period of time prior to locating another relevant treatment point. This was the beginning of what I refer to as the *advanced single point protocol*, as it utilizes one acupoint at a time and is not limited to the 14 acupoints used in thought field therapy.

---

* Energy diagnostic and treatment methods are also referred to as *energetic psychotherapy* or *Energetischen Psychotherapie* in German-speaking countries.

Some patients who did not respond adequately to the single point approach achieved significant results when a cluster or series of clusters were used. Therefore, the *advanced multi-point protocol* was the next logical step. In training programs, we start off by teaching the basic single point and basic multipoint protocols, which simply draw on the original 14 acupoints employed in thought field therapy. After this we bring in other treatment points that have been identified as therapeutically effective.

Additionally, if you will pardon the clichés, I have found that since nature abhors a vacuum, it is often helpful to accentuate the positive after eliminating the negative. Therefore, I developed the outcome projection procedure (OPP), which helps clients to increase the probability that the results will last (Gallo, 2000). After the subjective units of distress have been reduced to 0, the outcome projection procedure is done by having the client develop an image or other thought — a positive outcome projection (POP) — and then install it by reviewing the belief or new behavior in mind while tapping on tri-heater-3 (TH-3) on the back of a hand between the little and ring fingers (some other tapping points are also effective). The level of installation is intermittently assessed by using a positive belief score (PBS), which is a rating of how much the client believes that the results will last. For example: "On a scale of 0 to 10, with 10 the highest level of conviction, how much do you believe that you will be able to comfortably talk to strangers from now on?" Often it is beneficial to apply this procedure "microscopically" to various contexts in which the problem occurred. With smoking cessation, for example, various contexts might include smoking while driving, smoking and drinking coffee, the first cigarette in the morning, smoking while drinking a glass of beer, smoking when upset, and so on. Each of these distinct aspects of the overall problem needs to be neutralized and then replaced with a more desirable behavior through this procedure.

Another treatment approach incorporated in energy diagnostic and treatment methods includes orientation to origins (OTO), which utilizes muscle testing to determine the precise moments or traumas when a psychological problem began and then assisting the patient in altering the conclusion or decision, thus alleviating the problem. This is consistent with psychoanalytic findings and some kinesiology methods.

Other energy diagnostic and treatment methods include protocols for enhancing peak performance, altering pathological core beliefs, identifying and reducing the effects of energy toxins and some allergies, general energy balancing, and elevating consciousness or understanding of thought involved in psychological problems.

NEGATIVE AFFECT ERASING METHOD

During my study and application of Callahan's methods, I initially worked with specific algorithms in addition to various comprehensive treatments similar to the one developed by Gary Craig. For example, one of the first comprehensive algorithms I used involved alternating between each of Callahan's treatment points and the collarbone point (i.e., kidney-27). Besides applying energy diagnostics, in the early 1990s I developed a brief energy-based treatment, the negative affect erasing method

(NAEM),* which many therapists have found to be highly effective in the treatment of various psychological problems. This method has been used to effectively treat trauma, phobias, anxiety, depression, and a number of other affect-based conditions. I have also found it effective for neutralizing negative core beliefs and for instilling positive ones.

The negative affect erasing method is actually quite simple to learn, although expert utilization of the method requires practice and considerable clinical experience. It entails many of the same features that are common to other approaches described in this book. That is, various levels of psychological reversal, treatments for neurologic disorganization, and other ancillary treatments, such as the nine gamut treatments and floor-to-ceiling eye roll, can be incorporated in the overall treatment when needed.

The effectiveness of the negative affect erasing method can be easily accounted for in terms similar to those discussed by various energy theories, quantum theory, etc. However, more traditionally oriented theorists and therapists may be inclined to describe the effects in terms of desensitization, reciprocal inhibition, orienting reflex, pattern interruption and disruption, etc. Surely, the most important aspects of the negative affect erasing method are the therapeutic results that it produces and only secondarily, any theoretical position that it supports.

The four negative affect erasing method treatment points are as follows:

TE = Third eye point, located between the eyebrows. This is the GV-24.5 point on the governing vessel.
UN = Under nose. This point is also on the governing vessel at GV-26.
BL = Under bottom lip. This point is on the central vessel at CV-24.
CH = Chest. This point is also on the central vessel in the vicinity of CV-20, which is also over the thymus gland.

I chose these points after discovering that they were robustly effective in treating many psychological problems. After reading about the use of the third eye point in acupressure and among the Hindus, early on I discovered that this treatment point is effective in treating many psychological conditions. I especially found it helpful in relieving depression before I learned that Callahan frequently used the third point on the tri-heater meridian (i.e., gamut spot) to treat depression. The choice of the thymus point was based on my exploration of behavioral kinesiology, noting that Diamond saw this gland as important in the acupuncture meridians. Further, the treatment points on the governing vessel (under nose) and central vessel (under bottom lip) were chosen because of their use by Callahan as well as their application in applied kinesiology for treating neurologic disorganization. I found that treating these points appeared to treat the meridian system as a whole.

The essential negative affect erasing method protocol is as follows:

1. The client focuses on the issue for which treatment is desired, such as a trauma, phobia, depressed feelings, pain or other physical sensation, etc.

---

* This technique is referred to as the midline energy treatment (MET) in *Energy Tapping* (Gallo and Vincenzi, 2000).

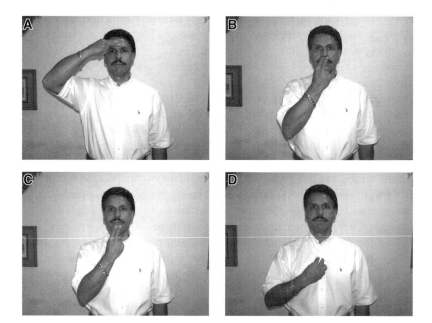

FIGURE 7.10 The four negative affect erasing method treatment points: (A) tapping the TE point, (B) tapping the UN point, (C) tapping the BL point, and (D) tapping the CH point.

A specific issue with a specific associated negative emotion is generally the target of treatment.

2. The client determines subjective units of distress rating using a range of 0 to 10, with 0 representing an absence of negative affect and 10 indicating the highest level feasible to the individual.

3. The client taps repeatedly with two fingers of either hand between the eyebrows at the TE point, continuing to monitor the level of distress (Figure 7.10A). Intermittently, the therapist requests a reevaluation of distress. (In some cases, especially with severe trauma, it is preferable not to have the client continue to think about the distressing issue while tapping at the treatment points. Rather, after an initial rating has been obtained, the entire series of treatment points is completed prior to reassessing the distress.)

4. When the distress level decreases by two or more points, the client taps several times under the nose, the UN point (Figure 7.10B).

5. Next, the client taps several times under the bottom lip, the BL point (Figure 7.10C)

6. Next, the client taps several times at the CH point on the chest (Figure 7.10D).

7. In some instances, effectiveness may be enhanced further by having the patient place the palm of one of the hands on the occipital region at the back of the head, similar to what is done in frontal/occipital holding.

8. After this phase of the treatment has been completed, another distress rating is obtained.

9. If the subjective units of distress are significantly decreased, but not down to a "0," the procedure can be repeated or the nine gamut treatments can be provided prior to repeating the procedure. However, in most instances the nine gamut treatments are not necessary.
10. When the distress is within the 0 to 2 range, the floor-to-ceiling eye roll (er) can be used to reduce the distress further or to solidify results. In this case the sequence notation is as follows: TE → UN → BL → CH → er.
11. If a client does not respond to the TE → UN → BLCH sequence, consider varying the treatment points. However, while a specific treatment point may be preferable depending on the client, in the vast majority of cases, a specific sequence appears to be irrelevant. However, various sequences can be explored depending on the individual client. It should be noted, however, that repeating the series of treatment points several times will often produce results without having to adjust the sequence.
12. Various psychological reversals, as well as switching (i.e., neurologic disorganization), can block progress with the negative affect erasing method, as they can with other treatment approaches. While this is rare, except with the most severe conditions, in such instances treatments for these facets must be provided to realize results.
13. Similar to any treatment procedure, this method is intended to alleviate the real-life problem. Therefore, even though the negative affect may be neutralized within the treatment session, performance in the person's everyday life is what counts. In this respect it is often beneficial after the distress has been reduced to "0," to have the subject think about (e.g., visualize if possible) various contexts in which the problem occurs and to repeat the procedure, again alleviating distress if present. However, even if there is not an elevation of distress when thinking about a specific context, another trial should be provided, as the affect may be repressed at the time of treatment.
14. It is often beneficial to introduce or instill a positive outcome or belief after the method has reduced the distress to "0." Often this occurs automatically, as negative cognitions and beliefs appear to be affect driven. That is, once the affect is discharged, the negative belief vanishes and is replaced by a positive or more neutral assessment. However, in instances where this does not occur to the satisfaction of both the therapist and client, having the client rehearse an antithesis while repeating the method will help to solidify results. For example, a rape victim may have concluded at the time of the trauma that he or she was "powerless." After alleviating the distress of the trauma, it may prove beneficial to have the client create an antithetical statement of his or her own choosing, such as "I'm strong and I survived," repeating this affirmation in the mind while repeating the process. If a phobia of dogs has been neutralized with the method, tapping the same points afterward can be used to install the vision and belief of being comfortable and even enjoying interaction with dogs.
15. In some instances it is beneficial for the negative affect erasing method to be done *in vivo* after it has been provided in the clinical setting. This can

be an aspect of treatment that is conducted by the client between sessions. Many clients find this self-treatment aspect to be quite empowering.

16. Another useful variation is to visualize the unwanted emotion and behavior disintegrating while exhaling and tapping the points in the descending direction (third eye to thymus point) and to visualize the desired emotion and behavior materializing while inhaling and tapping the points in the ascending direction. The materialization phase appears to be enhanced by producing a slight smile while inhaling and tapping. The smile occurs automatically with many clients, although recommending the smile probably enhances the effects that likely include a calming, pleasurable parasympathetic nervous system response and heart–brain coherence.

NAEM and Energy Diagnostics for the Treatment of Trauma

A 19-year-old female college student was referred to me because of post-traumatic stress disorder due to an automobile accident. The driver in the opposing car crossed over the medial strip and struck her vehicle head-on, killing him and both of his passengers. My patient was pinned under the dashboard for several hours while a rescue team cut her out of her car. She had incurred broken ankles, a broken arm and shoulder, and back injuries. She had been suffering frequent nightmares, flashbacks, panic, generalized anxiety, and guilt feelings and anger related to this event. She was also frequently abusing alcohol.

Initially, we chose to focus on the incident of being pinned under the dashboard. After she thought about the incident and rated the distress level as a 9, I then had her dismiss the memory from consciousness while following the negative affect erasing method, intermittently reassessing the distress level. (Rather than assuming the necessity of exposure to promote desensitization, this and other meridian-based therapies do not require detailed exposure.) After about five rounds of tapping, she was able to think about the event without experiencing distress. Follow-up sessions at 1 week, 2 weeks, and 2 months revealed that after the initial session, nightmares and flashbacks no longer occurred. Additionally, if she thought about the event, she could no longer experience emotional distress.

During the course of treatment, other aspects of the trauma were treated, including feelings of anger and guilt about the people who died. That distress was also successfully resolved in one session.

During intake she revealed that a relative molested her from age 5 to 12. After successfully treating the vehicular trauma, we treated several of her distressing memories of being molested. These were easily resolved by employing the negative affect erasing method and a more specifically focused energy diagnostic-treatment protocol involving manual muscle testing.

Even after treating the memories that she was conscious of, she reported a feeling of worthlessness, which entailed a "dirty and disgusting" feeling localized in the vicinity of the lower abdomen. Employing energy diagnostic and treatment methods, we were able to alleviate this sensation and thus the implications about personal worth in a single session as well. Follow-up several months later revealed ongoing relief of this and other issues treated with these modalities. Resolution of the traumas yielded many benefits, including alleviation of intrusive thoughts, flashbacks, and nightmares of the trauma, as well as resolution of clinical depression and a tendency to abuse alcohol.

HEALING ENERGY LIGHT PROCESS

The healing energy light process (HELP), used to globally address therapeutic issues, is covered in detail in a previous publication (Gallo, 2000), and is also available in an audiotape format (Gallo and Wheeler, 2000). In developing the healing energy light process, I incorporated procedures from educational kinesiology, the negative affect erasing method, diaphragmatic breathing, Qigong, an ancient yoga exercise of imaging healing light entering the body, and an aspect of a HeartMath protocol, which involves accessing "heart energy" to promote healing (Childre and Martin, 2000). In the place of tapping on meridian acupoints, acupressure holding is substituted for the most part because touching is less likely to interrupt the meditative experience that is an integral aspect of the process. Consistent with this meditative feature, the client is mindful of thoughts as they come and go without becoming absorbed in any of them. This is a highly relaxing process that corrects for switching or neurologic disorganization and many levels of psychological reversal and is also spiritually oriented. I have found this process to be beneficial in the treatment of a wide variety of psychological, relationship, and even some physical problems, including chronic pain. It is used as an aspect of a comprehensive treatment approach.

A gentleman in his mid-40s came to see me because of depression related to the fact that his 20-year-old daughter would have nothing to do with him. In the early days of his separation from her mother, she would visit with him, but that stopped sometime during early adolescence. He regularly tried to contact her — sending letters and cards, phone calls, presents on her birthday and at Christmas, etc. While she was in college, he attempted to visit her at the dormitory several times, but she would not receive him. To say the least, he was crushed.

We used the healing energy light process to assist him in resolving the distress about his daughter. After the initial treatment he felt much better, more at peace about his daughter and feeling that eventually things would work out for them. Perhaps it is a coincidence, but when I saw him in follow-up 2 weeks later, he reported that after all these years of alienation his daughter spontaneously contacted him and indicated a desire to see him. That was nearly 2 years ago and their relationship is good. They see each other regularly, and the previous falling out is a thing of the past.

Perhaps it is not a coincidence at all. Perhaps this effect is consistent with the positive results we sometimes find with prayer, distant healing, psychokinesis, and consistent Bell's theorem. Recall the physics experiments that demonstrated a non-local connection between related photons (Clauser et al., 1978; Aspect et al., 1982; Tittel et al., 1998). I would suggest that consciousness and energy are interrelated and that when you resolve a relationship problem in yourself, this promotes a resonating of energy that touches the other person in a positive way, even when that occurs at a distance.

Here are the steps for a version of the healing energy light process:

1. Hold in mind the purpose for which you are doing the healing energy light process. For example, purposes include any desirable outcome, such as to overcome depression, increase self-confidence and comfort in social situations, eliminate panic attacks, eliminate this migraine, improve your golf game, etc. Be sure that you are aligned with this intention. Notice how you feel. Do you feel congruent or is there some sense of conflict? If you feel congruent, go ahead with the remainder of the protocol. If not, it might be useful to do the HELP exercise with the intention of resolving the incongruence first.

2. Cross your left ankle over your right. Hold your hands out in front of you, arms extended, with palms facing. Turn your hands over so your thumbs point down and the back of the hands are touching. Raise your right hand up and over your left hand, and interlock the fingers. Turn your hands in and up so that your hands are resting on your chest under your chin.

3. Place the tip of your tongue at the roof of your mouth behind your teeth. Take some slow, deep diaphragmatic breaths in through your nose. Close your eyes and attend to your steady, slow breathing. Also sense that the breath is coming in through the bottom of your feet all the way up through your body. Comfortably hold in mind your intention while doing this.

4. Now become aware that there is a perpetual healing light shining down from the heavens onto your head. This light is a color of your choosing, a color that you associate with healing. This light comes in through the top of your head as you are breathing and then travels throughout your body, vibrating into every cell, every fiber of your body: from the top of your head all the way down your shoulders, into your chest and stomach, into your legs and arms, into your feet and hands. Simply continue to experience this for a little while, perhaps a minute or two. Comfortably hold in mind your intention while doing this.

5. Next unlock your fingers, arms, and legs and set your feet flat on the floor, placing your fingertips in a prayer-like position, the fingertips of the left hand touching the fingertips of your right hand. Your palms are not touching. While you maintain this position, continue to position the tip of your tongue at the roof of your mouth and to breathe slowly and steadily. Continue to sense the perpetual light glowing throughout your body. As you are breathing, continue to notice the breath coming in through the bottom of your feet. Maintain this position for perhaps a minute or two. Comfortably hold in mind your intention.

6. Now discontinue this position and notice how you feel. Next, with light pressure place the index and middle fingers of one hand on your forehead slightly above and between your eyebrows (the third eye point). Take in a deep breath from your diaphragm and then slowly exhale. If you are experiencing any tension or discomfort of any kind, imagine or think that the discomfort is dissipating. You might also think or verbalize this phrase: "Any remaining aspects of this problem are being eliminated from my whole being, from my *body, mind, and soul.*"

7. Now place two fingers under your nose while thinking or announcing, "Any remaining aspects of this problem are being eliminated from my whole being, from my *body, mind, and soul*." Take a slow deep diaphragmatic breath in and slowly exhale.

8. Next place two fingers under your bottom lip and take a diaphragmatic breath in and slowly exhale while thinking or verbalizing, "Any remaining aspects of this problem are being eliminated from my whole being, from my *body, mind, and soul*."

9. Next place the fingertips of one hand at the upper section of your chest and take a diaphragmatic breath in and slowly exhale while thinking or verbalizing, "Any remaining aspects of this problem are being eliminated from my whole being, from my *body, mind, and soul*." It may help to slowly tap on this section of your chest. Exhale and relax.

10. Now place the palm of one of your hands at the center of your chest over your heart and get in touch with the feeling of love, appreciation, or gratitude. Do this in any way that suits you best. Perhaps thinking about your love or gratitude for a particular person, an animal, the earth, a toy, etc. can facilitate this process. Center that feeling in the area immediately around your heart and focus on the healing moving to fulfill your intention. You might use a phrase to facilitate this. For example, "I am sending healing love to (specify)." Or "Healing love, appreciation, and gratitude is giving energy to this intention."

11. Finally, return your awareness to your surroundings and give yourself some time to reorient. Reconsider the issue for which you did this process. In most instances the symptom will be relieved or the issue will no longer carry a negative emotional charge. The process may need to be repeated a few times for you to realize substantial benefit. It should be noted that the process is often best considered to be part of an overall treatment approach.

NEURO-ENERGETIC SENSORY TECHNIQUES

Since practicing energy psychology for more than 12 years, I have found that many of my clients experience relief from a problem — that is, ongoing significant reduction of distress — simply by attuning the problem and then disrupting it through simultaneous stimulation of the body, which also involves dual focus of attention. These active ingredients are discussed earlier in this volume and in previous journal articles (Gallo, 1996a,b). Frequently, variability seems to add extra benefits — for example, tactile stimulation (tapping) at several locations on the body, not simply acupoints. Stimulation of different senses is also effective in this regard. We might even predict that olfactory stimulation would disrupt the unconscious synaptic patterns in the brain's amygdala even more profoundly, as smell more directly affects the limbic system. It should be noted that the olfactory pathways go directly to the limbic areas of the brain rather than being filtered along the way through the thalamus (Campbell and Jaynes, 1966; Dodd and Costellucci, 1991). However, it is probable that the effect of simultaneous stimulation is not limited to the brain but also affects the body as a whole, including energy fields that are integral to our makeup. In other words, it does not simply affect the hardware of the central nervous system but also the cells that communicate via biophotons (Popp and Beloussov, 2003) and psychological software.

If I may coin an acronym for identification purposes, this pattern interruption and disruption technique might be referred to as neuro-energetic sensory techniques (NEST). Essentially, it utilizes two or three variables that are found in many energy psychology approaches. This approach involves having the client think about the problem (exposure or subtle attunement), rate the subjective units of distress, and then stimulate one of the senses, such as by tapping at a physical location on the body (e.g., hands, feet, shoulders, head, etc.). Variable stimulation might involve tapping randomly at various locations. Alternatively, the stimulation can involve various visual or auditory effects (e.g., different colors or lights, different sounds, etc.), different physical movements (e.g., turning around, bending over, rocking, etc.), various smells, and so forth. Intermittently, the level of distress is assessed until no distress remains. After eliminating the distress, the outcome projection procedure can be used to increase the likelihood that the treatment effects remain stable. (See section on energy diagnostic and treatment methods for details about the outcome projection procedure.) Also, the client should be instructed to repeat the treatment procedures if the problem returns. Other treatments, such as correcting for psychological reversal and neurologic disorganization, can be incorporated when needed.

Given this approach, the question naturally arises about the necessity of using acupoints in treatment. Certainly, if there is no distinction between tapping at specific acupoints and tapping randomly at various locations on the body, then it makes little sense to learn about the acupoints and the various algorithms discussed in this text. While this is consistent with Occam's razor (*Non sunt multiplicanda extia praeter necessitatem*), which counsels us to be parsimonious in our assumptions and procedures, to dismiss the advantage of stimulating acupoints requires us to ignore the fact that acupuncture and acupressure effectively treat many conditions, that stimulating acupoints has been effective in treating psychological problems, and that there is research that supports the reality of acupoints. Additionally, when employing manual muscle testing to diagnose or therapy localize relevant acupoints to treat psychological problems, specificity of acupoints is generally found (Gallo, 2000, 2002). To draw the conclusion that treatment with acupoints is equivalent to simultaneous stimulation would be jumping to conclusions at this point in the absence of methodologically sound research; dismantling research is necessitated. Neuro-energetic sensory techniques and approaches that utilize acupoints may have distinct advantages. It is possible that research will demonstrate that both approaches work and that treatment with acupoints has unique therapeutic effects. Also the research must not be limited to demonstrating that subjective units of distress can be reduced with both methods; rather, it must determine which approach with which conditions produces ongoing improvements. At this point in time, it is advisable that the therapist have both clinical options available in the service of the client.

CONCLUSIONS

The methods covered in this chapter represent a sampling of what is available in this field of energy psychology. There are a number of energy psychology algorithms that are not covered here, and there are various approaches that do not focus on diagnosing specific acupoints and instead use a standardized treatment recipe. These include emotional stress release (ESR), frontal/occipital holding, negative affect erasing method (NAEM), healing energy light process (HELP), emotional freedom techniques (EFT), BE SET FREE FAST (BSFF), Tapas acupressure technique (TAT), and more.

There are various diagnostic approaches used to specify the characteristics of "imbalances" within the energy system, including Diamond's method (1985); Callahan's thought field therapy (1985); Durlacher's acu-power (1995), which focuses on single meridian points, several degrees of psychological reversal, and altering negative life beliefs and life issues; Gallo's energy diagnostic and treatment methods (EDxTM) (Gallo, 1997b, 2000), which includes various criteria-related reversals and delineates the single most relevant meridian acupoint or cluster of relevant meridian acupoints, as well as methods of elevating consciousness (energy consciousness therapy) and protocols for alleviating energy disruptions associated with negative core beliefs, energy toxins, etc.; Seemorg matrix work (Clinton, 2002), which utilizes chakras in the treatment of trauma, core beliefs, etc.; and Walker's neuro-emotional technique (NET), which is primarily used by physicians to treat the psychological components of a physical problem; and more. There are indications that, frequently, simply introducing variable physical stimulation while attuning a psychological problem can be used to successfully treat the problem.

Given this introduction to energy therapy or energy psychotherapy techniques and methods, we now turn to matters of research and additional clinical issues.

8 Beginnings

The glory of giving blessings to others is that the blessings don't go just to one person.
They spread like sparks of fire. They touch other beings and other parts of the earth, also.

— **Gurumayi Chidvilasananda**

The last chapter of a book should not be the final chapter, especially when it concerns a topic of such great importance. Energy psychology and energy psychotherapy open a plethora of possibilities, infusing new life into the field and making it possible to relieve suffering efficiently. The question now becomes, "Where do we choose to go from here?"

We have discussed various paradigms or models of psychology and psychotherapy, focused specifically on the energy paradigm, and reviewed some highly efficient therapies. We have explored the body's energy system and the origins of energy psychology in applied kinesiology and acupuncture, and we have also touched on some applied kinesiology offshoots, such as touch for health (TFH), clinical kinesiology (CK), and educational kinesiology (Edu-K). In the area of energy psychotherapy specifically, we have reviewed the approaches of Dr. John Diamond and Dr. Roger J. Callahan. Finally, an introductory energy psychotherapy manual has been provided, exploring methodology and techniques for the efficient treatment of a variety of clinical conditions. In this manual we have addressed issues such as client preparation and debriefing, manual muscle testing, neurologic disorganization/switching, psychological reversal and criteria-related reversals, a variety of therapeutic algorithms or recipes, and some related therapeutic approaches. The last has included emotional stress release (ESR), frontal/occipital holding (F/O holding), emotional freedom techniques (EFT), Tapas acupressure technique (TAT), negative affect erasing method (NAEM), energy diagnostic and treatment methods (EDxTM), neuro-energetic sensory techniques (NEST), and the healing energy light process (HELP).

There are other issues that need to be addressed if energy psychology is to gain a firm footing in the field and thus provide increasing numbers of patients and clients with the benefits this approach has to offer. We turn our attention now to matters of research and incorporating these methods into what we do.

CLINICAL AND RESEARCH MATTERS

While clinical reports and case studies can be informative, gratifying, and useful in charting a course, they merely represent the humble beginnings of a field that hopes to develop scientifically and to be accepted into the mainstream of psychological therapy. How do we ever really know what is operating within a technique or method if we simply listen to the opinions of its principal proponents? To paraphrase Immanuel Kant (1783), how can we accurately evaluate the flight of our theories in the absence of the air resistance that empirical studies have to offer? Our theories cannot hold up in a vacuum. While we may believe deeply in the methods and understandings that we employ to assist others and find that these methods are consistently effective and efficient, how can we know that it is not, rather, something about us and our enthusiasm or something else escaping our notice that truly produces the results? And how can we know what is essential to the approaches that we employ and what is not? Solid research studies, both laboratory and clinically oriented, are essential to advance the field and to verify what we do.

Some research has been conducted on energy psychology and more is in progress. Also, there have been a number of significant, well-executed studies on eye movement desensitization and reprocessing (EMDR). While eye movement desensitization and reprocessing is not purported to be energy psychotherapy, its uniqueness and effectiveness challenge the accepted treatment paradigms, as do energy psychotherapies, and provide well-defined protocols that can be readily researched.* This is a credit to Shapiro (1995), her vision, and those who have found the energy to conduct such studies. It will be to the credit of energy psychology to model this vision. Energy psychology will proliferate exponentially as soon as solid research demonstrates the effectiveness of this therapeutic approach.

RESEARCH IN ENERGY PSYCHOLOGY

Although more than a dozen studies have been completed in the area of energy psychology, most of them are methodologically deficient and only a few have been published in peer-reviewed journals. Several preliminary studies have supported the effectiveness of thought field therapy in the treatment of phobias and anxiety (Callahan, 1987; Leonoff, 1995), phobias and self-concept (Wade, 1990), post-traumatic stress disorder (Carbonell and Figley, 1995, 1996, 1999; Figley et al., 1999; Diepold and Goldstein, 2000; Johnson et al., 2001), acrophobia (Carbonell, 1997), blood-injection-injury phobia (Darby, 2001), public speaking anxiety (Schoninger, 2001), and a variety of other clinical problems (Sakai et al., 2001; Pignotti and Steinberg, 2001).

Although the Callahan (1987) and Leonoff (1995) studies revealed significant decreases in subjective units of distress (SUD) ratings, given the nature of the methodologies, which involved treating call-in subjects on radio talk shows, they could not include control groups, placebo treatments, follow-up evaluations, or other evaluative measures. Although the most demanding researcher would dismiss these studies since they merely demonstrate that the procedure was able to decrease the subjects' discomfort at the time, it is interesting that the same level of criticism is not invariably raised when a psychopharmacological study demonstrates that a benzodiazepine or a beta blocker is able to relieve anxiety or deter a phobic response. After the agent has been discontinued follow-up studies would seldom support the effectiveness of the psychotropic in relieving the phobia or anxiety disorder over time. Nonetheless, the ability of a treatment to afford even temporary relief is

---

* In view of the theory proposed in this book, any approach that rapidly and efficiently treats psychological problems must be effecting change at the most fundamental level and therefore at the level of energy.

TABLE 8.1
Telephone Therapy of Phobias and Anxiety on
Call-in Radio Programs

	Callahan (1985–1986)	Leonoff (1995–1996)
Programs	23	36
Subjects treated	68	68
Effectively treated	66	66
Success rate	97%	97%
Mean pre-SUD	8.35 (1–10 scale)	8.19 (0–11 scale)
Mean post-SUD	2.10	1.58
Mean SUD decrease	6.25	6.61
Mean treatment time[a]	4.34 min	6.04 min

[a] Treatment time included discussions with subjects in addition to providing treatments.

considered acceptable by the medical community and as far as the general public is concerned.*

The Callahan (1987) and Leonoff (1995) studies entailed the same number of subjects, 68, with various phobia and other anxiety complaints. All told, 132 of the 136 subjects were successfully treated with thought field therapy. This translated into a 97% success rate, which is really unheard of in the field of psychotherapy. What is perhaps even more significant in some respects is the fact that the total treatment times were exceptionally low, which is also uncommon in the field. Callahan's average treatment time was 4.34 min and Leonoff's was 6.04 min. Within those time frames, the mean decrease in the subjective units of distress was 6.25 for Callahan's subjects and 6.61 for those treated by Leonoff. Across both studies, an overall mean decrease in the subjective units of distress was 6.43. Table 8.1 presents a summary of those statistics.

The Carbonell and Figley (1996, 1999) study was a systematic clinical demonstration project, evaluating the effectiveness of thought field therapy and a number of other approaches, including visual/kinesthetic dissociation (V/KD), eye movement desensitization and reprocessing (EMDR), and traumatic incident reduction (TIR) in the treatment of post-traumatic stress disorder symptoms (see Chapter 2 for details). This study was sophisticated and detailed in evaluative measures and also included follow-along and follow-up assessments. Follow-up evaluations within the 4- to 6-month range revealed that all of the approaches yielded sustained reduction in subjective units of distress, although minimal rebound in subjective units of

---

* Obviously, there are advantages and disadvantages with treatments that afford only temporary symptomatic relief. Concerning the latter, if the client does not assist in alleviating the fundamental cause of the symptoms, the condition may worsen. Consider chronic utilization of tranquilizers. The medication affords immediate relief, but the anxiety remains until the fundamental cause has been addressed. Patients do not learn how to manage anxiety, since the tranquilizer "does it" for them. Also, immediate relief itself can be addicting and therefore, the client develops a compounded problem.

distress was evident in many cases. Although follow-up evaluation time frames and the number of subjects varied considerably across treatment conditions, notably imposing variables, respective mean group treatment times, and post-treatment follow-up subjective units of distress ratings are shown in Table 2.1 earlier in this book.

The Wade (1990) and Carbonell (1997) studies included control groups, randomization, paper-pencil measures, and SUD ratings. The Carbonell study also included double-blind procedures, placebo controls, and behavioral measures.

The Wade (1990) study was a doctoral dissertation. It included 28 experimental subjects and 25 controls. Two self-concept questionnaires were employed in the study, the Tennessee self-concept scale (TSCS) and the self-concept evaluation of location form (SELF). Approximately 1 month after these instruments were administered, the experimental subjects were treated in a group with the following thought field therapy treatment points: stomach-1 (ue or under the eye), spleen-21 (ua or under the arm), bladder-2 (eb or beginning of the eyebrow), and treatment for psychological reversal, which includes small intestine-3 in conjunction with the associated affirmation. Of the subjects, 16 evidenced a drop in subjective units of distress ratings of four or more points, while only 4 of the no treatment controls showed a decrease in the subjective units of distress of two or more points. At 2 months after treatment and 3 months after the original questionnaires were administered, the questionnaires were repeated. Analysis of variance revealed modest but significant improvements in three of the scales: the self-acceptance scale of the Tennessee self-concept scale and the self-esteem and self-incongruency scales of the self-concept evaluation of location form. Results support the effectiveness of a thought field therapy phobia treatment and the hypothesis that the treatment can affect one's self-concept.

The Carbonell (1997) study investigated the effectiveness of thought field therapy in the treatment of acrophobia or fear of heights. The 49 subjects of the study were college students, initially screened from a total subject pool of 156 students with the Cohen acrophobia questionnaire (Cohen, 1977). All subjects completed a behavioral measure, which involved approaching and possibly climbing a 4-ft ladder. A 4-ft path leading to the ladder was also calibrated in 1-ft segments. As the subject approached and climbed the ladder, subjective units of distress ratings using a 0 to 10 scale were taken at each floor segment and rung. Subjects were permitted to discontinue the task at any time. After these preliminary measures were obtained, the subject met with another experimenter in a separate room and a subjective units of distress rating was obtained while the subject thought about an anxiety-provoking situation related to height. Subjects were then randomly assigned to one of two groups: thought field therapy phobia treatment or placebo "treatment." While all of the subjects did the psychological reversal treatment at the onset, as far as the tapping sequence is concerned, the placebo group tapped on body parts not employed in thought field therapy. After these procedures were conducted, subjective units of distress measures were obtained again. If the subject did not obtain a rating of 0, the respective procedure (experimental or placebo control) was administered once again. Post-testing was invariably conducted after the second administration of the procedure. Afterward, the subject returned to the initial experimenter, who was "blind" to the treatment received by the subject, for post-testing. Post-testing was the same as pre-testing, which involved *in vivo* assessment of subjective units of distress ratings as the subject approached and possibly climbed the ladder. Prior to data analysis, comparison of the groups on pretreatment measures revealed that the groups were essentially equivalent. "Although both groups got somewhat better there was a statistically significant difference between those subjects who had received real thought field therapy and those who received placebo, with the thought field therapy subjects showing significantly more improvement. There was a significant difference when all the subjective units of distress scores were averaged for each subject and the difference was more pronounced when examining the subjective units of distress scores of the subjects while climbing the ladder" (Carbonell, 1997, p. 1). Unfortunately, this study has not yet appeared in a professional journal.

Darby (2001) reported on his doctoral dissertation, which involved the utilization of thought field therapy in the treatment of 20 patients with blood-injection-injury phobia. Measures included subjective units of distress and a fear inventory. Treatment time was limited to 1 hour with the diagnostic approach to thought field therapy. Although the study contains many methodological flaws (i.e., the experimenter collected the data and administered the treatments), 1-month follow-up measures yielded statistically significant treatment effects.

Diepold and Goldstein (2000) conducted a case study of thought field therapy with evaluation by quantitative electroencephalogram (QEEG). Statistically abnormal brain-wave patterns were recorded when the patient thought about a trauma compared to a neutral (baseline) event. Reassessment of the brain-wave patterns associated with the traumatic memory immediately after thought field therapy diagnosis and treatment revealed no statistical abnormalities. An 18-month follow-up indicated that the patient continued to be free of emotional upset regarding the treated trauma. This case study supports the hypothesis that negative emotion has a measurable effect and also objectively identified an immediate and lasting neuro-energetic change in the direction of normalcy and health after thought field therapy.

Johnson et al. (2001) reported on uncontrolled treatment of trauma victims in Kosovo with thought field therapy during five separate 2-week trips in the year 2000. Treatments were given to 105 Albanian patients with 249 separate violent traumatic incidents. The traumas included rape, torture, and witnessing the massacre of loved ones. Total relief of the traumas was reported by 103 of the patients and for 247 of the 249 separate traumas treated. Follow-up data averaging 5 months revealed no relapses. While these data are based on uncontrolled treatments, the absence of relapse ought to pique our attention, as a 98% spontaneous remission from post-traumatic stress is unlikely.

Sakai et al. (2001) reported on an uncontrolled study of 1594 applications of thought field therapy in the treatment of 714 patients with a variety of clinical problems including anxiety, adjustment disorder with anxiety and depression, anxiety due to medical condition, anger, acute stress, bereavement, chronic pain, cravings, panic, post-traumatic stress disorder, trichotillomania, etc. Paired *t*-tests of pre- and post-treatment subjective units of distress were statistically significant at the 0.01 level in 31 categories.

Pignotti and Steinberg (2001) reported on 39 uncontrolled cases that were treated for a variety of clinical problems with thought field therapy, observing that in most cases, improvement in subjective units of distress coincided with improvement in heart rate variability (HRV), which tends to be stable and placebo-free. The authors suggest that heart rate variability can be employed to objectively evaluate the effectiveness of psychotherapy treatment.

Several additional energy psychology approaches have been subjected to experimental tests. A recent trial compared diaphragmatic breathing with a meridian-based technique (emotional freedom techniques, or EFT) that involves tapping on several to all of the 14 meridian acupoints used in thought field therapy for the treatment of specific phobias of small animals (Wells et al., 2003). Subjects were randomly assigned and treated individually for 30 minutes with meridian tapping ($n = 18$) or diaphragmatic breathing ($n = 17$). Statistical analyses revealed that both treatments produced significant improvements in phobic reactions, although tapping on meridian points produced significantly greater improvement behaviorally and on three self-report measures. The greater improvement for the energy technique was maintained at 6- to 9-month follow-ups on the behavioral measure (i.e., avoidance behavior). These results were achieved in a single 30-minute treatment without inducing the anxiety typical of traditional exposure therapies and without *in vivo* exposure to the animals during the treatment phases. Since similar levels of imaginary exposure, experimental demand, and cognitive processing were present in the two treatment conditions, this suggests that additional factors contributed to the results achieved by the energy psychology treatment. It is postulated that intervening in the body's energy system through the meridian acupoints may have been the differentiating factor. While there is a need to corroborate these findings through comparing energy tapping to traditional behavior therapies and to investigate other clinical conditions in which this method may be of value, these results are certainly encouraging about the effectiveness of meridian-based therapies with specific phobias.*

Another study of emotional freedom techniques focused on subjects who had been involved in motor vehicle accidents and who experienced post-traumatic stress associated with the accident (Swingle and Pulos, 2000). All subjects received two treatment sessions and all reported improvement immediately following treatment. Brain-wave assessments before and after treatment indicated that subjects who sustained the benefit of the treatments had increased 13 to 15 Hz amplitude over the sensory motor cortex, decreased right frontal cortex arousal, and an increased 3 to 7 Hz/16 to 25 Hz ratio in the occipital region.

Waite and Holder (2003) conducted a study of emotional freedom techniques for phobias and other fears with 119 university students. An independent four-group design was used and subjects were treated in group settings. The treatment conditions included emotional freedom techniques, placebo (tapping sham points on the arms), modeling (tapping the acupoints on a doll) and no treatment controls. Although the difference between the emotional freedom techniques and control groups did not reach significance, a statistically significant decrease in subjective units of distress at post-treatment was evident with all three groups. Discomfort ratings decreased

---

* It should be noted that the article does not specify which acupoints were utilized with the subjects. The authors state that all 12 meridian points were used, whereas 14 acupoints can be employed in this comprehensive algorithm.

from baseline to post-treatment for the emotional freedom techniques ($p = .003$), placebo ($p < .001$), and doll tapping ($p < .001$) groups, but not for controls ($p = .255$). Although the authors suggest that the effects of emotional freedom techniques are related to systematic desensitization and distraction, it should be noted that the placebo and modeling groups also involved simultaneous physical stimulation, treatment for psychological reversal, a simplified collarbone breathing exercise, reminder phrases and the nine gamut treatments. I believe that these factors significantly minimized the distinction among the various treatment conditions and compromised the results. Additionally, the study was limited to subjective units of distress and did not involve follow-up evaluations as was the case with the Wells study (2003). The researchers conclude, "The clinical significance of EFT, including the duration of treatment effectiveness, still needs to be ascertained" (p. 26).

A doctoral dissertation experimental study of the original BE SET FREE FAST (BSFF) procedure, which involves a four-point tapping routine combined with statements regarding elimination of emotional distress, suggests that this approach is effective in the treatment of insect phobia (Christoff, 2003).* This research involved four single case design studies. Specifically, two of the subjects were phobic of crickets, one of ants, and one of caterpillars and worms. For each subject, extensive pre- and post-testing was done during six twice-weekly sessions to establish baselines followed by six treatment sessions and evaluation. Continued monitoring with psychological instruments was conducted at the following six sessions. Also, subjective units of distress and heart rate measures were obtained throughout the study. The major portion of phobic reduction occurred during the seventh session (i.e., the first treatment session), with some additional improvement in the next one to two sessions. In all four cases, the tests confirmed and the clients experienced sharp drops in their phobic experience and the subjects reported that they were no longer having difficulty or discomfort in the presence of the phobic object.

A pilot study examined the effects of energy psychology on claustrophobia with four claustrophobic subjects and four normal controls (Lambrou et al., 2001). All subjects were evaluated with pencil-paper tests, biofeedback measures, and subjective and behavioral measures before and after treatment and at approximately 2-week follow-up. A unique feature of this study is that the electrical properties in the acupuncture system were measured. Statistical analysis revealed significant differences before and after treatment between the control group and the group with claustrophobia. The researchers noted that the measures of autonomic functions included in the study are less susceptible to placebo or positive expectancy effects.

The most extensive preliminary clinical trial on the effectiveness of energy psychology was conducted in Uruguay, South America (Andrade and Feinstein, 2003). The study took place over a 5-year period with 5000 patients diagnosed with panic disorders, agoraphobia, social phobias, specific phobias, obsessive-compulsive disorder, generalized anxiety disorder, post-traumatic stress disorder, acute stress disorder, various somatoform and eating disorders, attention deficit hyperactivity disorder, addictive disorders, and more. Included in the study were only those

---

* BSFF originally involved tapping on four specific acupoints while making certain pronouncements. See Nims (2002).

disorders in which a treatment group ("tapping") and a control group (cognitive-behavioral therapy plus medication) could be used. The researchers report a 90% positive clinical response and a 76% complete remission of symptoms in the group with tapping alone ($p < 0.01$) and a 63% positive clinical response and a 51% complete remission of symptoms in the control group of medication plus cognitive-behavior therapy. Mean number of sessions in the tapping group was 3, and mean number of sessions in the cognitive-behavioral-medication group was 15. The principal researcher, Joaquin Andrade, concluded

> Whether serotonin, the calcium ion, or the energy field (or some combination) is the primary layer in the sequence by which tapping reconditions disturbed emotional responses to thoughts, memories, and events, early trials suggest that easily replicated procedures seem to yield results that are more favorable than other therapies for a range of clinical conditions. Based on the preliminary findings in the South American Treatment ceters, new and more rigorous studies by the same team are planned or underway. ... While much more investigation is still needed to understand and validate an energy approach, early indications are quite promising. (p. 198–199)*

CLINICAL ISSUES AND FUTURE RESEARCH

While these studies suggest that energy psychology is effective and efficient in many areas, more extensive, well-designed research is needed. This is an exceptionally fertile area of study, worthy of a deluge of surveys, dissertations, nonrandomized and randomized controlled trials, and eventually, systematic reviews of randomized controlled trials.

Research should investigate the various protocols (e.g., algorithms and diagnostic protocols) and eventually involve dismantling studies. As with any solid research, the methodologies should generally entail randomization, matching for relevant variables such as age and sex, and double-blind and placebo controls when feasible and ethical. When a placebo is not appropriate, the methods can be compared to standard therapies. At this point in research with patients, it is most appropriate to compare standard of care with energy therapies plus standard of care.

While subjective units of distress ratings correlate highly with a number of indices, other measures should be incorporated, including physiologic parameters, for example, galvanic skin response (GSR), blood pressure, heart rate variability (HRV), quantitative electroencephalographs (QEEG); standardized objective questionnaires; and behavioral measures. Additionally, because the issue of staying power is relevant, follow-up studies are indicated. Also, before the scientific and therapeutic community will wholly embrace energy psychology, independent replications of methodologically sound studies are essential.

Although this is not intended as a comprehensive overview, the following focuses on supplementing clinical information covered in the preceding chapters and providing some avenues for future research. This hope is that readers with sophisticated

---

* For updates on energy psychology research, intermittently visit my energy psychology homepage at www.energypsych.com.

research backgrounds will be inspired to improve on these suggestions and to carry out revealing studies.

Addiction and Addictive Urges

Any study or clinical work that focuses on the efficacy of energy psychology in the treatment of addiction and addictive urges will necessarily have to explore the hypotheses expressed by Callahan. These include the position that chemically dependent individuals generally are not psychologically reversed for alleviating the addictive urge but are psychologically reversed for getting over the addiction. This can be evaluated through manual muscle testing as well as studies that compare regular usage of the addictive urge algorithms as compared to such algorithms supplemented with treatments for specific and massive psychological reversals. In these instances, the researcher might also consider the relevance of various criteria-related reversals (see Chapter 7).

Another position of Callahan's is that addictive withdrawal is essentially a severe panic attack. This suggests that withdrawal can be efficiently treated with several energy psychology approaches. Studies of this nature must necessarily take place within appropriate medical facilities when treating severe dependence on alcohol, heroin, and other addictive substances that are associated with violent withdrawal. It would be of tremendous interest and benefit if these treatments were empirically proved to consistently alleviate physiologic dependence/withdrawal.

Additionally, considering the position that addiction signals the possibility of the addictive substance simultaneously being an energy toxin or allergen, treatments purported to alleviate the toxic effects of substances should be explored (Hallbom and Smith, 1988; Nambudripad, 1993; Fleming, 1996a,b; Gallo, 2000). See the following section and relevant sections in Chapter 7.

Allergies and Energy Toxins

Callahan has proposed that exogenous substances, referred to as energy toxins, can prevent an effective treatment from working or will otherwise cause successful therapeutic effects to degrade (Callahan and Callahan, 1996). While it has been recognized by others that many chemical substances can elicit negative affects that may be incorrectly assumed to be psychologically based (Rapp, 1986, 1991; Walther, 1988; Travis et al., 1989; Nathanson, 1992), this is actually a rather unique position in the field of psychotherapy.

Callahan's basic approach is to employ applied kinesiology procedures to track down the specific toxins involved and then to advise the patient to avoid them. Reportedly, abstinence then allows the previously ineffective treatments to work. Obviously, extensive experimental research is needed on this phenomenon. While we are exposed to thousands of new substances every year, "only a relative handful [has] ever been tested for their effects on behavior" (Travis et al., 1989).

A highly relevant series of studies could be conducted in this area. Validity studies correlating applied kinesiology tests of substances with other measures would be useful. Investigations of the relationship of chronic psychopathology and exposure to various toxins are needed. Additionally, some have proposed methods purported to be effective in curing allergies as well as possibly energy toxins (Nambudripad, 1993; Fleming, 1996a,b; Gallo, 2000). These methods should be closely investigated, especially as they involve noninvasive approaches to allergy relief.

Clinical Depression

Research in the area of clinical depression is also an area wide open to investigation with these methods. For example, many of these procedures, particularly thought field therapy (TFT), emotional freedom techniques (EFT), negative affect erasing method (NAEM), and energy diagnostic and treatment methods (ED×TM) have been found to be highly effective in alleviating a depressed affect within a few minutes and with sustained relief after a few sessions, according to client reports in addition to measures such as the Beck depression inventory (BDI-II), Hamilton depression inventory (HDI), and Minnesota multiphasic personality inventory (MMPI-2). It would also be valuable to have studies that compare energy psychotherapies with antidepressant medication, cognitive therapy, interpersonal therapy, etc. The eventual hope is to see a National Institute of Mental Health longitudinal study of this nature. Such an investigation could provide much clarification.

Dissociative Identity Disorder

Patients with dissociative identity disorder (DID) are generally assumed to be the victims of significant trauma, as a result of which the mechanism of splitting encapsulates aspects of their personality into distinct personalities, more or less dissociated from each other. In Aristotle's terms, the efficient cause of dissociative identity disorder is the specific traumas. We might look to the material cause in terms of neurochemistry and bioenergy, the formal cause as splitting and perturbations, and the final cause as related to the purpose for which dissociative identity disorder has been "created." Perhaps the latter is consistent with criteria such as those discussed in Chapter 7 under criteria-related reversals.

The process of alleviating dissociative identity disorder entails resolving the traumas that generated the condition in the first place. This can be done singularly or, in some instances, simultaneously. An especially receptive personality is assisted to painlessly neutralize a trauma while other parties observe or even simultaneously participate in the process with their own traumas. Generally, psychological reversals and criteria-related reversals are operating to maintain the dissociation and lack of integration. The clinician experienced in treating dissociative disorders will be most proficient in applying these tools. A comparison of this approach with other standard treatment approaches to treating these conditions should prove of inestimable value.

Generalized Anxiety Disorder

Studies of generalized anxiety disorder, as well as the treatment of this condition, will need to focus on treatment delivered in the clinical setting, as well as equipping the subject/patient with self-treatment procedures for regular use. Consistent with Callahan's position, chronic anxiety may be indicative of the presence of an energy toxin. Researchers and clinicians trained in energy diagnostics are at an advantage in this regard. Relevant studies would entail tracking down the culprit toxins and ensuring that the patients avoid them. These studies would also include regular treatment with relevant algorithms or by utilizing diagnosis or more global treatments such as negative affect erasing method, emotional freedom techniques, Tapas acupressure technique, etc.

In accordance with thought field therapy theory, it should be noted that generalized anxiety disorder and "free-floating" anxiety are essentially misnomers. There are invariably thought fields associated with these conditions, and if the relevant thought fields can be attuned and treated, it is proposed that these conditions can be alleviated.

Medical Conditions

There have been a number of clinical reports of patients being physically helped with various energy psychotherapies. Craig and Fowlie (1995) report on clients being helped by emotional freedom techniques for irritable bowel syndrome, constipation, premenstrual syndrome (PMS), migraines, allergic reactions, hiccups, and even leg weakness associated with multiple sclerosis.

Some time ago, I treated a patient with thought field therapy for her chronic pain condition; she also had a perforated bladder. The possibility of surgery was being considered. After a period of successful treatment for the pain, she returned to her physician, who was surprised to discover that the perforations were healed. Did our treatment accelerate the healing of the bladder?

Another patient with chronic back pain also had severe angina. After a period of successfully alleviating his back pain via thought field therapy, the angina was also relieved, and he was able to discontinue use of nitroglycerin. Did the treatment improve coronary circulation? Or was it the reduction in stress via alleviation of his chronic pain condition that resolved the angina?

Physicians and other health practitioners are encouraged to explore the possibilities of this approach as an aspect of complementary and alternative medicine (CAM). Studies in these areas are needed as we further explore the interface of energy and health.

Obsessive-Compulsive Disorder

Studies of obsessive-compulsive disorder, as treated by energy psychology, would naturally involve comparisons with selective serotonin reuptake inhibitors (SSRIs) such as Luvox and Paxil, the tricyclic Anafranil, exposure and response prevention (EARP), and cognitive therapy. Treatment targets for the energy psychotherapies should include any relevant traumas in addition to obsessive-compulsive disorder symptoms.

Panic Disorder and Agoraphobia

Many clinicians have reported the ability to rapidly assist patients in the throes of a panic attack with energy psychology. In most cases, alleviation of the panic has been a simple matter of employing one of the more complex algorithms (e.g., ue, ua, eb, cb, lf). A number of patients with these conditions also have been able to self-treat effectively when a panic attack occurs. Studies of panic disorder must take into account the same consideration noted with regard to generalized anxiety disorder. That is, in addition to being treated within the clinic, the patient/subject will regularly engage in self-treatment and the possibility of energy toxins must be taken into account. Studies of panic disorder and generalized anxiety disorder can compare the effectiveness of various energy treatments with relaxation training, biofeedback, pharmacotherapy, etc.

Additionally, it has been proposed that patients suffering from panic disorder and agoraphobia have been significantly traumatized by previous panic attacks, which result in their being hypervigilant about the next, possibly "self-fulfilling" episode around the corner.

According to Callahan (1990), complex anxiety conditions such as panic disorder result in a post-traumatic stress disorder. Alleviation of the traumas that catalyze panic disorder should result in significant improvement in the disorder as a whole. Further, therapist availability to provide treatments "on the spot," such as over the telephone and patient training in self-treatment, are imperative.

Specifically with regard to agoraphobia, the treatment necessarily involves targeting a wide range of the aspects involved in the disorder. In this respect, treatment is directed at the thought of distance from the home, distance from the "safe person" when in various phobic contexts, distance from the exit within a building, being in crowds of various sizes, fear of becoming "sick," and so forth. These features or thought fields are targeted within treatment, and the patient is equipped with self-treatment procedures to employ within the various contexts.

Phobias

Studies of this nature can be conducted on various specific and more complex phobias to determine the scope of treatment efficacy. For example, are the specified thought field therapy algorithms, emotional freedom techniques, and negative affect erasing method effective with acrophobia, driving and riding phobia, fear of flying, needle phobia, claustrophobia, agoraphobia, social phobia, and such? Are some types of phobias more effectively treated than others with these methods? How do these methods compare with standard treatments such as flooding, systematic desensitization, and cognitive-behavioral therapies?

Physical Pain

Also, the thought field therapy physical pain algorithm, along with relevant extensions (see Chapter 7), is highly effective in relieving headaches, migraines, and pain in other bodily locations. In instances of chronic pain, frequently the pain relief improves over time such that the treatments work faster and the treatment effects last longer. Pain clinics are encouraged to explore this area, which should prove beneficial to many patients. To hardly anyone's surprise, both clinical depression and physical pain are generally alleviated by the identical thought field therapy algorithms. In cases that do not respond to these therapeutic sequences, the effectiveness of energy diagnostics should be explored.

Psychological Reversal

Throughout the energy psychology literature, it is maintained that when psychological reversal is present, patients do not respond to treatment. A multitude of studies are needed to explore this phenomenon in the areas of psychotherapy, medical treatment, education, sports, etc. In the area of psychotherapy, a study might evaluate clients in terms of psychological reversal prior to their undergoing various therapeutic approaches to determine if the presence or absence of psychological reversal is a primary factor in therapeutic results. Such a study would be complex, as some psychologically reversed clients will benefit therapeutically without having to do a standard reversal correction. Similar studies in the areas of medicine and sports may prove "cleaner" in this respect.

Trauma and Acute and Post-Traumatic Stress Disorders

Trauma, acute stress disorder, and post-traumatic stress disorder are areas of tremendous importance, and each of the energy psychotherapies appears to be effective in these areas. Studies similar to those suggested for phobias can be conducted in this area as well. Given involvement of Veterans Administration hospitals, rape crisis centers, trauma centers, the Red Cross, the Green Cross, and other organizations that respond to crisis, research in this area could literally change the face of trauma. Many of these organizations already utilize specific protocols, which can be compared with these methods.

In this area, studies could also pose questions about therapeutic effectiveness and the length of time after a trauma. Are energy psychotherapies as effective immediately after the trauma has occurred as compared to after a significant passage of time? Here it is hypothesized that, given willingness on the part of the patient and the therapist, it makes little difference, even though this may not be the case with a number of other therapeutic approaches.

Another research question would compare the complex thought field therapy algorithm (eb, ue, ua, cb, lf, cb, if, cb → 9G → Sq → er) with emotional freedom techniques, negative affect erasing method, eye movement desensitization and reprocessing, and Tapas acupressure technique. The hypothesis offered here is that while all of these methods will prove effective, the thought field therapy, emotional freedom techniques, and negative affect erasing method will be significantly faster, albeit not as readily conducive to client conscious insights. A more extensive study could compare thought field therapy, emotional freedom techniques, eye movement desensitization and reprocessing, traumatic incident reduction, visual/kinesthetic dissociation, Tapas acupressure technique, and negative affect erasing method.

Miscellaneous Conditions

The clinician and researcher are referred to Chapter 7 for treatment algorithms for a variety of conditions including anger, rage, guilt, jealousy, fatigue, etc. A wide array of research possibilities exists in these areas as well.

Some clinicians have reported value in using the anger and rage algorithms, in addition to trauma protocols, with prison populations. Highly relevant studies and clinical opportunities exist in these settings for evaluating energy psychotherapies. Given that these therapies efficiently produce clinical and statistically significant results, it is possible that violence within prisons and recidivism can be significantly reduced. Similar studies and programs should be conducted within juvenile institutions as well. Assuming that the results are favorable, this would prove a valuable contribution to our societies.

Is Sequence Necessary?

A major debate among energy psychology practitioners is the question of sequence. Callahan has maintained that sequence of meridian points is of unquestionable importance, and he cites examples of conditions that are effectively treated with a specific sequence. For example, he reports that most specific phobias respond to the sequence ue, ua, cb; except for claustrophobia, fear of spiders, and fear of flight turbulence, which respond to ua, ue, cb. Emotional freedom techniques and the negative affect erasing method, on the other hand, entail a one-sequence-fits-all approach with sequence not relevant at all. Additionally, the Tapas acupressure technique, which simply activates the bladder meridian and governing vessel, entails no sequence and yet reportedly achieves appreciable results in many areas.

It is my opinion that it must be extremely rare that sequence is relevant. In the vast majority of instances, it appears that it is rather the cluster of treatment points and often only a single point that is necessary to produce clinically significant results. When a single-point protocol is employed, however, often extended percussion of the point is needed, as is the case when employing the thought field therapy algorithms for clinical depression and physical pain. That is, the back of hand point (tri-heater-3) is tapped extensively in that algorithm. On the other hand, sequences and cluster treatments generally produce results with less extended percussion of the individual points — only a few taps per point before moving on to the next point.

This question can be easily settled, given adequately designed studies. Of course, this is in the category of dismantling research. One possibility would be to have a four-group design for any thought field therapy algorithm: thought field therapy sequence, no treatment control, placebo control, and alternative sequences. If one chooses to evaluate the thought field therapy algorithm for specific phobias, ue, ua, cb could be compared to random assignments of ue, cb, ua; cb, ue, ua; ua, cb, ue; and so on. By including a placebo control (e.g., elbow, hip, knee), one can determine if a bogus sequence produces a therapeutic effect, if random alternative sequences are equivalent to bogus sequences, if clusters of meridian points are equivalent regardless of sequence, and if sequence is superior to simple cluster. (For purposes of research, the nine gamut treatments and the eye roll would be excluded.) The hypotheses proposed are that the clusters and established sequences will be essentially equivalent in therapeutic effect and that they will prove more effective than either bogus treatments or no treatment controls. However, the bogus treatments should result in a greater treatment effect than the no treatment controls. Possibly, the bogus treatments would at least provide the feature of keeping the patient focused on the present while the relevant thought field is attuned. Additionally, it may be that the "bogus treatments" would produce sufficient stimulation as to result in treatment effects. Let us see.

This design also can be applied to any number of treatment issues, including trauma, depression, physical pain, panic, etc. In this way, it can be determined if perhaps some conditions respond more favorably to sequence than others. The hypothesis offered at this time is that while the bogus treatments may produce lasting therapeutic effects with specific phobias and trauma, significance will not be evident with clinical depression, physical pain, or obsessive-compulsive disorder. Again, let us see.

ALGORITHMS VS. ENERGY DIAGNOSTICS

Algorithms appear to be effective means of treating a wide array of psychological conditions, and yet Callahan and others (Durlacher, 1995; Gallo, 1997b, 2000) offer diagnostic methods that delineate specific treatments tailored to the individual. Are these approaches really superior to treating algorithmically? Also, is there a difference in the effectiveness of the various diagnostic approaches? Callahan's approach involves diagnosing sequences of meridian points to neutralize the negative affect. Durlacher (1995) approaches diagnosis by determining a single treatment point and also provides protocols for alleviating "negative life beliefs" and "life issues." The method proffered by Gallo (1997b, 2000, 2002) provides several treatment points for each meridian and also includes single-point and multiple-point protocols, detection and elimination of negative core beliefs, and an "outcome projection procedure" to solidify therapeutic results by projecting into future contexts. As a number of professionals become well trained in these approaches, relevant comparisons can be made.

THE VOICE TECHNOLOGY™

Callahan describes his voice technology as "the proprietary technology which allows for the rapid and precise diagnosis of perturbations by telephone through an objective and unique voice analysis technology" (Callahan and Callahan, 1996). This method needs to be empirically researched to determine its effectiveness as compared to other diagnostic and treatment approaches. In this regard, a comparison of the effectiveness of voice technology with algorithms, various global energy treatments, and intuitive and surrogate testing should be explored.

Concerning voice technology itself, if the approach involves analyzing frequencies in the voice, there is the question of the actual sensitivity of this technology. Given that modern-day telephone signals are digitized, does a sufficient range remain available to decipher information about correlates with the various meridians?

A preliminary study suggested that reduction of subjective units of distress through voice technology is not significantly better than results obtained by random sequences of the treatment points used in thought field therapy (Pignotti, 2004). However, the methodology employed makes it difficult to draw definitive conclusions in several areas. For example, the researcher knew which treatments were administered to the clients and also administered the treatments herself.

Additionally, a reduction in distress can be achieved through various treatment approaches that target symptoms. Nonetheless, the study raises legitimate questions about the necessity of specific sequences of treatment points and also calls into question the value of voice technology. However, the question remains about the stability of treatment via each approach. Namely, is there no significant difference between reductions of distress via random sequences as compared to voice technology? Also, this study was limited to subjective units of distress and other more stable measures were not included.*

Even if voice technology is an effective approach, many practitioners have successfully helped clients via telephone consultations that incorporate energy psychology treatments. I have utilized comprehensive treatments such as the negative affect erasing method, as well as more specific algorithms, assumptions about the relationship between meridians and emotions, and intuitions about treatment needs. When treating in this manner, I write down the results that the client experiences with each treatment round, which in turn guides the treatment process. That is, the client attunes the issue and rates the level of emotional distress 0 to 10, after which the client is guided through a treatment series and then reevaluated. This feedback makes it possible to adjust the treatments as needed to eliminate distress. Additionally, I have sometimes found surrogate muscle testing useful in enhancing my intuitions about what is needed during telephone treatment. With this approach, the therapist self-muscle-tests to determine the specific treatment points needed. No doubt the ability to accurately perform a muscle test on oneself raises issues of validity and reliability, let alone the esoteric implications of being able to evaluate a client through a surrogate. Nonetheless, this approach has been widely employed in kinesiology and it appears to be of value. Surely, experimental studies in this area are needed as well.

INCORPORATING ENERGY METHODS INTO PRACTICE

In closing for now, we briefly discuss incorporating energy psychology methods into therapeutic practice. Specifically, we focus on the issues of combining these procedures with current methods; achieving a healthy balance of technique and understanding; and exploring the interface of energy, cognition, behavior, and health.

COMBINING WITH OTHER THERAPIES

These methods are so unique and so at variance with what most psychologists and psychotherapists do that initially, at least, we should not attempt to simply employ them independently of the approaches to which we are accustomed. While this may seem an obvious thing, for completeness sake it is put on the record.

---

* While subjective units of distress ratings are not necessarily stable, they are valuable clinical measures that assist in determining progress and guiding the therapeutic processes.

These procedures are best employed within a therapy context and as an aspect of a comprehensive treatment plan. Techniques are best not delivered in a vacuum. As a matter of fact, they never take place in a vacuum. Even if a person obtains information about a technique from an article, book, audio, or video program, a position is nonetheless conveyed, even if it is a less-than-desirable one. Thus, self-help products are frequently best employed as an aspect or adjunct of a comprehensive treatment plan. Many clients who enter therapy have initially attempted self-treatment, which was not quite satisfactory. The self-treating client brings to the procedure his or her own understandings, beliefs, and misunderstandings that significantly interact with the technique.

These cautions should not interfere with basic research. At one level it is entirely appropriate and necessary to separate out the techniques from practice to determine the power of the techniques themselves, independent of the confounding variables imposed by proper practice. However, clinical research should take a rather different course, assessing the power of the methodology as a whole in the hands of capable clinicians. At this level, we desire to know how this therapy plays out in the real world, in addition to the laboratory.

Although this book will assist experienced, capable clinicians in incorporating energy psychotherapy into their clinical practices, attendance at quality training, entailing supervised practice, and even ongoing supervision is recommended to develop expertise in this specialty area. As Marshall McLuhan (1964) observed several decades ago, "The medium is the message." Diverse qualities of information are obtainable, depending on the venue. A book can only provide so much information. There is no substitute for observing a qualified practitioner employ these methods and for receiving supervision.

TECHNIQUE VS. UNDERSTANDING

Techniques are at best procedures that produce specific results in specific contexts. In the therapy realm, not to the neglect of other areas of science and practice, they often emanate from an intuitive leap or studied inventiveness on the part of the creator. Really, they involve a packaging of steps that make it possible for others to reproduce the same quality of results obtained by the developer, assuming that the procedure has been adequately specified.

As mentioned, techniques are best delivered within a therapeutic context and nested within a therapeutic methodology, which includes "rules" about therapist–client interaction, ethics, when to apply which techniques, and so on. However, to simply follow the well-defined rules without being open to the rich information available moment-to-moment within the therapeutic context is to deprive oneself and the patient of valuable opportunities for growth and discovery. This implies a rule to which the other rules must be open.

This is an inclusive paradigm that recognizes that paradigms are forever being subsumed into a richer framework that hopefully parallels the ever-emerging truth. Therefore, this is a meta paradigm. Quantum mechanics has alerted us to the fact that observer-observed (the distinction between observer and object), certainty, and locality are merely illusions, namely, constructs of another paradigm that are useful under certain conditions but hardly the truth. Thus, we ought to be humble about the power of our techniques.

As a corollary to this, it is important that we not give our clients the wrong idea about these techniques. A technique used improperly can convey the position to the client that the client is somehow powerless: that the technique is where the true power lies and that the client is merely a machine that we program or deprogram. But the client is not a machine, not an object. It would be better not to employ techniques at all if we are to mistakenly convey this position. Rather, we should be open to the mystery and view the technique as a means of harnessing the power of life energy, the power within the person.

Consider the process by which one learns to dance. The instructor teaches the steps: "You put your right foot in, you take your right foot out, you put your right foot in and you shake it all about, then you do the Hokie Pokie and you turn yourself around; that's what it's all about." Well if you keep doing it that way, you will hardly ever be dancing, since that's not what it's really all about! But once you move beyond the steps, the steps were merely a way of getting to the real dancing that you already had inside of you. In a sense you are already there, even before you go through the steps of getting there.

When a patient achieves a beneficial result in therapy, the place to which the person arrives is a far cry from the technique that ushered in the change. The technique merely (no small thing) helped one arrive. Used properly, the technique puts the person in touch with the power within, and in various ways, it is proper to remind ourselves and the client of this.

As another example, while antidepressant medications may be beneficial in helping some patients to feel better, to simply depend on the antidepressant without achieving a higher level of understanding can be damaging. If the patient thinks that he or she has a chemical disorder and has no power or choice in the matter, other than to consume the antidepressant, this philosophical position can produce more harm than good. Here the person remains a patient, a victim of the "chemical imbalance." Many who prescribe these agents hold this reductionistic opinion themselves, and herein lies the real problem. The professional who understands the medication as a technique, as a means, is in the best philosophical position to prescribe.

So, too, the therapist who understands that the technique is only a means to the therapeutic end is in the best philosophical position to use the technique. Teaching the person to realize his or her capacity for health is an important aspect of what therapy should be about. The therapist who employs the technique should always have an eye on the power within the person, the god within. This assists the therapist in seeing through the distortions of the ego, which are frequently at the source of disrupted energy. This vision also helps to keep the therapist's energy in balance, which is not only good for the therapist, but this view and this balance in turn aid the client even more.

ENERGY, COGNITION, BEHAVIOR, AND HEALTH

There is an interface of energy, cognition, behavior, and health. When a negative affect predominates, this is consistent with energy disturbances and a perturbed thought field, which in turn are associated with negative cognition and negative behavior. Health is compromised.

But when energy is balanced and the thought field is not perturbed, the affect is pleasant and the cognition and behavior are positive. Health predominates.

There is a cybernetic relationship involved. Although directly balancing the energy system by targeting relevant meridian points can collapse perturbations in the thought field, dissolve duality, and concomitantly alleviate negative affect, cognition, and behavior, this is merely one means by which therapeutic change can occur. This method may surely be among the most efficient, but it is obviously not the only way to produce positive change. Positive change can also occur through higher awareness of thought and behavior, combined with creative choice. These approaches to meridian problems and psychological health are also most profound and intriguing (Gallo, 2001).

Thus said, we close for now with an eye and ear to the immediate future. We may easily predict that the realization of energy and energy fields will so advance psychology and psychotherapy that the fields will be difficult to recognize before long. These approaches will not only significantly advance the fields, more importantly they will help to relieve massive amounts of suffering and to elevate human consciousness as well.

Appendix: Manual Muscle Testing Uses and Abuses

MANUAL MUSCLE TESTING AND KINESIOLOGY

Manual muscle testing was developed by physical therapists Florence and Henry Kendall (Kendall and Kendall, 1949) to evaluate muscle functions for diagnostic, treatment, and insurance purposes. It is based in part on the self-evident fact that structural and nutritional deficits result in impaired muscle functioning, which can be assessed by physically assessing the strength of muscles. This method, variably adapted, is widely employed by physical therapists, chiropractors, osteopaths, physiatrists, some body workers, and some psychotherapists, especially those who practice energy psychology. When manual muscle testing is employed to evaluate psychological issues, it is based on the observation that muscle functioning often evidences distinct characteristics when the patient brings to mind a psychological problem. For example, neuromuscular functioning is generally facilitated when the subject experiences positive emotions, and muscular dysfunction is evidenced when the subject experiences distressing emotions. In other words, positive emotions generally result in a "strong" muscle response, whereas negative emotions, such as anxiety and guilt feelings, generally result in a "weak" muscle response.

Kinesiology is the study of muscles and muscular movement (*kinesis,* motion). It has been a field integral to physical education and sports since the early 1900s. Kinesiology is distinct from applied kinesiology, which was later developed by chiropractor George Goodheart, Jr. (Goodheart, 1987) as a result of his unique applications of manual muscle testing and therapy localization (TL). Therapy localization involves a combination of manual muscle testing with touching specific points on the body, which is purported to assist in disclosing information relevant to the treatment of a structural, chemical, or mental problem. The applied kinesiology approach to manual muscle testing is more subtle than that employed by followers of the method developed by Kendall and Kendall, who use it to evaluate the integrity of muscles and their nervous system supply. Walther (1988) describes the applied kinesiology approach as "functional neurology." In this regard, manual muscle testing is used to evaluate aspects of the nervous system, meridian system, neurolymphatic system, neurovascular reflexes, various organ systems, and more. It is assumed that what is being evaluated is the energy supply to the muscle and not the

211

muscle itself. Any controversy about manual muscle testing appears to be related to aspects of the applied kinesiology approach as compared to the fundamental approach proffered by Kendall and Kendall.

APPLIED KINESIOLOGY OFFSHOOTS

In addition to applied kinesiology, manual muscle testing is an integral aspect of offshoots such as touch for health (TFH), three in one concepts, educational kinesiology (Edu-K) or brain gym, health kinesiology (HK), behavioral kinesiology (BK), thought field therapy (TFT), and energy diagnostic and treatment methods (ED×TM) (Gallo, 1999, 2000, 2002). Many of the approaches that use manual muscle testing, other than traditional kinesiology and applied kinesiology, are often referred to as kinesiology as well. In this appendix, I refer to these approaches as *neo-kinesiology* to distinguish them from applied kinesiology and the original kinesiology. It should be noted that there is a significant distinction between applied kinesiology and neo-kinesiology. While the latter includes thought field therapy, three in one concepts, and several other approaches that employ manual muscle testing, many of these genres are considered by practitioners of applied kinesiology to be less professionally rigorous.

Although most practitioners of emotional freedom techniques (EFT) (Craig and Fowlie, 1995) do not utilize manual muscle testing to determine treatment needs, this approach nonetheless owes its development in part to the fact that Callahan (2001) employed manual muscle testing and other information from applied kinesiology to select the 15 treatment points (12 meridian points, 2 collector vessel points, and 1 neurolymphatic reflex) used in thought field therapy, emotional freedom techniques, and many other approaches. Since I have had the opportunity to work with many professionals who use manual muscle testing over the past 12 years, I have become quite impressed with its utility and its drawbacks.

EMPIRICAL RESEARCH ON MANUAL MUSCLE TESTING

There is some empirical support for interexaminer reliability among manual muscle testers (Scoop, 1978; Lawson and Calderon, 1997). In addition to supporting the reliability and validity of muscle testing as a clinical tool, the Lawson and Calderon (1997) study demonstrated significant interexaminer reliability for individual tests of the pectoralis major and piriformis muscles but not for the tensor fascia lata or hamstring muscles, which involve groups of muscles. This highlights the need for clinicians to be aware of potential inaccuracies when testing some muscle groups. There is also some empirical support that muscle testing by an experienced practitioner can accurately differentiate subjects' congruent from incongruent verbal statements (Monti et al., 1999). Further, a number of studies point to the value of manual muscle testing for allergy detection and regarding the relationship of manual muscle testing to nervous system function (Leisman et al., 1989, 1995; Perot et al., 1991; Schmitt and Leisman, 1998; Motyka and Yanuck, 1999; Schmitt and Yanuck, 1999;

Caruso and Leisman, 2000). Similar to studies with various psychometric techniques, studies on manual muscle testing must utilize accomplished evaluators, as skill with the method necessarily affects reliability and validity of the method. Also, the manual muscle testing technique can vary and this must be taken into account when assessing the meaning of the studies.

MUSCLE TESTING PROFICIENCY

Developing proficiency with manual muscle testing is achieved through attending training with qualified muscle testers and diligently practicing muscle testing. What constitutes a skilled muscle tester is similar to what constitutes a skilled pianist, dancer, singer, or skier; it is an art. Yet through this art we are attempting to discern relevant information. Certification in this technique is an important step along the way. That is what applied kinesiology training involves, and this skill is also taught in the energy diagnostic and treatment methods certification program.*

INTEGRITY AND MUSCLE TESTING

Manual muscle testing can be abused. The tester's intention and level of conscious-ness is important here. By this I mean that there are levels of consciousness that are not well suited to the accurate use of manual muscle testing. Consider shame, greed, striving for power, and other less-than-desirable ego states. These are states of consciousness or understanding that most humans enter at times. Some people appear to want to conduct the test incorrectly because of their own level of consciousness at the time. A position of disinterest in the results and humility is preferred. John Diamond expressed the opinion that therapists should not be allowed to muscle-test until they have achieved a profound level of integrity. This is along the lines of traditional psychoanalysis where the psychoanalyst undergoes treatment before being "certified" to provide the service.

THERAPY AND DIAGNOSIS

The question of the attitude required when conducting diagnosis as compared to therapy and the possible difficulties with combining the two approaches arises. In my experience, I learned how to use psychological testing as an aspect of therapy. There are humanistic ways of so doing that do not create a dual relationship and do not involve objectifying the client. Neutrality is both possible and not, depending on how we define neutrality. If we mean being open to whatever occurs without having a results bias, I find this is possible. These same considerations apply to manual muscle testing. Is it possible for a researcher to control for experimenter bias? I believe so, as long as one is aware that such a phenomenon as experimenter bias exists. Of course, the traditional experimenter has the luxury of creating double and triple blinds, but this is not possible within the context of manual muscle testing.

---

* Visit www.energypsych.com for listings of seminar offerings.

Nonetheless, diagnosis is an aspect of treatment. I think that one of the most important issues here is rapport. Can the therapist who conducts a diagnostic process with a client simultaneously maintain rapport with the client? As long as the therapist recognizes that rapport is ultimately important therapeutically and diagnostically, there is no conflict. Rapport is job number one. In most instances it enhances the quality of information obtained.

SELF-TESTING

What about self-manual-muscle-testing? For example, if you are experiencing distress and you want to locate a principal meridian that can be stimulated to relieve the distress, self-testing might involve therapy localizing various alarm points while testing a muscle on your own body. In self-testing you need to step "out of your mind" so to speak and assume a disinterested position. This is along the lines of mindfulness. You have to "clear" your mind and not engage expectations, although you will observe expectations along the way. However, it is difficult enough to test someone else, let alone yourself. Nonetheless, I think that good self-testing is equivalent to having accurate intuitions.

THERAPEUTIC ALGORITHMS VS. CAUSAL DIAGNOSTICS

While I believe that manual muscle testing is of great value in the area of psychological treatment, it is obviously not a necessary component of psychotherapy, let alone energy psychology approaches. In the field of energy psychology, initially I utilized and taught specific treatment algorithms and various comprehensive treatment algorithms that do not necessitate manual muscle testing. Comprehensive algorithms include emotional freedom techniques, Tapas acupressure technique (TAT), negative affect erasing method (NAEM), healing energy light process (HELP), and related approaches. Negative affect erasing method and the healing energy light process are treatment algorithms from energy diagnostic and treatment methods, which include an array of diagnostic and treatment protocols, many of which involve manual muscle testing (Gallo, 2000).

When manual muscle testing is used to derive the specific acupoints to stimulate during treatment, this is often referred to as *causal diagnosis*. In this respect it is assumed that the specific meridians are associated with or are the energetic cause of the disturbance. By diagnosing and treating acupoints that therapy localize in response to manual muscle testing, it is assumed that the basis of the problem has been addressed. This is distinct from a comprehensive algorithm approach, which does not assume that it is necessary to address the specific acupoints that are revealed during manual muscle testing.

Among the causal diagnostic approaches, thought field therapy includes the assumption that the meridians must be treated in the precise order in which they are diagnosed. However, because each meridian is treated with one standard acupoint, thought field therapy does not assume that specific acupoints are as relevant as the meridians themselves. The 14 thought field therapy acupoints are assumed to have a one-to-one relationship with the meridian as a whole. An interesting problem arises in that many of the points used in thought field therapy are not those that would be expected to affect the entire meridian according to traditional meridian theory. Energy diagnostic and treatment methods do not assume that linear order of acupoints is relevant, although distinctions among acupoints are frequently seen as relevant (Gallo, 2000). [As noted, similar to emotional freedom techniques, energy diagnostic and treatment methods include global algorithms. Energy diagnostic and treatment methods also include meridian and nonmeridian protocols for addressing core beliefs, temporal origins of problems, and elevating or expanding the client's consciousness.]

ENERGY PSYCHOLOGY AND MANUAL MUSCLE TESTING

Assuming that the therapist has developed proficiency, manual muscle testing can be valuable in causally diagnosing the most relevant meridians and specific acupoints that can be used to treat psychological and even many physical disorders. Depending on the practitioner's orientation, manual muscle testing can also be used to determine which neurovascular reflexes (NVR), neurolymphatic reflexes (NLR), chakras, nutritional supplements, flower essences, and homeopathic remedies can be used effectively in treatment.

Manual muscle testing can also be used to identify substances that are toxic to an individual and can help to determine if a treatment has alleviated the toxic reaction. In these areas, the tester is usually using an indicator muscle (IM) as compared to testing a specific muscle with respect to its various parameters (e.g., the muscles associated with certain meridians, neurovascular reflexes, neurolymphatic reflexes, etc.). Indicator muscle testing entails using one muscle in conjunction with therapy localization to draw specific inferences. For example, the middle deltoid muscle can be isolated as an indicator muscle, a distressing issue can be attuned, and then the client can therapy localize (or touch) various alarm or neurovascular points to determine which meridian or neurovascular reflex can be utilized to alleviate the distress. Involved meridians or neurovasculars are those that cause an indicator change from weak to strong, or vice versa. With meridians, the inquiry can be refined further by also therapy localizing specific acupoints (e.g., bladder-1, bladder-2, bladder-10, etc.). Again, the acupoints that result in an indicator change are those that can be effectively stimulated to alleviate the stress.

To some extent, manual muscle testing is based on the naturalistic observation that muscles tend to weaken when a person is experiencing significant psychological stress. Diamond (1985) refers to this as double-negative testing. Therapy localization is based on the assumption that whatever changes the response of the indicator muscle (from weak to strong, or vice versa) can be used to address the specific problem or stressor therapeutically. So if a person recalls a disturbing incident and an indicator muscle weakens in response to the memory, whatever overrides that weakening can be used to treat the distress (e.g., Bach rescue remedy, stimulating bladder-2 or bladder-10, a specific mudra, holding the emotional neurovasculars, etc.). In this respect, manual muscle testing is diagnostic and it is used to guide therapy.

Certainly manual muscle testing is a mechanical process and it requires skill with the technique and therapeutic finesse to maintain rapport and the flow of therapy. But that is seldom a problem for the experienced therapist. As the therapist becomes adept at manual muscle testing, intuitive skill and "flow" predominate in the same way that an accomplished skier or dancer no longer comes to rely on a prescribed routine. The process is conducted skillfully in such a way that the therapist and client are joined on a discovery mission to hear and observe what the body has to say. Obviously, this is a mind–body approach. Nonetheless, this process is distinct from other aspects of therapy. It is a diagnostic process but it is also therapeutic, as it assists therapist and client in observing the issue and therapeutic needs in a more refined way. George Goodheart advised that we should be diagnostic giants and then the therapy is a simple matter.

Manual muscle testing can be a consciousness-raising therapeutic ritual not unlike ideomotor signaling and biofeedback. As therapists practice manual muscle testing, their intuitive abilities are frequently enhanced. For example, the therapist will develop a hunch about what is needed therapeutically and the muscle test helps to corroborate or to refine the hunch. This same consciousness-raising feature assists clients in developing their intuitions, which essentially means that their internal communication network is operating to the fullest. Just as patients can learn to adjust blood pressure or muscle tension via biofeedback, as they observe their muscle response to various statements, consciousness and self-understanding can be enhanced.

I have found manual muscle testing helpful in locating the precipitating events and the client's decision, conclusion, and perception that perpetuates the psychological problem. I refer to this as orientation-to-origins (OTO), which has some similarity to Diamond's upsilon factor (Gallo, 1999), Goulding's redecision therapy (Goulding and Goulding, 1979), and other therapeutic approaches that attempt to pinpoint the historical origin of a problem and to assist the client in altering perceptions. The difference with orientation-to-origins is that muscle testing is employed, the energetic structure of the problem is assessed via therapy localization, and the patient is simply invited to alleviate the problem through any creative means, which is then assessed for effectiveness by the therapist. Of course, manual muscle testing is not always necessary in this respect, but it is frequently invaluable. Once we are attuned to the "deciding" event, the precise moment, the client can become aware of what he or she decided, concluded, perceived and is now free to shift the decision, conclusion, perception in a healthier direction. The original decision is consistent with a negative attachment, which may have been entirely accurate and needed at the time. But now things are different. It is time to release that negative attachment and to flow freely. To paraphrase T. S. Elliot, *as the client returns to this place from which this started, he comes to know it anew for the first time.* And now change becomes possible. Consciousness is elevated and the energetic disruption is alleviated.

In addition, when a comprehensive algorithm does not help the client find the core issue or relieve the distress, manual muscle testing can help us locate the most effective meridian points, diagnose the psychological reversal (PR) blocking treatment from working, find the treatment point or points that help to alleviate the reversal, etc. For example, a standard treatment for psychological reversal is to have the client tap on the side of the hand (small intestine-3) while sometimes making a statement about accepting oneself with the problem. However, that does not always work to correct the reversal. Sometimes the correction is achieved by stimulating another meridian acupoint, such as governing vessel-26, central vessel-24, kidney-27, etc. Manual muscle testing is helpful in making this determination.

I realize that discussing manual muscle testing in this way is not a "convincer" of the validity and reliability of manual muscle testing or the value of it in terms of deciding on which acupoints to stimulate. The only convincer in this area is clinical experience and refined research that demonstrate the effectiveness of manual muscle testing–guided treatment. At present, skeptics are on safe ground, since sufficient definitive research does not yet exist (and likely many skeptics have never seriously worked with or developed skill with manual muscle testing). However, in some respects, I think of manual muscle testing as similar to microscopes or stethoscopes, which hardly require statistical research to support their utility. Arguments against the value of manual muscle testing would be like arguing that a microscope is unreliable since many inexperienced students are unable to see through it. Obviously, there is a difference between the tool and one's proficiency at using it. Nonetheless, skeptics provide an important service in requiring such validation and we should welcome statistical research because there are a number of complications and questions that arise concerning the use of this tool.

ABUSES OF MANUAL MUSCLE TESTING
AND ALGORITHMS

One of the major problems involves the ways the manual muscle testing tool is used, which is the same with any tool. So there are the problems of overuse and inappropriate use. It is not always necessary to use manual muscle testing to determine what is therapeutically beneficial. For example, note the frequent effectiveness of emotional freedom techniques and negative affect erasing method in treating various categories of psychological problems. If a simple recipe can produce the desired result, it is undoubtedly more elegant and parsimonious to keep it simple. Also, this makes it easier for the client to self-treat, instead of having to rely on a therapist. As the old adage goes, rather than simply giving a man a fish, we want to teach him how to fish.

Even though this caution is warranted, we should keep in mind the possibility of a noteworthy difference between algorithm-based treatments and those derived from manual muscle testing or other diagnostic approaches that delineate specific treatment points. While some categories of problems generally can be treated with algorithms, they can also be successfully treated by stimulating acupoints derived via manual muscle testing (e.g., I have found that trauma can be successfully treated by using negative affect erasing method, the thought field therapy trauma algorithms, or emotional freedom techniques.). *If* it turns out (big if) that there is no substantial difference between the two approaches once the subjective units of distress (SUD) are neutralized, the interesting question then becomes why stimu-

lating bladder-10 vs. negative affect erasing method, for example, produces the
same result. Could it be that it does not necessarily matter where we tap? However,
could there be a relevant difference between the results achieved by stimulating
diagnostically derived treatment points as compared to using an algorithm? We
might not observe a difference reducing distress, but are the treatment effects more
substantial and longer lasting with one approach as compared to the other? In this
regard, perhaps there is a deeper or qualitative change when diagnostically derived
acupoints are addressed. That qualitative change might be the difference between
traumatic memories no longer bothering the person as compared to the person's
life changing substantially for the better. Neutralizing a trauma does not guarantee
substantial change. LeDoux (1996) notes that even when treatment alleviates the
conscious distress of a trauma, neuroimaging techniques demonstrate that the
amygdala, an integral structure in the brain's limbic system, continues to activate
when the person is exposed to cues associated with the traumatic event. This
suggests that the trauma continues to exist at a neuro-energetic level even when it
is not registered in awareness. Although LeDoux was not referring to energy
psychology approaches, the relationship might still apply and should not be overlooked with subsequent research.

MANUAL MUSCLE TESTING AND INTUITION

Inappropriate uses of manual muscle testing might undermine a client's ability to
develop deeper intuition about his or her psychological functioning. For example, a
misguided muscle tester might convince a client that the tester knows better than
the client and insist on the absolute accuracy of a conclusion drawn from an inac-
curate test. This might confuse the client's ability to focus. Note the research by
Gendlin (1978) on the client's ability to improve via focusing, regardless of the
therapeutic approach used. Obviously, we should use manual muscle testing humbly,
with integrity and respect. That is, the test is an *indicator* and it is always possible
that we have not conducted the test accurately. Of course, if we are in accord with
reality, the results derived from manual muscle testing will be the "proof." If the
client becomes better as a result of treatments derived from our test, then we have
some indication of the value of manual muscle testing. Accurate manual muscle
testing should help the client to change and to develop deeper awareness.

UNWARRANTED USES

Essentially manual muscle testing should not be used to evaluate something that we
have no way of corroborating. For example, if we were to use muscle testing to
determine if there is life on a specific distant planet or to determine if muscle testing
taps into the wisdom of God, we have no way to determine if we are correct — or
at least not for a long, long time. Similarly, although manual muscle testing might
be used by some to determine the level of truth of a book, religion, political ideology,
etc., what would such a conclusion really mean? Would this be *the truth* or rather
the beliefs of the subject or the evaluator?

Manual muscle testing is not a test of truth but rather an indicator in the same way that any test is an indicator. It is acceptable to state that muscle testing *indicated* or *suggested* (and maybe even *showed*) as long as we are not implying that the testing *proved* anything beyond a shadow of a doubt. As a psychologist, I have applied psychometrics and projective techniques extensively over the years. Any tester worth his or her salt knows that a variety of measures are important in assessing any situation: history, interview, observations, different types of tests, and so on. In professional applied kinesiology, manual muscle testing is one measure taken into account in the process of developing an effective treatment approach. Manual muscle testing should not be considered to be the single most important piece of information to the neglect of other relevant information.

Manual muscle testing is based on certain assumptions, as all tests are. One of the principal assumptions is that challenging acupoints, neurovascular reflexes, and some verbal statements can provide relevant therapeutic information. This is often information that neither the therapist nor the client has in conscious awareness. However, the final test is the behavioral change. Both muscle responses and behavioral change are behavior, but obviously the latter is of a higher quality. Perhaps manual muscle testing would be more accurately referred to as a technique, or manual muscle technique. It has been referred to as "muscle checking" by many practitioners. It is merely a method that assists in the gathering of pragmatic therapeutic information.

Surely this will be obvious to many readers — we cannot accurately use muscle testing to evaluate the effectiveness of manual muscle testing. For example, the evaluator tests a muscle and has the subject say, "Muscle testing is valid." Or "Muscle testing is invalid." If the indicator muscle tests strong in response to the first statement and weak in response to the latter, this cannot serve as proof that muscle testing is valid. To draw conclusions on the basis of such an "experiment" is a confusion of logical levels. The same holds true for using muscle testing to determine if the information from muscle testing comes from heaven above. I emphasize this fallacy because I have observed muscle testing used incorrectly in this way.

WHEN WE'RE STUMPED

I frequently use manual muscle testing when we are stumped. In this respect, it can be used when an algorithm does not work or when we need to discern the origins of a problem. We can also use muscle testing to diagnose a toxin that causes an emotional reaction or that reverses a therapeutic result. However, even in this area, abuses can arise. For example, if a substance tests as toxic to a client, does this invariably mean that the substance is the cause of the problem or the reason for the resurrection of a problem? Some so-called toxic substances might have little or nothing to do with the psychological problem in question. Also in some cases the concept of energy toxins can become a garbage bin to explain away therapeutic failures, thus interfering with the advancement of our therapeutic models. Again, manual muscle testing is an indicator that can be usefully applied in conjunction with other information.

SYSTEMIC MANUAL MUSCLE TESTING

Although there are conceivably many other aspects involved, briefly I would like to touch on one additional feature of manual muscle testing. Manual muscle testing has many systemic qualities, as do all interactions. When the therapist and client interact in this way, some very powerful messages are delivered. It seems impossible to separate this interaction from the underlying assumptions that the parties entertain.

If we assume that manual muscle testing accesses *the absolute truth*, what message is being conveyed? Does this serve to enhance or to undermine the client? Surely, we therapists prefer to undermine whatever it is that causes our clients' distress. However, we do not want to demoralize or to lead the client's consciousness astray in the process, and inappropriate use of manual muscle testing can sway in this way. If we assume, on the other hand, that the test has the same validity and reliability constraints of all other tests, then our interaction and our utilization of the results are quite different. I prefer the latter approach, since it is more in line with what we know about tests, quality therapeutic interaction, and "the truth." And we should not want to interfere with the client's sense of self-efficacy, which is one of the most powerful therapeutic forces we have.

Recommended Reading and Other Resources

Here are some recommended books, products, and information and training sites on energy psychology and other areas discussed in this book.

BOOKS AND MANUALS

Arenson, G. (2001). *Five Simple Steps to Emotional Healing*. New York: Fireside.

Bandler, R. and Grinder, J. (1979). *Frogs into Princes*. Moab, UT: Real People Press.

Becker, R. O. and Selden, G. (1985). *The Body Electric*. New York: Morrow.

Bohm, D. (1980). *Wholeness and the Implicate Order*. Boston: Routledge & Kegan.

Burr, H. S. (1972). *Blueprint for Immortality: The Electric Patterns of Life*. Essex, U.K.: Saffron Walden.

Callahan, R. J. (1985). *Five Minute Phobia Cure*. Wilmington, DE: Enterprise.

Cameron-Bandler, L. (1978). *They Lived Happily Ever After*. Cupertino, CA: Meta Publications.

Craig, G. and Fowlie, A. (1995). *Emotional Freedom Techniques: The Manual*. The Sea Ranch, CA: Author.

Diamond, J. (1985). *Life Energy*. New York: Dodd, Mead.

Diepold, J., Britt, V., and Bender, S. (2004). *Evolving Thought Field Therapy*. New York: Norton.

Dossey, L. (1993). *Healing Words: The Power of Prayer and the Practice of Medicine*. San Francisco, CA: Harper.

Durlacher, J. V. (1995). *Freedom from Fear Forever*. Tempe, AZ: Van Ness.

Eden, D. (with Feinstein, D.). (1998). *Energy Medicine*. New York: Jeremy P. Tarcher/Penguin/Putnam.

Feinstein, D. (2004). *Energy Psychology Interactive*. Ashland, OR: Innersource.

Fleming, T. (1996). *Reduce Traumatic Stress in Minutes: The Tapas Acupressure Technique (TAT) Workbook*. Torrance, CA: Author.

Flint, G. A. (2001). *Emotional Freedom: Techniques for Dealing with Emotional and Physical Distress*. Vernon, BC, Canada: NeoSolTerric Enterprises.

Furman, M. and Gallo, F. (2000). *The Neurophysics of Human Behavior: Explorations at the Interface of Brain, Mind, Behavior, and Information*. Boca Raton, FL: CRC Press.

Gallo, F. (2000). *Energy Diagnostic and Treatment Methods*. New York: Norton.

Gallo, F., Ed. (2002). *Energy Psychology in Psychotherapy: A Comprehensive Source Book*. New York: Norton.

Gallo, F. and Vincenzi, H. (2000). *Energy Tapping: How to Rapidly Eliminate Anxiety, Depression, Cravings, and More Using Energy Psychology*. Oakland, CA: New Harbinger.

Goodheart, G. J. (1987). *You'll Be Better*. Geneva, OH: Author.

Goswami, A. (1993). *The Self-Aware Universe: How Consciousness Creates the Material World*. New York: Jeremy P. Tarcher.

Hartmann-Kent, S. (2000). *Adventures in EFT.* Eastbourne, U.K.: DragonRising.com.

Hartung, J. and Galvin, M. (2003). *Energy Psychology and EMDR: Combining Forces to Optimize Treatment.* New York: Norton.

Hover-Kramer, D. (2002). *Creative Energies: Psychotherapy for Self-Expression and Healing.* New York: Norton.

Kuhn, T. S. (1962). *The Structure of Scientific Revolutions.* Chicago: University of Chicago Press.

Lambrou, P. and Pratt, G. (2000). *Instant Emotional Healing.* New York: Broadway.

Mills, R. (1995). *Health Realization.* New York: Sulburger & Graham.

Pransky, G. S. (1992). *The Relationship Handbook.* Blue Ridge Summit, PA: HIS and TAB Books.

Rapp, D. (1991). *Is This Your Child?: Discovering and Treating Unrecognized Allergies in Children and Adults.* New York: William Morrow.

Shapiro, F. (1995). *Eye Movement Desensitization and Reprocessing: Basic Principles, Protocols, and Procedures.* New York: Guilford.

Sheldrake, R. (1988). *The Presence of the Past.* New York: Times Books.

Thie, J. F. (1973). *Touch for Health.* Pasadena, CA: T. H. Enterprises.

Tiller, W. A. (1997). *Science and Human Transformation: Subtle Energies, Intentionality and Consciousness.* Walnut Creek, CA: Pavior.

Walther, D. S. (1988). *Applied Kinesiology: Synopsis.* Pueblo, CO: Systems DC.

Zukav, G. (1979). *The Dancing Wu Li Masters: An Overview of the New Physics.* New York: Bantam.

AUDIOTAPES AND CDS

Feinstein, D. (2004). *Energy Psychology Interactive CD.* Ashland, OR: Innersource: www.innersource.net.

Gallo, F. and Wheeler, M. (2002). *Healing Energy Light Process* (HELP) Audiotape: www.energypsych.com, 724-346-3838.

INFORMATION, CONTINUING EDUCATION, TRAINING, CERTIFICATION

Association for Comprehensive Energy Psychology (ACEP): Provides annual conferences and other relevant support to energy psychology, 800-915-3606 (ext. 21), www.energypsych.org.

Energy Psychology Homepage: Covers free information on energy psychology, training in energy diagnostic and treatment methods (EDxTM) and energy consciousness therapy (ECT), certified EDxTM Practitioners and Trainers, and more: 724-346-3838 Fax: 724-346-4339, www.energypsych.com, fgallo@energypsych.com.

ENERGY PSYCHOLOGY APPROACHES

Acupower: 800-529-8836, freedomfromfearforever.com.

BE SET FREE FAST: 714-771-1866, www.BeSetFreeFast.com.

Callahan Techniques/TFT: 800-359-2873, www.tftrx.com.

Emotional Freedom Techniques: www.emofree.com.

Energy Consciousness Therapy (ECT): 724-346-3838, www.energypsych.com.

Energy Diagnostic and Treatment Methods (EDxTM): 724-346-3838, www.energypsych.com.

Evolving Thought Field Therapy (EvTFT): 973-746-5959, www.tftworldwide.com.
Healing from the Body Level Up (HBLU): 781-453-0737, www.jsswack.com.
Seemorg Matrix Work: www.matrixwork.org.
Tapas acupressure technique: 310-378-7381, www.tat-intl.com.
Thought Energy Synchronization Therapies: 412-683-8378, www.thoughtenergy.com.

ENERGY PSYCHOLOGY TRAINING LOCATIONS

Brooks & Shaler Conference Partners, Vancouver, BC: info@theconferencepartners.com, www.theconferencepartners.com.
Georgia Bay NLP, Toronto, Canada: gbnlp@gb-nlp.com, www.gb-nlp.com, 519-538-1194.
Institut für Angewandte Kinesiologie–IAK GmbH, Kirchzarten bei Freiburg, Germany: info@iak-freiburg.de, www.iak-freiburg.de, 0049-7661-98710.
Institut für Coaching, Bildung und Gesundheit, Hamburg, Germany: www.coaching-und-bildung.de, institut@dr-karin-hauffe.de, 0049-40-32527923.
Milton-Erickson-Institut, Berlin, Germany: mail@erickson-institut-berlin.de, www.erickson-institut-berlin.de, 0049-3078-17795.
Milton-Erickson-Institut, Heidelberg, Germany: office@meihei.de, www.meihei.de, 0049-6221-410941.
Southeast Institute for Group and Family Therapy, Chapel Hill, NC: vjoines@seinstitute.com, 919-929-1171.

RELATED TRAINING AND INFORMATION

Colorado Consulting Group: DrGalvin@earthlink.net, 719-634-4444.
David Baldwin's trauma information pages: www.trauma-pages.com.
Edu-K Foundation: www.braingym.org, 800-356-2109.
EMDR International Association (EMDRIA): www.emdria.org, 512-451-5200.
Energy Kinesiology Association: www.energyk.org, energyk@sunwave.com, 888-749-6464.
Energy therapy homepage: home.att.net/~tom.altaffer/index.htm.
International College of Applied Kinesiology: www.icakusa.com.
Nambudripad allergy elimination technique: www.naet.com, 714-523-8900.
PsychInnovations: www.psychinnovations.com/y1inner.htm.
Three in One Concepts: www.3in1concepts.net, 818-841-4786.
Touch for Health Kinesiology Association: www.tfh.org, admin@tfh.org, 800-466-8342.

E-MAIL DISCUSSION GROUPS

EnerGym Email List (moderated by Fred Gallo, Ph.D.): Subscribe by sending an e-mail to: energym-subscribe@yahoogroups.com.
Energyspirit1 e-mail discussion list (moderated by Phil Friedman, Ph.D.): Subscribe by sending an e-mail to: PilF101@aol.com.
Institute for Meridian Psychotherapy and Counseling list: Send blank e-mail to IMPC.Forum-subscribe@listbot.com.

Glossary

Acupoint: "Acupuncture point." Points on the surface of the skin, many of which evidence lower electrical resistance relative to other skin surfaces. It is thought that subtle energy from the environment enters the body through these portals. The acupoints interconnect along hypothesized meridians. Acupoints are the locations where acupuncture needles are inserted to balance energetic flow (chi) through the meridians. In many energy psychology approaches, the acupoints are employed in treatment to reduce subjective distress related to specific psychological issues.

Acupuncture meridian system (AMS): Diagnostic and treatment system employed in traditional Chinese medicine, applied kinesiology, and many approaches to energy psychology. This system includes the concepts of meridians, vessels, acupoints, and chi.

Alarm point: Also referred to as test point, these diagnostic acupoints are located bilaterally and along the midline of the torso. There are 12 bilateral and 6 midline alarm points. Alarm points are associated with specific acupuncture meridians and can also be used as treatment points. The governing and central vessels do not have alarm points, although therapy localizing points at the end of these vessels serve as test points.

Algorithm: A procedure or formula for solving a problem. In mathematics and computer science, an algorithm refers to a small procedure that solves a recurrent problem. In energy psychology, an algorithm often refers to a specific sequence of acupoints for treating a problem.

Amygdala: An almond-shaped brain structure within the limbic system, instrumental in emotional expression.

Applied kinesiology (AK): This holistic health system, developed by George J. Goodheart, Jr., D.C., involves utilizing manual muscle testing as functional neurology. AK is concerned primarily with neuromuscular function as it relates to the structural, chemical, and mental physiologic regulatory mechanisms. AK has multidisciplinary applications.

Attunement: Tuning in or accessing a thought field. A therapist can assist the client in attuning a thought field by instructing the client to think about it.

Aura: The energetic field that surrounds and permeates the body, also referred to as biofield. It is hypothesized that the aura is composed of several distinct layers.

BE SET FREE FAST (BSFF): Therapeutic approach developed by Larry Nims, Ph.D. There are two forms of BSFF. The original approach involves a brief acupoint algorithm in addition to the client making statements regarding the elimination of various aspects of the presenting problem. The most recent approach is referred to as instant BSFF and involves using a cue word or phrase to treat the presenting problem.

Behavioral kinesiology (BK): Therapeutic approach developed by John Diamond, M.D., which addresses acupuncture meridians in the diagnosis and treatment of psychological problems. This is one of the earliest approaches that can be referred to as energy psychology.

Biofield: The electromagnetic and subtle energetic field that surrounds and permeates the body, also referred to as aura.

Chakra: Body energy centers that serve as transformers of subtle energies. The chakras are assumed to convert subtle energy into chemical and cellular forms. *Chakra* is from the Sanskrit, meaning "wheel."

Chi: Also written as Qi, this is a traditional Chinese medicine concept that refers to subtle energies or life force. The term can also be translated as power, influence, and mind.

Clinical kinesiology (CK): Also referred to as human biodynamics (HBD), this complex methodology employed by health professionals, is an extension of applied kinesiology that was developed by Alan Beardall, D.C. An assumption of CK is that health is a function of good communication among the body's various systems. There are more than 70 therapeutic procedures germane to CK, including handmodes; Nutri-West® Core-Level™ nutrients; pause lock; cumulative two-pointing, three-pointing, and four-pointing to determine priorities among associated symptoms, meridians, neurolymphatic reflexes, and other bodily systems; etc.

Cranial faults: Failure of the skull bones to move in their normal, rhythmic manner. Neurologic disorganization may be associated with cranial faults.

Cross-crawl exercises: Exercises developed by Doman and Delacato and elaborated further in applied kinesiology and various AK offshoots such as educational kinesiology. These exercises are often useful in the treatment of neurologic disorganization, learning disabilities, and as an adjunct to various energy psychology procedures.

Educational kinesiology (Edu-K): Developed by Paul Dennison, Ph.D., educational kinesiology entails a number of techniques to enhance hemispheric communication and functioning. Brain Gym®, an aspect of this approach, entails a series of easily performed activities to prepare children and adults for learning and coordination skills. Some of the techniques include Cook's hook-ups, homolateral crawl and cross-crawl, positive points, crazy eights, elephant ears, educational anchoring, and assisting the learner in establishing clear and positive goals.

Emotional freedom techniques (EFT): An energy psychology approach developed by Gary Craig. This approach involves a comprehensive treatment algorithm that is used to treat all problems. Additionally, EFT involves various protocol considerations to treat the problem's aspects without causing undue distress for the client.

Emotional stress release (ESR): A treatment approach that utilizes the emotional neurovasculars located on the forehead on frontal eminences to treat emotional issues.

Energy consciousness therapy (ECT): Psychotherapeutic approach developed by Fred P. Gallo, Ph.D. that combines principles of consciousness and energy psychology. ECT emphasizes the energetic interaction between therapist and client, teaching healthy psychological functioning, and addressing relevant principles to assist the client in elevating consciousness.

Energy diagnostic and treatment methods (EDxTM): Comprehensive psychotherapeutic approach developed by Fred P. Gallo, Ph.D. that includes various energy-based protocols for treating conditions such as trauma, anxiety, depression, limiting core beliefs, physical pain, peak performance obstacles, etc.

Energy psychology (EP): The branch of psychology that studies the effects of energy systems, such as the acupuncture meridians, chakras, and morphic resonance on emotions and behavior.

Energy psychotherapy: Psychotherapeutic approaches that specifically address bioenergy systems in the diagnosis and treatment of psychological problems.

Energy toxin: Substance that deleteriously affects the bioenergy system. When an energy toxin is significantly affecting the patient's energy system, therapeutic results can be hampered.

Frontal/occipital holding: A treatment approach that involves holding the forehead and the occipital region of the head to treat emotional issues.

Healing energy light process (HELP): An energy psychology technique that integrates intention, progressive relaxation, diaphragmatic breathing, imagery, acupressure, the negative affect erasing method (NAEM), and elements of HeartMath to treat various psychological issues.

Healing from the body level up (HBLU): Treatment approach developed by Judith Swack, Ph.D. that addresses the somatic, psychological, and spiritual aspects of an issue and involves a synthesis of biomedical science, psychology, applied kinesiology, neurolinguistic programming, and energy psychology with original research on the structure and healing of complex damage patterns.

Hemisphere dominance test (HDT): A therapy localization procedure that assists the examiner in discerning relative cerebral hemispheric dominance and in localizing affected meridians and treatment points.

In the clear: Testing a muscle without concurrent therapy localization or introducing factors that can otherwise influence the muscle to respond as either "weak" or "strong."

Indicator change: A change in an indicator muscle response in response to stimuli or therapy localization from "strong" to "weak," or vice versa.

Indicator muscle (IM): A muscle that is isolated to gauge change in strength or in response to a stimulus.

Meridian: A hypothesized channel that carries subtle energy through the body, interconnected with acupoints. There are 12 primary meridians, 2 collector vessels, and 6 additional extraordinary channels.

Muscular units of distress (MUD): Similar to subjective units of distress (SUD), MUD is a measure of an indicator muscle's response to an inquiry of the subject's level of distress in a particular context. A comparison of the SUD and MUD measures provides additional information that is not available from either alone.

Neuro-emotional technique (NET): Originated by Scott Walker, D.C., this approach utilizes muscle testing to pinpoint the source of the patient's distress, after which the practitioner locates the associated points on the bladder meridian on the spine that abolish the weakness. NET addresses the mental leg of the triad of health, as it is believed that many structural adjustments that do not hold are a function of the mental-emotional factors.

Neuro-energetic sensory techniques (NEST): Pattern interruption techniques that involve tuning in an emotionally charged issue while simultaneously stimulating one or more sensory modalities.

Neurologic disorganization: Also referred to as switching, partially this condition involves the central nervous system misinterpreting and misconstruing nerve impulses. When this condition is present, the effectiveness of manual muscle testing is impaired.

Neurolymphatic reflex (NLR): Originally identified by Chapman, these reflexes are located between and under the ribs and in the pelvic region. Stimulation of the reflexes promotes lymphatic drainage. Some of these reflexes can be used in the treatment of psychological reversal.

Neurovascular reflex (NVR): Originally identified by Bennett, stimulation of these reflexes actuates circulation in various locations throughout the body. Some of these reflexes, especially those on the frontal eminences, can be used to treat psychological issues.

Ocular lock: A useful screening indicator of neurologic disorganization, characterized by the failure of the eyes to work together, often evidenced by a saccadic movement of the eyes at some point along a 360° rotation.

Perturbation: In physics this term refers to a secondary influence that causes deviation in a system. Correlated with specific acupoints, in thought field therapies a perturbation is the hypothesized fundamental subtle energetic catalyst of negative emotions. The term also applies to the fundamental energetic cause of any emotion that disrupts homeostasis.

Professional kinesiology practitioner (PKP): Developed by Bruce Dewe, M.D., this is a training program for kinesiologists who have completed the touch for health training, leading to certification as professional kinesiology practitioner (PKP). The program is a synthesis of findings from applied kinesiology, clinical kinesiology, and other branches of kinesiology.

Psychological reversal (PR): A term coined by Roger J. Callahan, Ph.D., referring to an energetic state that blocks healing. PR is often associated with negative attitudes and self-sabotage. When manual muscle testing is used to diagnose PR, the indicator muscle response generally will be contrary to the subject's expressed intention. For example, in response to the statement "I want to get over this problem," reversed subjects generally muscle test as though they want to keep the problem (i.e., a weak indicator muscle response to this statement). The same subject will test strong to the statement, "I want to keep this problem." Alternatively, I have found that some reversed subjects muscle test that they both want to get over the problem *and* do not want to get over the problem (i.e., both strong or weak indicator muscle responses). There are several categories of PR: massive, specific, mini or intervening, deep level, recurrent, and criteria related.

Pulse testing: A method of testing the hypersensitivity of an individual to an exogenous substance.

Seemorg matrix work: Therapeutic approach developed by Asha Nahoma Clinton, Ph.D., that involves a synthesis of several energy psychology techniques, trauma work, analytical psychology, self-psychology, psycho-neuroimmunology, and spiritual principles.

"Strong" muscle: During muscle testing, the indicator muscle functions neuro-logically to its capacity and immediately locks.

Subjective units of distress (SUD): A subject-reported measure of distress level on a scale such as 0 to 100, 0 to 10, 1 to 10, etc.

Switching: A condition in which the body is neurologically disorganized. (*See* neurologic disorganization.) When a subject is switched, the muscle testing response generally will be equally strong such that no distinction can be made.

Temporal sphenoidal (TS) line: The line on the cranium that begins in front of the auditory canal along the upper border of the zygomatic process and progresses along the anterior superior surface of the zygomatic process to the temporal bone before turning superiorly and coursing along the temporal border of the zygomatic bone. Upon reaching the level of the frontal bone, it continues in a posterior direction along the superior edge of the great wing of the sphenoid and the temporoparietal suture to approximately 1 in. behind the external auditory meatus. The TS line is percussed (temporal tap) in applied kinesiology for treatment purposes.

Temporal tap: A method for interrupting the brain's sensory filtering so as to assess therapeutic effectiveness, improve muscle responsiveness, modify habitual patterns, or install beliefs. The temporal sphenoidal (TS) line is the area utilized for this procedure.

Therapy localization: A diagnostic procedure whereby the subject is directed to place the hand or fingers at a specific location on the body while an indicator muscle is tested to determine changes in muscle responsive-ness. Therapy localization is an aspect of the diagnostic process and must be combined with additional clinical and empirical tests to arrive at a valid conclusion.

Thought field: While thoughts entail sensory, linguistic, neurologic and chemical features, the term *thought field* indicates that thought also entails an energetic field. Although the term was introduced by Callahan in relation to thought field therapy, the term had already been used somewhat differently in *Psychiatry and Mysticism,* an edited book by Stanley Dean, M.D. In his introductory chapter, "Metapsychiatry: The confluence of psychiatry and mysticism," Dean writes, "Thought is a form of energy: it has universal field properties which, like gravitational and magnetic fields, are amenable to scientific research. Thought fields, like the theoretical tachyon, can interact, traverse space, and penetrate matter more or less instantaneously" (1975, p. 15).

Thought field therapy (TFT): Therapeutic approach developed by Roger J. Callahan, Ph.D. that is based on diagnosing and treating energetic aspects of psychological problems as associated with the acupuncture meridians by percussion on acupoints.

Three-in-one concepts: Also referred to as one brain, this approach to stress reduction was developed by Gordon Stokes, D.C. and Daniel Whiteside, D.C. It involves light touch manual muscle testing to identify the client's stresses with their specific emotional characteristics (behavioral barometer) and to pinpoint the origins of the stress through the process of age recession.

Touch for health (TFH): Approach developed by John Thie, D.C. that involves a synthesis of early material from applied kinesiology. Thie's vision was to make it possible for others without medical training or manipulative skills to apply kinesiological methods to enhance self-health and the health of family members. As it turns out, while the lay public has been receptive to touch for health, many professionals have also taken this training and applied it to the treatment of psychological, educational, and health issues.

Triad of health: Structural, chemical, and mental/emotional factors that can result in health consequences when not in balance. The health triad is an essential consideration in holistic approaches.

"Weak" muscle: During muscle testing, the indicator muscle does not function neurologically to its capacity and weakens. This is a measure of muscle responsiveness, not muscle integrity.

Bibliography and References

Agar, W. E., Drummond, F. H., and Tiegs, O. W. (1942). Second report on a test of McDougall's Lamarkian experiment on the training of rats. *Journal of Experimental Biology*, 19, 158–167.

Agar, W. E., Drummond, F. H., Tiegs, O. W., and Gunson, M. M. (1954). Fourth (final) report on a test of McDougall's Lamarkian experiment on the training of rats. *Journal of Experimental Biology*, 31, 307–321.

American Psychiatric Association. (1994). *Diagnostic and Statistical Manual of Mental Disorders,* 4th ed., Washington, D.C.: American Psychiatric Association.

Andrade, J. and Feinstein D. (2003). Energy psychology: theory, indications, evidence. In D. Feinstein, *Energy Psychology Interactive.* Ashland, OR: Innersource.

Andreas, C. and Andreas, S. (1995). Eye movement integration (applied with a Vietnam Veteran who has been experiencing intrusive memories) [Videotape]. Boulder, CO: NLP Comprehensive.

Ashby, R. W. (1956). *An Introduction to Cybernetics.* London: Chapman & Hall.

Aspect, A., Grangier, P., and Roger, G. (1982). Experimental realization of Einstein-Podolsky-Rosen-Bohm Gedanen experiment: a new violation of Bell's inequalities. *Physical Review Letters*, 48, 91–94.

Astin, J. A., Harkness, E., and Ernst, E. (2000). The efficacy of "distant healing": a systematic review of randomized trials. *Annals of Internal Medicine*, 132, 903–910.

Aviles, J. M., Whelan, E., Hernke, D. A., Williams, B. A., Kenny, K. E., O'Fallon, W. M., and Kopecky, S. L. (2001). Intercessory prayer and cardiovascular disease progression in a coronary care unit population: a randomized controlled trial. *Mayo Clinic Proceedings*, 76, 1192–1198.

Bach, E. (1933). *The Twelve Healers and Other Remedies.* London: C. W. Daniel.

Bandler, R. (1985). *Using Your Brain for a Change.* Moab, UT: Real People Press.

Bandler, R. and Grinder, J. (1979). *Frogs into Princes.* Moab, UT: Real People Press.

Barry, J. (1968). General and comprehensive study of the psychokinetic effect on a fungus culture. *Journal of Parapsychology*, 32, 237–243.

Bassett, C. A. L. (1995). Bioelectromagnetics in the service of medicine. In Blank, M., Ed., *Electromagnetic Fields: Advances in Chemistry Series 250.* American Chemistry Society, Washington, D.C., 261–275.

Bassett, C. A. L., Mitchell, S. N., and Gaston, S. R. (1982). Pulsating electromagnetic field treatment in ununited fractures and failed arthrodeses. *Journal of the American Medical Association*, 247, 623–628.

Beardall, A. G. (1982). *Clinical Kinesiology Instruction Manual.* Lake Oswego, OR: Author.

Beardall, A. G. (1995). *Clinical Kinesiology Laboratory Manual.* Portland, OR: Human Bio-Dynamics, Inc.

Becker, R. O. (1990). *Cross Currents.* New York: G. P. Putnam's Sons.

Becker, R. O. and Selden, G. (1985). *The Body Electric.* New York: Morrow.

Benveniste, J., Aïssa, J., and Guillonnet, D. (1998). Digital biology: specificity of the digitized molecular signal. *FASEB Journal*, 12, A412.

Blaich, R. (1988). Applied kinesiology and human performance. *Selected Papers of the International College of Applied Kinesiology*, Winter, 7–15.

Bohm, D. (1980). *Wholeness and the Implicate Order.* London: Routledge & Kegan Paul.

Bohm, D. (1986). A new theory of the relationship of mind and matter. *Journal of the American Society for Psychical Research,* 80(2), 113–135.

Bohm, D. and Hiley, B. J. (1993). *The Undivided Universe: An Ontological Interpretation of Quantum Theory.* London: Routledge & Kegan Paul.

Boudewyns, P. A. and Hyer, L. (1990). Physiological response to combat memories and preliminary treatment outcome in Vietnam veteran PTSD patients treated with direct therapeutic exposure. *Behavior Therapy,* 21, 63–87.

Brom, D., Klebar, R. J., and Defares, P. B. (1989). Brief psychotherapy for posttraumatic stress disorders. *Journal of Consulting and Clinical Psychology,* 57, 607–612.

Brown, G. L., Ballenger, J. C., Minichiello, M. D., and Goodwin, F. K. (1979). Human aggression and its relationship to cerebrospinal fluid 5-hydroxy-indolacetic acid, 3-methoxy-4-hydroxy-phenyl-glycol, and homovannilic acid. In Sandler, M., Ed., *Psychopharmacology of Aggression.* New York: Raven Press.

Burr, H. S. (1972). *Blueprint for Immortality: The Electric Patterns of Life.* Essex, U.K.: Saffron Walden.

Callahan, R. J. (1981). Psychological reversal. In *Collected Papers of the International College of Applied Kinesiology.* Shawnee Mission, KS: International College of Applied Kinesiology, 79–96.

Callahan, R. J. (1983). *It Can Happen to You.* New York: New American Library.

Callahan, R. J. (1985). *Five Minute Phobia Cure.* Wilmington, DE: Enterprise.

Callahan, R. J. (1987). Successful psychotherapy by radio and telephone. *International College of Applied Kinesiology,* Winter.

Callahan, R. J. (1990). *The Rapid Treatment of Panic, Agoraphobia, and Anxiety.* Indian Wells, CA: Author.

Callahan, R. J. (1994a). *Thought Field Therapy Glossary.* Indian Wells, CA: Author.

Callahan, R. J. (1994b). The five minute phobia cure: a reproducible revolutionary experiment in psychology based upon the language of negative emotions. Paper presented at the International Association for New Science, Fort Collins, CO.

Callahan, R. J. (1995). A thought field therapy (TFT) algorithm for trauma: a reproducible experiment in psychology. Paper presented at the Annual Meeting of the American Psychological Association, New York, August.

Callahan, R. J. (1992–1997). Personal communications.

Callahan, R. J. (2001). The impact of thought field therapy on heart rate variability. *Journal of Clinical Psychology,* 57(10), 1153–1170.

Callahan, R. J. and Callahan, J. (1996). *Thought Field Therapy and Trauma: Treatment and Theory.* Indian Wells, CA: Author.

Callahan, R. and Callahan, J. (1997). Thought field therapy: aiding the bereavement process. In C. R. Figley, Ed., *Death and Trauma: The Traumatology of Grieving.* London: Taylor & Francis, 249–268.

Callahan, R. J. and Perry, P. (1991). *Why Do I Eat When I'm Not Hungry?* New York: Doubleday.

Callahan, R. J. (with Turbo, R.). (2001). *Tapping the Healer Within.* Chicago: Contemporary.

Cameron-Bandler, L. (1978). *They Lived Happily Ever After.* Cupertino, CA: Meta Publications.

Campbell, S. and Jaynes, J. (1966). Reinstatement. *Psychological Review,* 73, 478–480.

Carbonell, J. (1997). An experimental study of TFT and acrophobia. *The Thought Field,* 2(3), 1–6.

Carbonell, J. and Figley, C. R. (1996). The systematic clinical demonstration: methodology for the initial examination of clinical innovations. *TRAUMATOLOGYe,* 2(1), article 1. Available from www.fsu.edu/~trauma/.

Carbonell, J. L. and Figley, C. (1999). A systematic clinical demonstration project of promising PTSD treatment approaches. *TRAUMATOLOGYe*, 5(1), article 4. Available from www.fsu.edu/~trauma/.

Caruso, B. and Leisman, G. (2000). A force/displacement analysis of muscle testing. *Perceptual and Motor Skills*, 91:683–692.

Chang, S. T. (1976). *The Complete Book of Acupuncture*. Berkeley, CA: Celestial Arts.

Christoff, K. M. (2003). Treating Specific Phobias with BE SET FREE FAST: A Meridian Based Sensory Intervention, doctoral dissertation. Anaheim, CA: Trinity College of Graduate Studies.

Chuang, Yu-min. (1972). *Chinese Acupuncture*. New York: Oriental Publications.

Clauser, J., Horne, M. A., and Shimony, A. (1978). Bell's theorem: experimental tests and implications. *Reports on Progress in Physics*, 41, 1881–1927.

Clinton, A. N. (2002). Seemorg matrix work. In Gallo, F., Ed., *Energy Psychology in Psychotherapy: A Comprehensive Source Book*. New York: Norton.

Coccero, E. F., Siever, L. J., Klar, H. M., and Maurer, G. (1989). Serotonergic studies in patients with affective and personality disorders. *Archives of General Psychiatry*, 46, 597–598.

Cohen, D. C. (1977). Comparisons of self-report and overt-behavioral procedures for assessing acrophobia. *Behavior Therapy*, 18, 17–23.

Collipp, P. J. (1969). The efficacy of prayer: a triple blind study. *Medical Times*, 97, 201–204.

Condon, W. S. (1970). Method of microanalysis of sound films of behavior. *Behavior Research Methods and Instruments*, 2(2), 51–54.

Cook, A. and Bradshaw, R. (1999). *Toward Integration: One Eye at a Time*. Vancouver, CA: One-Eye Press.

Cooper, N. A. and Clum, G. A. (1989). Imaginal flooding as a supplementary treatment for PTSD in combat veterans: a controlled study. *Behavior Therapy*, 20, 381–391.

Craig, G. (1993). *The Callahan Techniques: Eliminate the Fears, Phobias and Anxieties (Addictive Cravings) That Are Lodged in Your Energy System*. The Sea Ranch, CA: Author.

Craig, G. (1993–1997). Personal communications.

Craig, G. and Fowlie, A. (1995). *Emotional Freedom Techniques: The Manual*. The Sea Ranch, CA: Author.

Crew, F. A. E. (1936). A repetition of McDougall's Lamarkian experiment. *Journal of Genetics*, 33, 61–101.

Darby, D. (2001). The Efficiency of Thought Field Therapy as a Treatment Modality for Individuals Diagnosed with Blood-Injection-Injury Phobia, doctoral dissertation. Minneapolis, MN: Walden University.

Darras, J. C., de Vernejoul, P., and Albarede, P. (1992). Nuclear medicine and acupuncture: a study on the migration of radioactive tracers after injection at acupoints. *American Journal of Acupuncture*, 20, 245–256.

Davidson, J. R. T., Morrison, R. M., Shore, J., Davidson, R. T., and Bedayn, G. (1997). Homeopathic treatment of depression and anxiety. *Alternative Therapies*, 3(1), 46–49.

Dean, S. R. (Ed.) (1975). *Psychiatry and Mysticism*. Chicago, IL: Nelson-Hall.

De Chardin, T. (1955). *Le Phenomene Humain*. Paris: Editions du Seuil.

Delacato, C. H. (1966). *The Diagnosis and Treatment of Speech and Reading Problems*. Springfield, IL: Charles C Thomas.

Dennison, P. E. and Dennison, G. (1989). *Brain Gym Handbook*. Ventura, CA: Educational Kinesiology Foundation.

Depue, R. A. and Spoont, M. R. (1989). Conceptualizing a serotonin trait: a behavioral model of constraint. *Annals of the New York Academy of Science*, 12, 47–62.

Diamond, J. (1977). *The Collected Papers of John Diamond, MD*. New York: Archaeus.
Diamond, J. (1978). *Behavioral Kinesiology and the Autonomic Nervous System*. New York: The Institute of Behavioral Kinesiology.
Diamond, J. (1979). *Behavioural Kinesiology*. New York: Harper & Row.
Diamond, J. (1980a). *The Collected Papers of John Diamond, MD*, Vol. II. New York: Archaeus, 249–268.
Diamond, J. (1980b). *Your Body Doesn't Lie*. New York: Warner Books.
Diamond, J. (1981a). *The Remothering Experience: How to Totally Love*. New York: Archaeus.
Diamond, J. (1981b). *Life Energy in Music,* Vol. I. New York: Archaeus.
Diamond, J. (1983). *Life Energy in Music,* Vol. II. New York, Archaeus.
Diamond, J. (1985). *Life Energy*. New York: Dodd, Mead.
Diamond, J. (1986). *Life Energy in Music,* Vol. III. New York: Archaeus.
Diamond, J. (1988). *Life-Energy Analysis: A Way to Cantillation*. New York: Archaeus.
Diamond, J. (1997a). *A Prayer on Entering: The Healer's Hearth a Sanctuary*. New York: Creativity Publishing.
Diamond, J. (1997b). Personal communications.
Diepold, J. H., Jr. and Goldstein, D. (2000). *Thought Field Therapy and QEEG Changes in the Treatment of Trauma: A Case Study*. Moorestown, NJ: Author.
Diepold, J. H., Britt, V., and Bender, S. S. (2004). *Evolving Thought Field Therapy: The Clinician's Handbook of Diagnosis, Treatment, and Theory*. New York: Norton.
Dodd, J. and Costellucci, V. F. (1991). Smell and taste: the chemical senses. In Kandel, E. R., Schwartz, J. H. and Jessell, T. M., Eds. *Principles of Neural Science*. Norwalk, CT: Appleton-Lange, 518.
Dossey, L. (1993). *Healing Words: The Power of Prayer and the Practice of Medicine*. San Francisco: Harper.
Dossey, L. (2001). *Healing beyond the Body: Medicine and the Infinite Reach of the Mind*. Boston: Shambhala.
Durlacher, J. V. (1995). *Freedom from Fear Forever*. Tempe, AZ: Van Ness.
Durlacher, J. V. (1997). Personal communications.
Epston, D. and White, M. (1992). *Experience, Contradiction, Narrative and Imagination*. Alelaide, Australia: Dulwich Centre.
Erickson, M., Rossi, E., and Rossi, S. (1976). *Hypnotic Realities*. New York: Irvington.
Feldenkrais, M. (1972). *Awareness through Movement: Health Exercises for Personal Growth*. New York/London: Harper & Row.
Feldenkrais, M. (1981). *The Elusive Obvious*. Cupertino, CA: Meta Publications.
Figley, C. R. and Carbonell, J. L. (1995). The "Active Ingredients" Project: The systematic clinical demonstration of the most efficient treatments of PTSD, a research plan. Tallahassee, FL: Florida State University Psychosocial Stress Research Program and Clinical Laboratory.
Figley, C. R., Carbonell, J. L., Boscarino, J. A., and Chang, J. A. (1999). Clinical demonstration model of asserting the effectiveness of therapeutic interventions: an expanded clinical trials method. *International Journal of Emergency Mental Health*, 2(1), 1–9.
Fleming, T. (1996a). Personal communication.
Fleming, T. (1996b). *Reduce Traumatic Stress in Minutes: The Tapas Acupressure Technique (TAT) Workbook*. Torrance, CA: Author.
Foa, E. B., Rothbaum, B. O., Riggs, D., and Murdock, T. (1991). Treatment of posttraumatic stress disorder in rape victims: a comparison between cognitive-behavioral procedures and counseling. *Journal of Consulting and Clinical Psychology*, 59, 715–723.
Foundation for Inner Peace. (1975). *A Course in Miracles*. New York: Viking.

Freedman, S. and Clauser, J. (1972). Experimental test of local hidden variable theories. *Physical Review Letters*, 28, 938–941.

Furman, M. E. and Gallo, F. P. (2000). *The Neurophysics of Human Behavior: Explorations at the Interface of Brain, Mind, Behavior, and Information.* Boca Raton, FL: CRC Press.

Gach, M. R. (1990). *Acupressure's Potent Points.* New York: Bantam.

Gallo, F. (1994a). *Thought Field Therapy Level 1 (and Associated Methods): Training Manual.* Hermitage, PA: Author.

Gallo, F. (1994b). *Thought Field Therapy Level 2 (and Associated Methods): Training Manual.* Hermitage, PA: Author.

Gallo, F. (1996a). Reflections on active ingredients in efficient treatments of PTSD, Part 1. *Electronic Journal of Traumatology,* 2(1). Available from www.fsu.edu/~trauma/.

Gallo, F. (1996b). Reflections on active ingredients in efficient treatments of PTSD, Part 2. *Electronic Journal of Traumatology,* 2 (2). Available from www.fsu.edu/~trauma/.

Gallo, F. (1996c). Therapy by energy. *Anchor Point,* June, 46–51.

Gallo, F. (1997a). A no-talk cure for trauma: thought field therapy violates all the rules. *The Family Therapy Networker,* 21(2), 65–75.

Gallo, F. (1997b). *Energy Diagnostic and Treatment Methods (EDxTM): Basic Training Manual.* Hermitage, PA: Author.

Gallo, F. P. (1999). *Energy Psychology: Explorations at the Interface of Energy, Cognition, Behavior, and Health,* 1st ed. Boca Raton, FL: CRC Press.

Gallo, F. P. (2000). *Energy Diagnostic and Treatment Methods.* New York: Norton.

Gallo, F. P. (2001). *Energy Consciousness Therapy: Training Manual.* Hermitage, PA: Author.

Gallo, F. P. (2002). *Energy Psychology in Psychotherapy: A Comprehensive Source Book.* New York: Norton.

Gallo, F. P. (2003). Meridian-based psychotherapy. In Leskowitz, E., Ed., *Complementary and Alternative Medicine in Rehabilitation.* New York: Churchill Livingstone, 215–225.

Gallo, F. P. and Vincenzi, H. (2000). *Energy Tapping: How to Rapidly Eliminate Anxiety, Depression, Cravings, and More Using Energy Psychology.* Oakland, CA: New Harbinger.

Gallup, G. J. and Lindsay, D. M. (1999). *Surveying the Religious Landscape: Trends in U.S. Beliefs.* Harrisburg, PA: Morehouse.

Garten, H. (1996). (Revised by F. Annunciato, Neurobiology Laboratory, Department of Histology, University of Sao Paulo, Brazil). The mechanism of muscle test reactions and challenge in applied kinesiology: an attempt to explain the test phenomena. *Townsend Letter for Doctors and Patients,* December.

Gazzaniga, M. (1967). The split brain in man. *Scientific American,* 217, 24–29.

Gazzaniga, M. (1985). *The Social Brain.* New York: Basic Books.

Gendlin, E. T. (1978). *Focusing.* New York: Everest House.

Gerber, R. (1988). *Vibrational Medicine.* Santa Fe, NM: Bear.

Gerbode, F. (1989). *Beyond Psychology: An Introduction to Metapsychology.* Palo Alto, CA: IRM Press.

Gerson, S. C. and Baldessarini, R. J. (1980). Motor effects of serotonin in the central nervous system. *Life Science,* 27, 1435–1451.

Goodheart, G. J. (1975). *Applied Kinesiology 1975 Workshop Procedure Manual,* 11th ed. Detroit: Author.

Goodheart, G. J. (1987). *You'll Be Better.* Geneva, OH: Author.

Goswami, A. (1993). *The Self-Aware Universe: How Consciousness Creates the Material World.* New York: Jeremy P. Tarcher.

Goulding, M. and Goulding, R. (1979). *Changing Lives through Redecision Therapy.* New York: Brunner/Mazel.

Hahnemann, S. (1982). *Organon of Medicine.* Torrance, CA: J. P. Tarcher (Original work published 1810).

Hallbom, T. and Smith, S. (1988). *Eliminating Allergies Video.* Boulder, CO: NLP Comprehensive.

Harris, W. S., Gowda, M., Kolb, J. W., Strychacz, C. P., Vacek, J. L., Jones, P. G., Forker, A., O'Keefe, J. H., and McCallister, B. D. (1999). A randomized, controlled trial of the effects of remote, intercessory prayer on outcomes in patients admitted to the coronary care unit. *Archives of Internal Medicine,* 159, 2273–2278.

Hartung, J. G. and Galvin, M. D. (2003). *Energy Psychology and EMDR: Combining Forces to Optimize Treatment.* New York: Norton.

Holmes, E. (1938). *The Science of Mind.* New York: R. M. McBride.

Hover-Kramer, D. (2002). *Creative Energies: Integrative Psychotherapy for Self-Expression and Healing.* New York: Norton.

Jenike, M. A., Baer, L., Summergrad, P., Minichiello, W. E., Holland, A., and Seymour, K. (1990). Sertroline in obsessive-compulsive disorder: a double blind study. *American Journal of Psychiatry,* 147, 923–928.

Johnson, C., Shala, M., Sejdijaj, X., Odell, R., and Dabishevci, K. (2001). Thought field therapy — soothing the bad moments of Kosovo. *Journal of Clinical Psychology,* 57(10), 1237–1240.

Johnson, R. (1994). *Rapid Eye Technology.* Salem, OR: RainTree Press.

Joyce, C. R. B. and Wellson, R. M. C. (1965). The objective efficacy of prayer: a double-blind clinical trial. *Journal of Chronic Disease,* 18, 367–377.

Kant, I. (1950). *Prolegomena to Any Future Metaphysics.* New York: Howard W. Sams (Original work published 1783).

Keane, T. M. (1998). Psychological and behavioral treatments for post-traumatic stress disorder. In Nathan, P. E. and Gorman, J. M., Eds., *A Guide to Treatments That Work.* New York: Oxford, 398–407.

Keane, T. M., Fairbank, J. A., Caddell, J. M., and Zimmering, R. T. (1989). Implosive (flooding) therapy reduces symptoms of PTSD in Vietnam combat veterans. *Behavior Therapy,* 20, 245–260.

Kendall, H. O. and Kendall, F. M. P. (1949). *Muscles — Testing and Function.* Baltimore, MD: Williams & Wilkins.

Kendall, H., Kendall, F., and Wadsworth, G. (1971). *Muscle Testing and Function,* 2nd ed. Baltimore, MD: Williams & Wilkins.

Koestler, A. (1967). *The Ghost in the Machine.* London: Hutchinson.

Korzybski, A. (1958). *Science and Sanity,* 4th ed. Lakeville, CT: International Aristotelian Library.

Kuhn, T. S. (1962). *The Structure of Scientific Revolutions.* Chicago: University of Chicago Press.

La Tourelle, M. and Courtenay, A. (1992). *Thorsons Introductory Guide to Kinesiology.* London: Thorsons.

Lambrou, P. T., Pratt, G. J., Chevalier, G., and Nicosia, G. (2001). Thought energy therapy: quantum level control of emotions and evidence of effectiveness of energy psychotherapy methodology. In *Proceedings of the Eleventh Annual Conference of the International Society for the Study of Subtle Energy & Energy Medicine,* June 15, 2001, Boulder, CO. Arvada, CO: ISSSEEM.

Langman, L. (1972). The implications of the electro-metric test in cancer of the female genital tract. In Burr, H. S., Ed., *Blueprint for Immortality: The Electric Patterns of Life.* Essex, U.K.: Saffron Walden, 137–154.

Lashley, K. S. (1950). In search of the engram. *Society for Experimental Biology.* Symposium 4, 454–482.

Lawlis, G. F. (2003). Transpersonal medicine. In Leskowitz, E., Ed., *Complementary and Alternative Medicine in Rehabilitation.* New York: Churchill Livingstone, 236–246.

Lawson, A. and Calderon, L. (1997). Interexaminer reliability of applied kinesiology manual muscle testing. *Perceptual and Motor Skills*, 84, 539–546.

LeDoux, J. E. (1994). Emotion, memory and the brain: the neural routes underlying the formation of memories about primitive emotional experiences, such as fear, have been traced. *Scientific American*, June, 50–57.

LeDoux, J. (1996). *The Emotional Brain: The Mysterious Underpinnings of Emotional Life.* New York: Simon & Schuster.

LeDoux, J. (2002). *Synaptic Self: How Our Brains Become Who We Are.* New York: Penguin.

LeDoux, J. E., Romanski, L. M., and Xagoraris, A. E. (1989). Indelibility of subcortical emotional memories. *Journal of Cognitive Neuroscience*, 1, 238–243.

Leisman, G., Shambaugh, P., and Ferentz, A. (1989). Somatosensory evoked potential changes during muscle testing. *International Journal of Neuroscience*, 45, 143–151.

Leisman, G. et al. (1995). Electromyographic effects of fatigue and task repetition on the validity of estimates of strong and weak muscles in applied kinesiology muscle testing procedures. *Perceptual and Motor Skills*, 80, 963–977.

Leonoff, G. (1995). The successful treatment of phobias and anxiety by telephone and radio: a replication of Callahan's 1987 study. *TFT Newsletter*, 1(2).

Levy, S. L. and Lehr, C. (1996). *Your Body Can Talk.* Prescott, AZ: Hohm Press.

Lockie, A. and Geddes, N. (1995). *The Complete Guide to Homeopathy.* New York: Dorling Kindersley.

Ma, W., Tong, H., Xu, W., Hu, J., Liu, N., Li, H., and Cao, L. (2003). Perivascular space: possible anatomical substrate for the meridian. *Journal of Alternative and Complementary Medicine*, 9(6), 851–859.

Maltz, M. (1960). *Psychocybernetics.* Englewood Cliffs, NJ: Prentice Hall.

Mann, F. (1964). *The Meridians of Acupuncture.* London: William Heinemann Medical Books.

McDougall, W. (1927). An experiment for the testing of the hypothesis of Lamark. *British Journal of Psychology*, 17, 267–304.

McDougall, W. (1930). Second report on a Lamarkian experiment. *British Journal of Psychology*, 20, 201–218.

McDougall, W. (1938). Fourth report on a Lamarkian experiment. *British Journal of Psychology*, 28, 321–345.

McLuhan, M. (1964). *Understanding Media.* Toronto: University of Toronto Press.

Meichenbaum, D. (1997). A conversation with Donald Meichenbaum. *Behavior OnLine*, 1–7.

Menzies, R. G. and Clarke, J. C. (1993). The etiology of childhood water phobia. *Behavior Research & Therapy*, 31(5), 499–501.

Menzies, R. G. and Clarke, J. C. (1995a). The etiology of phobias: a nonassociative account. *Clinical Psychology Review*, 15(1), 23–48.

Menzies, R. G. and Clarke, J. C. (1995b). Individual response patterns, treatment matching, and the effects of behavioural and cognitive interventions for acrophobia. *Anxiety, Stress & Coping: An International Journal*, 8(2), 141–160.

Mills, R. (1995). *Health Realization.* New York: Sulburger & Graham.

Monti, D. A., Sinnott, J., Marchese, M., Kunkel, E. J., and Greeson, J. (1999). Muscle test comparisons of congruent and incongruent self-referential statements. *Perceptual and Motor Skills*, 88, 1019–1028.

Motyka, T. and Yanuck, S. (1999). Expanding the neurological examination using functional neurologic assessment. Part I: Methodological considerations. *International Journal of Neuroscience,* 97, 61–76.

Nadeau, R. and Kafatos, M. (1999). *The Non-Local Universe: The New Physics and Matters of the Mind.* New York: Oxford University Press.

Nambudripad, D. S. (1993). *Say Goodbye to Illness.* Buena Park, CA: Delta.

Nash, C. B. (1982). Psychokinetic control of bacterial growth. *Journal of the American Society of Psychical Research,* 51, 217–221.

Nathanson, D. L. (1992). *Shame and Pride: Affect, Sex, and the Birth of the Self.* New York: W. W. Norton.

Nims, L. (2002). BE SET FREE FAST: an advanced energy therapy. In Gallo, F., Ed. *Energy Psychology in Psychotherapy: A Comprehensive Source Book.* New York: Norton, 77–92.

Nordenstrom, B. (1983). *Biologically Closed Electric Circuits: Clinical, Experimental and Theoretical Evidence for an Additional Circulatory System.* Stockholm: Nordic.

Overskeid, G. (1995). Cognitivist or behaviourist: who can tell the difference? The case of implicit and explicit knowledge. *British Journal of Psychology,* 86(4), 517–522.

Penfield, W. and Perot, P. (1963). The brain's record of auditory and visual experiences — a final summary and discussion. *Brain,* 86, 595–696.

Perot, C., Meldener, R., and Gouble, F. (1991). Objective measurement of proprioceptive technique consequences on muscular maximal voluntary contraction during manual muscle testing. *Agressologie,* 32(10), 471–474.

Philips, D. C. (1969). Systems theory — a discredited philosophy. *Abacus,* September, 3–15. (Reprinted in Schoderbek, P. P., Ed., *Management Systems,* 2nd ed. New York: Wiley, 1971, 55–65.)

Pignotti, M. (2004). Personal communication.

Pignotti, M. and Steinberg, M. (2001). Heart rate variability as an outcome measure for thought field therapy in clinical practice. *Journal of Clinical Psychology,* 57(10), 1193–1206.

Pitman, R. K., Altman, B., Greenwald, E., Longpre, R. E., Macklin, M. L., Poire, R. E., and Steketee, G. S. (1991). Psychiatric complications during flooding therapy for post-traumatic stress disorder. *Journal of Clinical Psychiatry,* 52, 17–20.

Pomeranz, B. (1996). Acupuncture and the raison d'etre for alternative medicine. *Alternative Therapies,* 2(6), 84–91.

Popp, F.-A. and Beloussov, L. (2003). *Integrative Biophysics: Biophotonics.* Amsterdam: Kluwer Academic.

Pransky, G. S. (1992). *The Relationship Handbook.* Blue Ridge Summit, PA: HIS and TAB Books.

Pribram, K. H. (1962). Interrelations of psychology and the neurological disciplines. In Koch, S., Ed. *Psychology: A Study of a Science,* Vol. IV. New York: McGraw-Hill.

Pribram, K. H. (1969). The neurophysiology of remembering. *Scientific American,* January.

Pribram, K. H. (1986). The cognitive revolution and mind/brain issues. *American Psychologist,* 41, 507–520.

Pulos, L. (1990). *Beyond Hypnosis.* San Francisco: Omega Press.

Pulos, L. and Richman, G. (1990). *Miracles and Other Realities.* San Francisco: Omega Press.

Radin, D. L. and Nelson, R. D. (1989). Consciousness-related effects in random systems. *Foundations of Physics,* 19, 1499–1534.

Rapp, D. (1986). *The Impossible Child.* Buffalo, NY: Practical Allergy Research Foundation.

Rapp, D. (1991). *Is This Your Child?: Discovering and Treating Unrecognized Allergies in Children and Adults.* New York: William Morrow.

Reichmanis, M., Marino, A.A., and Becker, R.O. (1975). Electrical correlates of acupuncture points. *IEEE Transactions on Biomedical Engineering*, 22, 533–535.

Reilly, D. T. (1986). Is homeopathy a placebo response? *Lancet*, October, 881–886.

Rochlitz, S. (1995). *Allergies and Candida*. Mahopac, NY: Human Ecology Balancing Sciences.

Rogers, C. (1942). *Counseling and Psychotherapy*. Boston: Houghton-Mifflin.

Rogers, C. (1957). The necessary and sufficient conditions of therapeutic personality change. *Journal of Consulting Psychology*, 21(2), 95–103.

Rosen, R. (1991). *Life Itself: A Comprehensive Inquiry into the Nature, Origin and Fabrication of Life*. New York: Columbia University Press.

Rosenthal, D. and Frank, J. D. (1956). Psychotherapy and the placebo effect. *Psychological Bulletin*, 53(4), 294–302.

Rubik, R. (1995). Energy medicine and the unifying concept of information. *Alternative Therapies*, 1(1), 34–39.

Sakai, C., Paperny, D., Mathews, M., Tanida, G., Boyd, G., Simons, A., Yamamoto, C., Mau, C., and Nutter, L. (2001). Thought field therapy clinical application: utilization in an HMO in behavioral medicine and behavioral health services. *Journal of Clinical Psychology*, 57, 1215–1227.

Sartre, J. P. (1957). *The Transcendence of the Ego: An Existential Theory of Consciousness*. New York: Noonday Press. (Original French version appeared as La Transcendance de L'Ego: Esquisse d'une description phenomenologique, *Recherches Philo-sophiques*, 6, 1936.)

Schmitt, R., Capo, T., and Boyd, E. (1986). Cranial electrotherapy stimulation as a treatment for anxiety in chemically dependent persons. *Alcoholism: Clinical and Experimental Research*, 10, 158–160.

Schmitt, W. and Leisman, G. (1998). Correlation of applied kinesiology muscle testing findings with serum immunoglobulin levels for food allergies. *International Journal of Neuroscience*, 96, 237–244.

Schmitt, W. and Yanuck, S. (1999). Expanding the neurological examination using functional neurologic assessment. Part II: Neurologic basis of applied kinesiology. *International Journal of Neuroscience*, 97, 77–108.

Schoninger, B. (2001). [Thought Field Therapy] in the Treatment of Speaking Anxiety, doctoral dissertation. Cincinnati, OH: Union Institute.

Scoop, A. L. (1978). An experimental evaluation of kinesiology in allergy and deficiency disease diagnosis. *Orthomolecular Psychiatry*, 7(2), 137–138.

Shapiro, F. (1995). *Eye Movement Desensitization and Reprocessing: Basic Principles, Protocols, and Procedures*. New York: Guilford.

Sheinkopf, S. J. and Siegel, B. (1998). Home based behavioral treatment of young autistic children. *Journal of Autism and Developmental Disorders*, 28(1): 15–23.

Sheldrake, R. (1981). *A New Science of Life*. Los Angeles: J. B. Tarcher.

Sheldrake, R. (1988). *The Presence of the Past*. New York: Times Books.

Sicher, F., Targ, E., Moore, D., and Smith, H. S. (1998). A randomized, double-blind study of the effects of distant healing in a population with advanced AIDS. *Western Journal of Medicine*, 169, 356–363.

Simonton, O. C. and Creighton, J. (1982). *Getting Well Again*. New York: Bantam.

Stux, G. and Pomeranz, B. (1995). *Basics of Acupuncture*, 3rd ed. New York: Springer.

Sullivan, H. S. (1954). *The Psychiatric Interview*. New York: W. B. Norton.

Swingle, P. G. and Pulos, L. (2000). Neuropsychological correlates of successful EFT treatment of posttraumatic stress. Paper presented at the Second International Energy Psychology Conference, Las Vegas, NV, May 12.

Talbot, M. (1991). *The Holographic Universe*. New York: HarperCollins.

Tedder, W. and Monty, M. (1981). Explorations of a long distance PK: a conceptual replication of the influence on a biological system. In Roll, W. G. et al., Eds., *Research in Parapsychology, 1980*. Metuchen, NJ: Scarecrow Press, 90–93.

Thie, J. F. (1973). *Touch for Health*. Pasadena, CA: T. H. Enterprises.

Tiller, W. A. (1978). A lattice model of space. *Phoenix*, 2, 27–48.

Tiller, W. A. (1997). *Science and Human Transformation: Subtle Energies, Intentionality and Consciousness*. Walnut Creek, CA: Pavior.

Tittel, W., Brendel, J., Zbinden, H., and Gisin, N. (1998). Violations of Bell inequalities more than 10 km apart. *Physical Review Letters*, 81, 3563–66.

Travis, C. B., McLean, B. E., and Ribar, C., Eds. (1989). *Environmental Toxins: Psychological, Behavioral, and Sociocultural Aspects, 1973–1989*. Washington, D.C.: American Psychological Association.

Truax, C. B. (1963). Effective ingredients in psychotherapy: an approach to unravelling the patient-therapist interaction. *Journal of Counseling Psychology*, 10(3), 256–263.

Valentine, T. and Valentine, C. (1985). *Applied Kinesiology: Muscle Response in Diagnosis, Therapy and Preventive Medicine*. Rochester, VT: Healing Arts Press.

van der Kolk, B. A. (1994). The body keeps the score: memory and the evolving psychobiology of posttraumatic stress. *Harvard Review of Psychiatry*, 1(5), 253–265.

van der Kolk, B. A. and van der Hart, O. (1991). The intrusive past: the flexibility of memory and the engraving of trauma. *American Imago*, 48(4), 425–454.

Vernejoul, P. de, Darras, J. C., Beguin, C., Cazalaa, J. B., Daury, G., and De Vernejoul, J. (1984). Approche isotopique de la visualisation des meridiens d' acupuncture. [Isotopic approach to the visualization of acupuncture meridians]. *Agressologie*, 25(10):1107–1111.

Vernejoul, P. de, Albarede, P., and Darras, J. C. (1985). Etude des meridiens d'acupuncture par les traceurs radioactifs. [Study of the acupuncture meridians with radioactive tracers.] *Bulletin of the Academy of National Medicine* (Paris), 169, 1071–1075.

Wade, J. F. (1990). *The Effects of the Callahan Phobia Treatment Techniques on Self Concept*. San Diego, CA: Professional School of Psychological Studies.

Waite, W. L. and Holder, M. D. (2003). Assessment of the emotional freedom technique: An alternative treatment for fear. *The Scientific Review of Mental Health Practice*, Spring/Summer, 2(1), 20–26.

Walther, D. S. (1981). *Applied Kinesiology, Vol. I: Basic Procedures and Muscle Testing*. Pueblo, CO: Systems DC.

Walther, D. S. (1988). *Applied Kinesiology: Synopsis*. Pueblo, CO: Systems DC.

Walther, D. S. (1997). Personal communication.

Weiner, N. (1948). *Cybernetics*. New York: Wiley.

Weiner, N. (1954). *The Human Use of Human Beings*. New York: Doubleday.

Wells, S., Polglase, K., Andrews, H., Carrington, P., and Baker, A. H. (2003). Evaluation of a meridian-based intervention, emotional freedom techniques (EFT), for reducing specific phobias of small animals. *Journal of Clinical Psychology*, 59(9). 943–966.

Whisenant, W. F. (1990). *Psychological Kinesiology: Changing the Body's Beliefs*. Austin, TX: Monarch Butterfly Productions.

Wolpe, J. (1958). *Psychotherapy by Reciprocal Inhibition*. Stanford, CA: Stanford University Press.

Wolpe, J. (1961). The systematic desensitization treatment of neuroses. *Journal of Nervous and Mental Disorders*, 132, 189–203.

Wylie, M. S. (1996). Going for the cure. *The Family Therapy Networker*, 20(4).

Young, A. (1976a). *The Reflexive Universe: Evolution of Consciousness*. Lake Oswego, OR: Robert Briggs Associates.

Young, A. (1976b). *The Geometry of Meaning*. Mill Valley, CA: Robert Briggs Associates.
Young, A. (1984). *The Foundations of Science: The Missing Parameter.* San Francisco: Robert
    Briggs Associates.
Yourell, R. A. (1995). *The Reprocessing Manual.* Denver, CO: Author.

Index

A

Abuses, manual muscle testing, 217–218
Acquired immunodeficiency syndrome (AIDS),
        44–45
Acrophobia
    behavioral-environmental paradigm, 5
    biochemical paradigm, 9
    case study, 194–195
    cognitive paradigm, 6
    future research, 202
Active ingredients project, 18–24
Acupoints, 33, 57, 237
Acupressure holding points, 60, 185
Acupuncture
    acupoint stimulation, 33
    basics, 31–32
    chi, 33–38
    meridians, 32–38
    Nei ching, 32–33
Acupuncture meridian system (AMS), 237, *see*
        also Meridians
Acute stress disorder (ASD), 90, 203
Addictions and addictive urges
    algorithm and application method, 154–157
    electrical neurotransmission, 11
    generalized anxiety disorder, 162
    research, 199
Affirmations
    basics, 23n
    Diamond method, 70–73
    psychological reversal, 96–97, 138–139
    rage, 167
Agar studies, 39
Agoraphobia, 165, 201–202
AK, *see* Applied kinesiology (AK)
Alarm point, 237
Alberts, James, 54–55
Alcohol, *see* Addictions and addictive urges
Alder, Alfred, 4
Algorithms
    application methods, 152
    basics, 237
    manual muscle testing, 118–121, 214–215,
        217–218

research, 205
    thought field therapy, 90–91
Allergies, 157, 199–200
Alternative scaling, 118
American Psychiatric Association, 153, 159
AMS, *see* Acupuncture meridian system (AMS)
Amygdala, 237
Ancillary treatments, 97–99
Andrade and Feinstein studies, 197–198
Andreas and Andreas studies, 22
Anger, *see also* Rage
    algorithm and application method, 157–158
    cover-up emotion, 78n
    research, 203–204
Anticipatory and performance anxiety, 158–159
Anxiety disorder, generalized
    algorithm and application method, 162
    electrical neurotransmission, 11
    research, 193, 200–201
Apex problem, 121–123
Applied kinesiology (AK)
    basics, 237
    cranial-sacral primary respiratory mechanism,
        55–56
    energy psychology, origins, 51–58
    intervertebral foramen, 57
    meridians, 56–57
    muscle testing, 51–53
    neurolymphatic reflexes, 53–54
    neurovascular reflexes, 54–55
    origin-insertion technique, 51–53
    triad of health, 58
Archaeus, 69
ASD, *see* Acute stress disorder (ASD)
Ashby studies, 8
Aspect, Alain, 14, 185
Asthma, 54–55
Astin studies, 45
Attention-deficit/hyperactivity disorder, 159–160
Attunement, *see also* Transmodal reattunement
    algorithm and application method, 113–115
    basics, 237
    highly efficient therapies, 24–25
Audiotapes, 222
Aura, 237

Life energy, 33, 69–70, *see also* Chi
Lindsay, Gallup and, studies, 40n
Liver meridian, *74, 127,* 157
Lockie and Geddes studies, 47, 49
Lund, Elmer J., 12
Lung meridian, *74,* 126–127, *127*

M

Major treatment points, 130–131
Maltz, Maxwell, 169
Mann, Felix, 56–57
Manual muscle testing
  abuses, 217–218
  algorithms, 118–121, 214–215, 217–218
  application method, 118–121
  applied kinesiology, 51–53
  basics, 211–212
  casual diagnostics, 214–215
  diagnosis, 213–214
  empirical research, 212–213
  energy psychology, 215–217
  failure, 219
  integrity, 213
  intuition, 218
  legal action, 61
  offshoots of applied kinesiology, 212
  proficiency, 213
  self-testing, 214
  straight arm, *69*
  systemic testing, 220
  therapy, 213–214
  thought field therapy, 91
  unwarranted uses, 218–219
Marsh, G., 12
Martin, Childre and, studies, 185
Massive psychological reversal, 93–94, 134–135
Ma studies, 34
McDougall, W.
  case study, 85n
  morphogenetic fields, 38–39
  specific phobias, 153
McLuhan, Marshall, 207
Medical conditions, 201
Megbe, 32n
Meichenbaum studies, 6
Melzak-Wall pain treatment, 165
Menzies and Clarke studies, 5, 153
Meridians
  algorithm and application method, 152
  applied kinesiology, 56–57
  basics, *74,* 89–90, 152, 239
  Diamond method, 73–74
  discovery, 32

evidence, 33–38
  guilt, 162–163
  touch for health, 60
Mills studies, 7
Mini psychological reversal, 95–96, 135–136
Minnesota multiphasic personality inventory
  (MMPI-2), 200
MMPI-2, *see* Minnesota multiphasic personality
  inventory (MMPI-2)
Monti studies, 119, 212
Monty, Tedder and, studies, 41–42
Morphogenetic fields, 12, 38–40
Mother Teresa (of Calcutta), 41
Motyka and Yanuck studies, 212
MUD, *see* Muscular units of distress (MUD)
Muscle, adding to therapy, *see* Energy
  psychology, origins
Muscle testing, *see* Manual muscle testing
Muscular units of distress (MUD), 239
Music, 70

N

Nadeau and Kafatos studies, 14
NAEM, *see* Negative affect erasing method
  (NAEM)
Nambudripad studies
  addiction and addictive urges, 199
  allergies and energy toxins, 200
  energy toxins, 126
  Tapas acupressure technique, 176–177
Narrative therapy, 17
Nasal stuffiness and congestion, 164
Nasal tap, 144
Nash studies, 42
Nathanson studies, 199
Needles, *see* Acupuncture
Negative affect erasing method (NAEM)
  algorithm and application method, 180–184
  attention-deficit/hyperactivity disorder, 160
  depression, 200
Negative thoughts, 7
Nei ching, 32–33
Nelson, Radin and, studies, 42
Neo-cognitive approach, 7
NEST, *see* Neuro-energetic sensory techniques
  (NEST)
NET, *see* Neuro-emotional technique (NET)
Neuro-emotional technique (NET), 63–64, 64n,
  240
Neuro-energetic sensory techniques (NEST),
  187–188, 240
Neurolinguistic programming (NLP), 21, 101, *see
  also* Language

physical pain, 165
thought field therapy, 85
triad of health, 58
War trauma, 105–106
"Weak" muscle, 242
Wellson, Joyce and, studies, 42
Wheeler, Gallo and, studies, 185
Whisenant, William F., 65
White, Epston and, studies, 6
Whitehead, Alfred North, 31
Whiteside, Daniel, 63
Wiener studies, 8

Williams, Robert M., 65
Wolpe, Joseph, 5
Women, cervical electrical charges, 13, 77

Y

Yanuck, Motyka and, studies, 212
Yanuck, Schmitt and, studies, 212
Yesod, 32n
Young studies, 10, 38
Yourell studies, 26